Nervous System

Diseases of the Nervous System

W. B. MATTHEWS
DM, FRCP
Professor of Clinical Neurology
University of Oxford

FOURTH EDITION

Distributed in the USA and Canada by
BLACKWELL / YEAR BOOK MEDICAL PUBLISHERS • INC.

BLACKWELL SCIENTIFIC PUBLICATIONS
OXFORD LONDON EDINBURGH
BOSTON MELBOURNE

© 1972, 1975, 1979, 1982 by
Blackwell Scientific Publications
Editorial offices:
Osney Mead, Oxford, OX2 0EL
8 John Street, London, WC1N 2ES
9 Forrest Road, Edinburgh, EH1 2QH
52 Beacon Street, Boston
  Massachusetts 02108, USA
99 Barry Street, Carlton
  Victoria 3053, Australia

All rights reserved. No part of this
publication may be reproduced, stored
in a retrieval system, or transmitted,
in any form or by any means,
electronic, mechanical, photocopying,
recording or otherwise
without the prior permission of
the copyright owner

First published 1972
Second edition 1975
Reprinted 1976
Third edition 1979
Fourth edition 1982

Photoset by Enset Ltd,
Midsomer Norton, Bath, Avon
and printed in
Great Britain by
William Clowes (Beccles) Limited,
Beccles and London

DISTRIBUTORS

USA
  Blackwell Mosby Book Distributors
  11830 Westline Industrial Drive
  St Louis, Missouri 63141

Canada
  Blackwell Mosby Book Distributors
  120 Melford Drive, Scarborough
  Ontario, M1B 2X4

Australia
  Blackwell Scientific Book Distributors
  214 Berkeley Street, Carlton
  Victoria 3053

British Library
Cataloguing in Publication Data

Matthews, W.B.
  Diseases of the nervous system—4th ed.
  1. Nervous system—Diseases
  I. Title
  616.8   RC346

ISBN 0-632-00832-6

Contents

Preface to the Fourth Edition   viii

1 **The Form and Functions of the Nervous System**   1
Neurone and Nerve Impulse. Neuroglia. Metabolism. The
Afferent System. Special Senses. The Motor System.
Integration. Reflex Activity. The Cerebellum. The
Extrapyramidal System. The Cerebral Cortex. Speech.
Consciousness. The Autonomic System. Blood Supply.
Meninges. The Cerebrospinal Fluid.

2 **Examination of the Nervous System**   35
The Adult. The Cranial Nerves. The Upper Limbs. The
Lower Limbs. Sensation. Speech. Intellectual Function.
Stupor and Coma. The Infant. Lumbar Puncture.

3 **Neurological Symptoms**   50
Headache. Numbness. Dizziness. Weakness. Cramp.
Unsteadiness. Double Vision. Blackouts.

4 **The Syndromes of the Cranial Nerves**   58
The Olfactory Nerve. The Optic Nerve. The Oculomotor
Nerve. Diplopia and Nystagmus. The Trigeminal Nerve.
The Facial Nerve. The Acoustic Nerve. The
Glossopharyngeal Nerve. The Vagus. The Accessory Nerve.
The Hypoglossal Nerve.

5 **Traumatic Lesions of the Peripheral Nervous System and Spinal Cord**   82
The Lower Motor and Sensory Neurones. Acute Trauma of
Peripheral Nerves. Pressure Palsies. Irritative and
Entrapment Syndromes. Brachial Plexus Injuries.
Cervical Ribs. Root Lesions. The Spinal Cord.
The Upper Motor Neurone. The Sensory Tracts.
The Brown–Séquard Syndrome. The Sphincters. Trauma to
the Cord. Management. Myelopathy due to Spondylosis.

6 Peripheral Neuropathy 108
Clinical Features. Pathogenesis. Causes.
External Toxins. Alcohol. Wernicke's Encephalopathy.
Drugs. Heavy Metals. Industrial Hazards.
Nutritional Causes. Intrinsic Disease. Diabetes.
Carcinoma. Collagen-Vascular Disease. Amyloidosis.
Porphyria. Genetic Forms. The Guillain–Barré Syndrome.
Neuralgic Amyotrophy. Neuropathy of Unknown Cause.
Restless Legs Syndrome.

7 Diseases of Voluntary Muscle 123
Progressive Muscular Dystrophy. Polymyositis.
Myasthenia Gravis. The Non-Dystrophic Myopathies.
Congenital Myopathy and the Floppy Baby. Metabolic
Myopathies. Endocrine Myopathies. Toxic Myopathy.
Carcinoma.

8 Head Injury 137
Extradural Haematoma. Chronic Subdural Haematoma.
Sequelae of Head Injury. Traumatic Epilepsy.
Traumatic Cerebrospinal Rhinorrhoea and Otorrhoea.

9 Vascular Disease of the Nervous System 147
Ischaemic Vascular Disease. Pathology. Transient Cerebral
Ischaemia. Cerebral Infarction. Hemiplegia. Apraxia.
Carotid Artery Occlusion. Vertebrobasilar Syndromes.
Cerebral Haemorrhage. Pathology. Clinical Features.
Cerebrovascular Dementia. Investigation and Treatment.
Venous Thrombosis. Subarachnoid Haemorrhage.
Unruptured Aneurysms. Giant Cell Arteritis.
Other Forms of Arteritis. Vascular Disease of the Spinal Cord.

10 Space-occupying Lesions of the Central Nervous System 169
Intracranial Pressure. Cerebral Tumour. Clinical
Features. Diagnosis of Cerebral Tumours. Treatment.
Cerebral Abscesses. Benign Intracranial Hypertension.
Tumours of the Spinal Cord. Chronic Compression.
Acute Compression. The Cauda Equina.

11 Infections 189
Meningitis. Purulent Meningitis. Tuberculous Meningitis.
Aseptic Meningitis. Encephalomyelitis. Poliomyelitis.
Herpes Simplex Encephalitis. Herpes Zoster. Other
Virus Infections. Neurosyphilis. Tetanus.

CONTENTS

12 The Demyelinating Diseases — 210
Multiple Sclerosis. Acute Disseminated Encephalomyelitis. Neuromyelitis Optica.

13 Diseases of the Basal Ganglia — 221
Parkinson's Disease. Chorea and Athetosis. Other Forms of Involuntary Movement. The Nature of Basal Ganglia Syndromes.

14 Metabolic Disease — 235
Deficiency Diseases. Inborn Errors of Metabolism. Systemic Metabolic Disease.

15 Developmental Diseases — 247
Congenital Hydrocephalus. Syringomyelia. Cerebral Palsy. Congenital Dyslexia. Cranial Nerve Anomalies.

16 Degenerative Diseases of Genetic or Unknown Origin — 258
The Spinocerebellar Ataxias. Peroneal Muscular Atrophy. Huntington's Chorea. Tuberose Sclerosis. Neurofibromatosis. Motor Neurone Disease. Presenile Dementia. Progressive Supranuclear Palsy. Idiopathic Orthostatic Hypotension.

17 Epilepsy, Syncope and Narcolepsy — 271
Diagnosis of Epilepsy. Diagnosis of the Cause. Mental Changes. Treatment. Status Epilepticus. Flicker-induced Epilepsy. Infantile Spasms. Management. Syncope. Narcolepsy.

18 Migraine — 289
Clinical Features. Clinical Variants. Causation. Diagnosis. Treatment. Migrainous Neuralgia. Cough Headache.

19 Neurological Aspects of Psychiatry — 297
Depression. Anxiety. Delirium and Confusional States. Hysteria. Epilepsy.

Index — 304

Preface to the Fourth Edition

In the ten years since the first edition of this book time and change have eroded the original contributions of the late Henry Miller and I have felt it best no longer to append his name to a work that he might have found unrecognizable.

Many have believed or feared that the advent of computer-assisted tomography would reduce clinical neurology to a simple mechanical exercise. The CT scan has greatly improved the lot of many patients with neurological disease and has rendered many formerly agonizing decisions far more simple. New problems have, however, arisen and provide new opportunities for the use of essential and far from obsolete clinical skills.

I am indebted to Dr Andrew Molyneux and the Department of Medical Illustration at the John Radcliffe Hospital for help with illustrations.

CHAPTER 1
The Form and Functions of the Nervous System

The functions of the nervous system are infinitely more varied than those of any other organ or system and are served by many thousands of millions of neurones, interlinked in an orderly but inconceivably complex manner. The student who has mastered the essentials of the comparatively simple pumping action of the heart or the rather more involved regulating functions of the kidney is naturally daunted by the prospect of exploring the impact of disease on this labyrinth, whose functions range from the control of sweating to those of memory, speech and consciousness. A further obstacle is that while other organs vary in no important respect throughout the mammalian kingdom, the human brain is very different from that of even the most advanced of other primates. Partly for this reason, much that has been learnt from animal experiments has no immediate application to the understanding of the normal or diseased nervous system in man. These limitations, imposed on student and professor alike, obscure our understanding of neurological disease, but also permit some simplification of the necessary basic knowledge. It is, for example, unnecessary to memorize all that is known or surmised about the connections of the red nucleus in the cat, since this has no certain clinical application. Nevertheless, it is impossible to embark on the study of neurology without a sound understanding of those elements of neuro-anatomy and physiology currently known to be clinically relevant. In the following account it will be assumed that the student has already received considerable instruction on the structure and function of the nervous system, but insufficient enlightenment on those aspects likely to prove useful in clinical medicine.

NEURONE AND NERVE IMPULSE

The neurone, the basic element of nervous tissue, consists of a cell body containing the nucleus, a variable number of branching dendrites, and an axon. The intense metabolic activity of the cell is reflected in the numerous mitochondria in the cytoplasm, and by the presence of basophilic Nissl granules containing ribose nucleoproteins. The axon, which varies in length from a few millimetres to almost a metre, is maintained by the continuous synthesis of axoplasm by the cell body, and therefore degenerates if the cell body is destroyed. The dendrites and the cell body receive synaptic connections from other neurones, often in enormous numbers, and the axon conveys the nerve impulse, sometimes to effector organs but more often to other neurones.

The interior of the neurone is electrically negative relative to the exterior. This actively excludes sodium (the sodium pump) while maintaining a relatively high concentration of potassium within the cell. The energy necessary for the metabolism of the cell is derived from oxidative phosphorylation and the generation of phosphocreatine and adenosine triphosphate. The nerve impulse originates in the region of the cell body adjacent to the axon, and is induced by a brief loss or reversal of the resting electrical gradient, a process known as depolarization. Stimuli reaching the neurone through the synapses may have either an excitory or inhibitory effect, the former tending to depolarize the membrane and the latter to maintain the resting potential. The nerve impulse does not cross the synapse, but transmission is effected by the liberation from minute vesicles of a chemical that then acts on the cell membrane. The nature of the stimulus, whether inhibitory or excitatory, depends on the chemical liberated and on the post-synaptic receptor sites.

We may picture the neurone exposed to conflicting impulses at high frequency and fluctuating intensity, and discharging along its own axon only when the balance swings so far towards excitation as to cause depolarization of the cell membrane. Propagation of the nerve impulse is quite unlike the conduction of an electric current along a wire. Depolarization, involving a brief reversal of the resting electrical gradient, spreads along the axon and both this active process and the maintenance of the resting state require the expenditure of energy and the consumption of oxygen. Many axons are surrounded by lipid sheaths of myelin. In peripheral fibres this is laid down spirally by the neurilemma or Schwann cells, while in the central nervous system the oligodendroglia perform a similar function. Many fine peripheral fibres have no myelin sheath, but are surrounded by a layer of Schwann cell processes. In all myelinated peripheral fibres the myelin sheath is interrupted at intervals of less than a millimetre by the nodes of Ranvier, the junctions between successive Schwann cells. Although much more difficult to demonstrate, similar nodes are present in the central nervous system. It is thought that active propagation takes place at the nodes, causing successive depolarization of each segment of axon and more rapid and economical transmission. Loss of the myelin sheath prevents efficient propagation of the impulse. Conduction velocity also varies with the diameter of the fibre and in large peripheral myelinated fibres may reach 60 metres per second (125 m.p.h.).

NEUROGLIA

The electron microscope has revealed that the central nervous system consists of an astonishing interlacing of branching processes of neurones and glial cells with little or no recognizable extracellular space, a finding in conformity with its lack of any lymphatic system. The glial cells are not merely supportive tissue, but are undoubtedly involved in the metabolism of the nervous system. Tissue culture studies have thrown some doubt on the original rigid classification, but the microglia appear to be phagocytic histiocytes and the oligodendroglia concerned with the formation of the myelin sheath. The astrocytes are often closely related to capillaries, but their precise metabolic role is not well understood.

METABOLISM

In the complex metabolism of the nervous system certain main streams can be identified. The most immediate is the provision of energy to maintain the relative exclusion of sodium and the electrical potential without which a neurone ceases to function. This is provided by the breakdown of high-energy phosphate compounds that must be constantly renewed by the catabolism of glucose. The process of glucose breakdown, glycolysis, is essentially similar in all tissues and proceeds through the citric acid cycle, catalysed by the agency of enzyme chains. Vitamin B_1 (aneurin) has been identified as a coenzyme concerned in the breakdown of pyruvate, an essential stage in the cycle, and it was the observed effect of deficiency of this vitamin that led to the important concept of the biochemical lesion. This implies that function is disturbed by a potentially reversible disorder of metabolism, in this instance a block in glycolysis leading to accumulation of pyruvate and failure to provide cellular energy. The importance of such lesions is being increasingly recognized. The lack of an enzyme or its inactivation by abnormal metabolites leads not only to failure of the normal step in the metabolic chain, but to accumulation of 'toxic' concentrations of normal tissue constituents. These in turn may block other enzymes, leading to a spreading chemical and functional disorder. If this is sufficiently prolonged permanent neuronal damage ensues, but if the original metabolic block can be recognized and corrected the adverse effects can be mitigated or reversed.

The nervous system differs from muscle in that anaerobic glycolysis does not occur and the removal of hydrogen ions linked with oxygen to form water is continuously necessary. The brain is therefore peculiarly vulnerable to any interruption of its supply of oxygen, wthout which the neurone rapidly dies, apparently consuming its own substance as a final source of energy. A continuous supply of glucose is also essential, for although glycogen is present in the brain there is no provision for carbohydrate storage comparable to that of muscle or liver. In conditions of rest the adult brain, comprising little more than 2% of the body weight, is responsible for one-fifth of the total consumption of oxygen and two-thirds of the consumption of glucose.

Glucose is indeed virtually the sole source of energy, as although brain slices can be induced to utilize other substrates this does not occur in life. Other potential sources of energy are prevented from accumulating in the central nervous system by the operation of the blood–brain and blood–cerebrospinal fluid barriers. These are homeostatic mechanisms ensuring that the neurones enjoy a relatively stable biochemical environment, shielded to some degree from fluctuations in the general metabolism. The walls of capillaries within the nervous system do not have the channels present in other organs and active processes operate in the transport of metabolites or their exclusion.

Surprisingly, the rate of protein synthesis in the adult brain is comparable to that in the liver. Much of this must be accounted for by the continuous synthesis of axoplasm in the cell body and its extrusion down the axon. There are suggestions from animal experiments that the physical basis for the storage of information may lie not in reverberating electrical circuits, but in the elaboration of specific proteins. The clinical significance of this intense metabolic activity is quite uncertain.

Knowledge of the chemistry of synaptic transmission is only beginning to contribute to our understanding of disease, partly because there is no certainty about the agents involved. There is evidence that acetylcholine, dopamine, noradrenaline, gamma-amino butyric acid and possibly glycine and serotonin play some role in transmission. Gamma-amino butyric acid appears to be a universal neuronal depressant but other probable transmitter substances have been shown to be capable of both inhibition and excitation, depending on the receptor mechanisms of the individual neurone. It is probable that many of the very numerous drugs that act on the nervous system exert their effect by modifying the release of, or response to, transmitter substances. Even the most complicated pharmacological action on the brain must result either from excitation or inhibition of neurones, but a drug may exert opposing effects at different anatomical sites or even on different populations of cells at a single site such as the descending reticular formation. The mode of action even of simple sedative drugs is imperfectly known, and nearly all therapeutic actions have been discovered by trial and error.

The metabolism of amino-acids is of central importance, being linked with the synthesis of transmitter substances, with protein metabolism, and with the citric acid cycle. The principal free amino-acid in the brain is glutamic acid, probably derived from glucose, and capable of combining with ammonia to form glutamine. The conversion of glutamic acid to gamma-amino butyric acid requires the coenzyme pyridoxal phosphate which has been shown to be absorbed as pyridoxine or vitamin B_6. The functions of glutamic acid that have been partially unravelled therefore include the detoxification of ammonia and almost certainly an important part in the regulation of neuronal excitability.

The ionic equilibrium involving the relative concentrations of potassium and sodium on either side of the cell membrane is influenced by the concentrations of other electrolytes. Calcium stabilizes the cell membrane, preventing depolarization, and a lack of extracellular ionic calcium has the opposite effect, causing repeated spontaneous firing of the neurone. Carbon dioxide, produced in the brain by glycolysis or conveyed in the blood stream, has a similar stabilizing effect on the membrane and therefore a depressant action on neuronal activity. Its accumulation is prevented by the action of the enzyme carbonic anhydrase which catalyses the combination of carbon dioxide with water to form carbonic acid.

About half the dry weight of the brain consists of lipids, many of which are specific for nervous tissue and apparently synthesized there. Cholesterol and the cerebrosides, containing a carbohydrate radical, and sphingomyelin which contains phosphorus, are all relatively concentrated in the white matter. The metabolism of these substances is only slowly being elucidated but their function in the formation of the myelin sheath is established. Once formed the myelin complex appears to be stable in health and is relatively little involved in active metabolism. Disorders of lipid metabolism are therefore particularly important in the early years of life when myelin is being laid down, and in those disease processes in which the myelin sheath is destroyed. Abnormal accumulation of lipids may therefore result from breakdown of myelin, or from disturbance of the normal lipid metabolic pathways during the period of development.

Investigation of the biochemistry of the brain in health and disease is rendered difficult by the operation of the blood–brain barrier and the inaccessibility of the central nervous system. Little is so far known of the different metabolic activities of specific organs and systems in the brain.

Biopsy techniques must necessarily be of limited value, permitting little more than an estimate of the metabolites present in the specimen at the moment it was taken. This can be but a poor reflection of the dynamic processes whose distortion must cause or accompany most forms of cerebral disease.

For purposes of description it is conventional to write of the sensory and motor aspects of the nervous system almost as if they existed in isolation. This is entirely artificial. The function of the nervous system is the reception, integration and perception of sense data, external or internal, and the organization of the appropriate response. This may indeed be motor but may also be secretory or concerned with such mental processes as memory or thought. The mechanisms underlying these integrative functions are naturally complex and but partially understood. When considering the impact of disease on the nervous system the traditional approach beginning with the ostensibly simpler functions of movement and sensation has much to commend it.

THE AFFERENT SYSTEM

A large proportion of the afferent impulses reaching the central nervous system do not give rise to any conscious 'sensation'. Of those that do it is convenient to speak of fibres conveying sensations of touch or pain, but it must be remembered that such fibres simply convey nerve impulses no different from others, and that there can be no sensation of touch or pain, unless these are interpreted as such by the brain.

Numerous specialized receptor organs are present in the skin, hair follicles, muscles, tendons, joints, connective tissue and viscera. In the skin some receptors appear to be structurally adapted to respond to specific stimuli, and it is well known that sensitivity to pain and thermal stimuli varies greatly from point to point within small areas. However, attempts to demonstrate that one type of receptor is specific for a given type of stimulus have proved inconclusive. Areas containing nothing but a network of bare nerve fibres may be exquisitely sensitive to all forms of stimulus.

One specialized receptor organ must be described in more detail. It is the muscle spindle—the spiral sensory organ that encircles a group of small specialized muscle fibres, the so-called intrafusal fibres. These fibres have a motor supply distinct from that of the bulk of the muscle, conveyed by fine fibres which, because of their size, fall into the gamma group. They are better referred to as the fusimotor fibres. Although further refinements are constantly being described, the essence of the muscle spindle is that the two ends of the intrafusal fibre can contract, while the centre, surrounded by the primary sensory receptor, cannot. When the fusimotor fibres discharge, the central portion including the receptor, is consequently stretched by the contraction of the two ends of the intrafusal muscle fibres. The sensitivity of the receptor organ is therefore variable and is increased by discharge of the fusimotor fibres. When the muscle itself is stretched, either by passive movement as in a neurological examination or as the result of contraction of antagonistic muscles, the spindles are also stretched and initiate afferent impulses which pass up fast-conducting fibres to the spinal cord. Spindles have been identified in nearly all of the voluntary muscles, and they play a most important part in all aspects of movement.

The afferent fibres originate in the cell bodies in the posterior root ganglia, and in similar ganglia related to the cranial nerves. On leaving the ganglion the axon divides, one branch being directed peripherally to the sense organ and the other centrally to the spinal cord or brain. The fibres vary greatly in diameter and thus in conduction velocity. The central branches of the spinal afferent fibres form the posterior roots, which divide into smaller rootlets and enter the spinal cord on its postero-lateral aspect.

Each posterior root receives fibres from a more or less well-defined area of skin, the dermatome (Fig. 1). These areas overlap and there is certainly some individual variation. The important landmarks can be summarized as follows: the first cervical root (C1) has no sensory component, and the C2 area extends over the back of the scalp almost to the vertex; C3 and 4 include the neck and upper part of the shoulder, while C5 to T1 supply the upper limb. Classically the C5 area is the outer side of the shoulder and upper arm; C6 the lateral aspect of the forearm to the thumb and index; C7 a strip down the centre of the forearm to the middle finger; C8 the inner side of the forearm and the ring and little fingers, and T1 the medial aspect of the upper arm to the axilla. On the chest wall, therefore, T2 is contiguous with C4 above.

Thereafter the root distribution on the trunk follows an orderly descending pattern. The nipple is at the T5 level, the rib margin at T8, the umbilicus at T10 and the symphysis pubis at T12.

This orderly pattern is again interrupted in the lower limb. The anterior aspect of the thigh is supplied by L1–3, the medial aspect of the calf by L4, and the lateral aspect and dorsum of the foot by L5. S1 supplies the sole and little toe, and S2 a strip up the back of the calf and thigh. The medial half of the buttock and the perineum are supplied by the lower sacral roots.

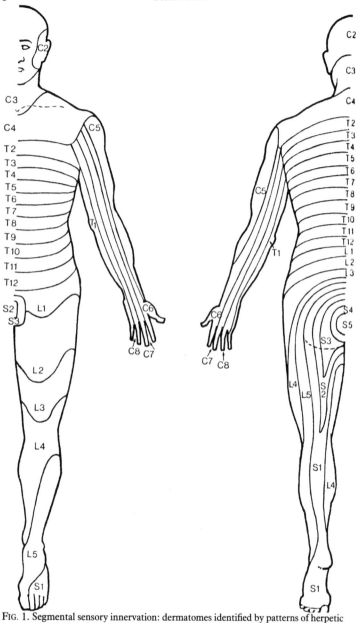

FIG. 1. Segmental sensory innervation: dermatomes identified by patterns of herpetic eruption and of remaining sensation after surgical division of posterior roots and below the relevant segment.

The spinal cord terminates at the lower border of the first lumbar vertebra and is much shorter than the spinal column. Below the cervical region the roots descend in the spinal canal for an increasing distance before passing through the intervertebral foramina. Thus, although T6 leaves the canal between the 6th and 7th thoracic vertebrae it originates opposite the 4th vertebra. The posterior root ganglia lie in the intervertebral foramina.

On entering the spinal cord some afferent fibres form direct synapses with motor cells in the anterior horns of the grey matter, or with other neurones whose axons run a short distance up or down the cord, known as the spinal interneurones. Those concerned with sensations of posture and vibration pass up the spinal cord in the posterior columns on the same side (Fig. 2). After ascending a short distance, fibres serving pain and thermal sensation synapse with cells in the posterior horn. The secondary fibres cross to the other side, close to the central canal, and pass up the cord in the lateral and anterior columns as the spinothalamic tracts. Whether a stimulus is felt as painful depends on many factors peripherally. Large-calibre fibres, synapsing locally, appear to inhibit the excitatory effect of small fibre activity on cells in the posterior horn concerned with pain. Whatever the mechanism an intact spinothalamic tract is an essential component. The discharge of the cells of origin of the tract is also controlled by brain stem centres from which axons descend to the posterior horns of the spinal cord. This is one site of liberation of endorphins, endogenous substances with an analgesic action. Fibres concerned with touch almost certainly ascend both in the posterior columns and in the spinothalamic tracts. In the posterior columns fibres from the lowest segments of the cord lie medially, while in the spinothalamic tracts the position is reversed as a result of the crossover, and fibres from the lowest segments are placed laterally.

Many fibres from the muscle spindles end in synaptic connection with cells at the base of the posterior horns, the secondary neurones ascending on the same side as the spinocerebellar tracts.

At the lower end of the medulla the posterior column fibres terminate in the gracile and cuneate nuclei. The second sensory fibres cross immediately, and ascend in the centre of the medulla as the medial lemniscus. The spinothalamic tract, joined by fibres from the sensory trigeminal nuclei on the opposite side, lies lateral to the medial lemniscus in the medulla, but the two sensory pathways converge as they pass up the brain stem.

The sensory supply of the face is derived entirely from the trigeminal (Vth cranial) nerve with the exception of the angle of the jaw supplied by the cervical roots. The cell bodies are in the Gasserian ganglion lying on the petrous temporal bone, and the central processes pass as a thick nerve trunk to enter the pons. The peripheral branches form the three main divisions of the nerve. The mandibular branch supplies an area of skin approximately overlying the lower jaw and also the lower teeth and the tongue. The maxillary division supplies the skin over the cheek and upper lip and the structures of the upper jaw including the mucosa of the hard palate. The ophthalmic division is distributed to the skin of the forehead up to the vertex, the conjunctiva, and part of the skin over the

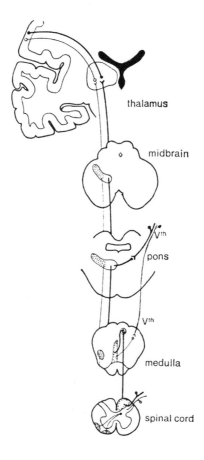

FIG. 2. Central sensory pathway: the diagram shows the separation of the two major sensory pathways within the spinal cord. The precise central connections of the trigeminal nerve remain controversial.

nose. The upper division supplies the pain-sensitive structures inside the cranium, and the meninges at the base of the skull and around the main blood vessels. The mucosa of the pharynx and back of the tongue is supplied by the glossopharyngeal nerve (IX) with its ganglion lying in the jugular foramen and its central processes entering the medulla.

The central connections of the sensory fibres of the trigeminal nerve are complex. The fibres mediating pain and thermal sense descend on the same side of the pons and medulla to the upper segments of the spinal cord. Here a synaptic connection is made and the secondary neurones cross the mid-line to join the spinothalamic tract. Fibres serving other forms of sensation terminate the principal nucleus in the pons, the secondary fibres ascending on the same side to the mid-brain before crossing.

The spinocerebellar tract enters the inferior cerebellar peduncle. In addition to these well-defined tracts there are many ascending fibres, less obviously grouped, that convey impulses from the spinal cord to the reticular formation in the brain stem and to other important structures.

The sensory fibres, united after their separation into two distinct pathways, terminate in the ventro-posterior nucleus of the thalamus, from which arise the third sensory neurones. Their axons pass through the internal capsule to the post-central gyrus and more diffusely to a wide area of the parietal lobe. Whether fibres mediating all forms of sensation are distributed in this way is uncertain, partly because we are no longer concerned simply with relaying nerve impulses but with their interpretation. The crude idea that pain and thermal sensations are 'felt' in the thalamus and other sensations in the cortex is much too simple. It is undoubtedly true that marked loss of the ability to interpret sensory stimuli may result from lesions of the parietal cortex with comparatively little impairment of ordinary sensation.

In the post-central gyrus there is a definite localization of function, the upper part being concerned with sensation from the lower limb, and the lower part with that from oral and facial structures, with a wide intermediate area concerned with the hand and arm. Since nearly all such information is derived from studying the effects of disease or of applying highly artificial stimuli under experimental conditions the more precise diagrams once so popular must be regarded with reserve.

SPECIAL SENSES

Smell

The receptor organs for smell, which includes the greater part of what is appreciated as taste, are in the mucosa of the upper part of the nasal cavity, and are extraordinarily and selectively sensitive to molecules in the inspired air. The afferent fibres originate in the olfactory sensory cells in the mucosa, and pass through the cribriform plate in a number of small bundles to enter the olfactory bulb on the inferior surface of the frontal lobe. The central connections are highly complex, no doubt reflecting the great importance of the sense of smell in our evolutionary ancestors. The main termination appears to be in the uncus of the temporal lobe.

Taste

The taste buds of the tongue respond to only four stimuli, appreciated as sweet, salt, acid and sour. The afferent impulses converge on the nucleus solitarius in the medulla by strangely devious routes. Those from the anterior two-thirds of the tongue, the only part that can easily be tested, enter the lingual nerve, a branch of the trigeminal, and leave it in the chorda tympani which passes through the middle ear and joins the sensory portion of the facial nerve. Those from the back of the tongue follow a simpler course in the glossopharyngeal nerve. Central connections from the nucleus solitarius follow those concerned with somatic sensation.

Vision

The optic nerve is formed of a very large number of fine fibres that originate in the ganglion cells of the retina. The receptor organs, the rods and cones, are not evenly distributed, there being an immense concentration of cones at the macula or fixation point, accounting for the enormously enhanced visual acuity at this point. The optic disc, where the nerve leaves the eye, is devoid of receptor organs and therefore forms a blind spot in the temporal half of the field of vision. The nerve passes backwards and medially through the optic foramen, and is then in close relationship with the internal carotid artery on its lateral side. It fuses with the nerve from the other eye to form the optic chiasma, which lies below the anterior end of the third ventricle and above the pituitary gland. The optic tract leaves the chiasma, and passes round the cerebral peduncle to terminate in the lateral geniculate body, where the visual fibres form synaptic connections. The optic radiation, formed by fibres originating in the lateral geniculate body, enters the internal capsule and then spreads out to form a wide band, the lower part of which sweeps round the temporal horn of the lateral ventricle. The radiation then runs posteriorly deep in the temporal lobe to reach the calcarine cortex. This lies almost entirely on the medial aspect of the occipital lobe.

The fibres are so arranged that light coming from the right and falling on the left side of each retina eventually excites the left calcarine cortex and, of course, vice versa. This is effected by means of a partial crossing over of fibres in the optic chiasma. Fibres from the temporal half of each retina receive light from the nasal visual fields and proceed to the optic tract without crossing. Those from the nasal halves receive light from the temporal fields, cross at the chiasma and proceed in the opposite optic tract. Thus the left tract contains fibres from the temporal half of the left retina and the nasal half of the right, both being responsive to stimuli in the right visual field.

Each point in the retina is connected with a strictly defined area of cortex and indeed this localization of function is preserved throughout the entire visual system. Experimental work is also now beginning the exciting task of relating specific cortical neurones to specific forms of stimulation but these results have not yet greatly influenced clinical neurology.

Binocular vision and the interpretation of what is seen is not, of course, merely a matter of retinal stimuli being conveyed to the calcarine cortex. Among other important factors is the coordination of movement of the eyes, and the optic nerves contain many fibres not directly concerned with vision. These do not enter the lateral geniculate body, but continue to the superior colliculus on the posterior aspect of the midbrain.

Hearing

The fibres of the cochlear branch of the VIIIth nerve originate in the spiral ganglion in close relationship to the cochlea. The central processes run in the internal auditory meatus with the vestibular and facial nerves, and enter the pons to terminate in the cochlear nuclei. The central pathways include at least two synapses, in the inferior colliculus and medial geniculate body, but other pathways are certainly involved. The cortical termination in the superior temporal gyrus is highly organized, and each area of cortex is stimulated by sounds of a different frequency. In striking contrast to the visual system precise clinical localization of lesions of the auditory cortex is not possible.

The cochlear nuclei form numerous other connections with brain stem nuclei concerned with reflex action.

Equilibrium

Among the numerous afferent stimuli involved in the maintenance of posture are those from the vestibular apparatus. In contrast with the special senses we have already considered, these vestibular afferents do not give rise to consciously appreciated sensations but are extremely important in reflex activity. In a very approximate way the semicircular canals can be regarded as receptor organs for changes in the position of the head, while impulses from the utricle and saccule reflect the actual position of the head relative to gravity.

The fibres of the vestibular division of the VIIIth nerve originate in ganglion cells in the internal auditory meatus, and the central processes accompany the cochlear nerve and enter the pons. Many of the fibres terminate in a large group of vestibular nuclei lying beneath the floor of the fourth ventricle. From here important connections are formed with the cerebellum, the centres controlling eye movements, and, via the vestibulo-spinal tract, with the anterior horn cells and spinal interneurones. Little is known of any direct or indirect connections with the cerebral cortex.

THE MOTOR SYSTEM

The motor nerve supply to skeletal muscles is derived from large nerve cells in the anterior horns of the spinal grey matter and in the motor nuclei of the brain stem. The axons of these lower motor neurones are of large diameter, falling into the alpha group. They leave the spinal cord on its antero-lateral aspect as a continuous series of rootlets which merge to form the anterior spinal roots. Each fibre divides to supply a number of muscle fibres, varying from 100 in muscles responsible for fine movements such as those of the hand, to 2000 in muscles controlling large joints. The neurone and its group of muscle fibres form a motor unit. Anatomically the muscle fibres of each unit are only relatively concentrated, and there is much overlap between neighbouring units.

The axon terminates in a motor end-plate applied in an intricate manner to the muscle fibre, and in some ways resembling a synapse. The nerve impulse liberates acetylcholine, which acts on the cell membrane of the muscle fibre to produce spreading depolarization. This in turn produces a physical change in the molecules of actin and myosin in the muscle fibrils that is responsible for the actual shortening or contraction of the muscle. This reaction is dependent on the entry of ionic calcium during the period of depolarization of the membrane. The energy for muscular contraction is ultimately derived from glucose, but, in contrast with conditions in the nervous system, both aerobic and anaerobic oxidation are possible, and carbohydrate can be stored as glycogen. The motor end-plates are usually concentrated in a comparatively restricted zone of the muscle, which is therefore the point at which it can most easily be stimulated electrically, the motor point. An important element in neuro-muscular transmission is the presence of the enzyme cholinesterase that permits rapid destruction of acetylcholine and prevents the prolonged depolarization of the membrane. The cell bodies of the fusimotor fibres to the intrafusal muscle fibres are less easy to identify anatomically but are also in the anterior horns. The intrafusal fibres play no part in the contractile force of the muscle.

It is usual to speak of the spinal cord as organized into segments, each segment corresponding to a pair of anterior and posterior roots. This is not strictly true of the anterior horn cells, since those supplying a particular muscle are not arranged in neat segmental groups, but in longitudinal columns which may extend over several segments. The roots themselves are, however, arranged in a more or less standardized segmental pattern. As with the sensory roots there is much overlap and some individual variation. The important features of motor root distribution are as follows:

Diaphragm	C4
Shoulder muscles and flexors of elbow	C5, 6
Triceps and extensors of wrist and fingers	C7
Flexors of wrist and fingers	C7, 8
Hand muscles	C8, T1
Intercostals and lumbar and abdominal muscles	T2 to L3
Quadriceps and adductors	L3, 4
Ilio-psoas	L1 to 5
Glutei	L4, 5
Hamstrings	L4 to S1
Muscles controlling the ankle	L5, S1
Foot muscles	S1, 2
Bladder	S2, 3, 4

The motor nuclei of the cranial nerves supplying skeletal muscle are analogous to the anterior horn cells. The hypoglossal (XII) nucleus lies in the floor of the fourth ventricle and provides the motor supply to the muscles of the tongue. The accessory nerve (XI) has a more complex origin from a medullary nucleus and from the third and fourth cervical roots. It supplies the sternomastoid and trapezius muscles. The somatic motor fibres of the vagus (X) nerve arise in the nucleus ambiguus in the medulla and supply the palate, pharynx and larynx. The nerve leaves the skull through the jugular foramen accompanied by the accessory nerve and after supplying the palate and pharynx, descends to the upper thorax before giving off the recurrent laryngeal nerves to the larynx. The right recurrent nerve arises at a higher level than the left, which passes behind the aortic arch.

Apart from its small sensory component the main function of the facial (VII) nerve is to supply the numerous muscles of the face, including the platysma. The motor nucleus is in the lower part of the pons, and the nerve emerges at that level and enters the internal auditory meatus. It pursues a course in close relation to the middle ear to emerge from the stylomastoid foramen, and divides into numerous branches within the substance of the parotid gland.

The motor fibres of the trigeminal (V) nerve supply the muscles of mastication, and originate in a nucleus in the pons at a higher level than the facial nucleus. All the motor fibres enter the mandibular division and leave the skull through the foramen ovale.

The abducent (VI), trochlear (IV) and oculo-motor (III) nerves are the motor nerves of the eyeball. The abducent nucleus is in the pons, closely related to the fibres of the facial nerve, and the nerve leaves the brain at the lower border of the pons. It supplies a single muscle, the lateral rectus, which abducts the eye. The trochlear nucleus is in the midbrain, and the nerve supplies only the superior oblique muscle which depresses the eyeball when it is in the adducted position. The oculomotor nucleus is more complex and consists of columns of cells close to the aqueduct in the midbrain. It supplies the other four external ocular muscles and the levator of the upper lid, and is therefore wholly responsible for adduction and elevation of the eyeball and for depressing the eyeball when it is in the abducted position. The nerve also contains fibres to the constrictor of the pupil and to the ciliary muscle. These arise from a separate centrally placed nucleus. All three nerves enter the orbit through the superior orbital fissure after having traversed the cavernous sinus lateral to the carotid artery.

The corticospinal or pyramidal trace (Fig. 3) originates chiefly in the cells of the pre-central gyrus, but receives contributions from a wide area of the frontal and parietal cortex. The fibres converge on the internal capsule, where fibres destined for the lower part of the spinal cord lie posteriorly. The trace then forms the central third of the cerebral peduncle, descends in a less compact manner through the pons, giving off fibres to the motor nuclei of the cranial nerves, and then forms the prominent 'pyramid' on the front of the medulla. At the lower end of the medulla most of the fibres cross and descend in the lateral column of white matter of the spinal cord. Probably most of the fibres do not terminate directly on anterior horn cells but on spinal interneurones. A small proportion of the corticospinal fibres descends uncrossed.

It is traditional to ascribe the cortical control of movement to the

FORM AND FUNCTIONS

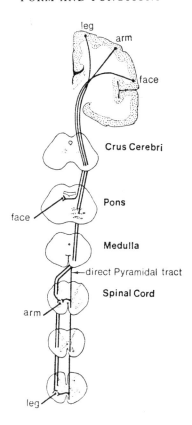

FIG. 3. Central motor pathway.

pyramidal tract and the upper motor neurones of the pre-central gyrus. From a clinical point of view this is perfectly valid but there is experimental evidence that movement that could certainly be termed voluntary and even skilled can persist after complete degeneration of the pyramidal tract. The relationship of cortical area to part moved closely parallels that of the sensory cortex in the post-central gyrus. It is certain that the relationship between a specific cortical point and a specific movement is much less precise than that existing between the retina and the visual cortex. With this qualification the upper part of the gyrus and the area on the medial surface of the hemisphere are concerned with movement of the lower limb, and the lower end, approaching the Sylvian fissure, with movements of the face and tongue. Movement of the hand and arm can be elicited from a wide area between two extremities of the gyrus.

While it is true that contraction of single muscles can be produced experimentally by suitable stimulation of the cortex, the organization of the cortical motor neurones is quite different from that of the anterior horn cells. Contraction of a single muscle is neither useful nor perhaps even physiologically possible, and the role of the cortex is certainly that of initiating movements and not merely muscular contractions.

INTEGRATION

The principal pathways by which stimuli reach the central nervous system and the outflow to the muscles have now been described in bare outline. The artificial nature of such a subdivision has already been mentioned. Even the simplest movement demands the coordinated response to a multitude of stimuli, not only to effect the movement but to maintain the equilibrium of the body while doing so. No oversimplified account can conceal our ignorance of many of the events that transmute stimulus or volition into effective action, but the basis for much of this integrative function is reflex activity.

REFLEX ACTIVITY

The reflex arc consists of an effective stimulus, a receptor organ, an afferent pathway leading through one or several synapses to the efferent pathway, and the effector organ. The reflexes concerned with the avoidance of harmful stimuli that seem so important in the physiology laboratory have curiously little relevance to clinical neurology. However, the corneal reflex furnishes such an example. When the cornea is touched, afferent impulses pass up the ophthalmic division of the trigeminal nerve and stimulate motor fibres in both facial nuclei. Both eyes blink and the stimulus is swept from the cornea. The reflex is a simple one with very little central synaptic delay. It can readily be interrupted by destruction of either the afferent or efferent limbs of the arc, but is little influenced by the activity of the rest of the nervous system. The gag reflex is a similar reaction to a noxious stimulus. When the back of the tongue or the pharyngeal mucosa is touched with a spatula, the pharyngeal muscles contract. The reflex arc is formed by the afferent fibres of the glossopharyngeal nerve and the motor fibres of the vagus.

Vestigial remnants of other protective reflexes can be elicited by stimulation of the skin. Although apparently without any useful function they are of some clinical value. The abdominal muscles contract when the skin overlying them is lightly stroked, the superficial abdominal reflexes. The cremaster muscle retracts the testis when the skin on the inner side of the thigh is scratched, though too slowly to afford it much protection from any immediate menace. The complex central pathways of these cutaneous reflexes suggest that they may have been more important at an earlier stage of evolution. Of more obvious use is the anal reflex, the contraction of the anal sphincter induced by pricking the peri-anal skin with a pin.

The plantar reflex is of far greater clinical importance and yet its physiological significance is obscure. When the outer side of the sole of the foot is firmly stroked the toes flex towards the sole. The stimulus bears little relation to any natural phenomenon and the response appears to be functionless; it is not even a withdrawal from the stimulus. Whatever its physiological meaning the importance of the reflex is that it is greatly influenced by activity of areas of the nervous system quite remote from the first sacral segment of the spinal cord, the source of the afferent and efferent fibres to the sole of the foot. Isolation from central impulses apparently from the corticospinal pathway causes a reversal of the normal response so that the toes dorsiflex and abduct, resembling a fragment of a withdrawal reflex. This abnormal reflex is the extensor plantar or Babinski reflex.

The reflex integrative actions so far considered have been comparatively simple and some are not even essential for the efficiency of the organism. The *stretch reflex* is, however, of paramount importance and interest. In any abbreviated account it is easy to describe the reflex activity of the spinal cord as something quite apart from the rest of the nervous system. Nothing could be further from the truth, and it is precisely at this point that we have the most vivid impression of the interplay of excitation and inhibition, arising from many regions of the nervous system and from the periphery, and all eventually concentrated on the anterior horn cells—the final common pathway.

This is not immediately obvious from the classical description of the stretch reflex in the spinal animal. When a muscle is stretched, even minutely, it contracts to restore its previous length. If stretch is continued the muscle will eventually lengthen and adapt itself to the new posture. The mechanisms underlying these apparently simple events are to a large extent responsible for all controlled movement. Stretch stimulates the sensory organs of the muscle spindles and the afferent fibres synapse, either directly or through interneurones, with the anterior horn cells to excite contraction of the muscle. This contraction must, however, be of exactly the correct degree to restore the previous length, and is limited by the spindles ceasing to discharge as soon as contraction of the muscle removes the stretch. At the same time contraction of antagonistic muscles must be inhibited. If stretch is continued, impulses arise from receptor organs in the tendons and also probably from secondary sensory endings in the spindles that inhibit the firing of the motor neurones and allow the muscle to lengthen; the lengthening reaction. If the new posture is to be maintained there must be simultaneous adjustment of the firing of the fusimotor fibres that control the sensitivity of the spindles.

The simplest form of stretch reflex is the phasic reflex, the response of the muscle to a sudden increase in tension. The *tendon jerks* are phasic reflexes and although apparently of little physiological importance they are of great clinical value. They are monosynaptic reflexes, the afferent fibres directly exciting the anterior horn cells, and the reflex arc is largely confined to a single segment of the spinal cord. The tendon jerks normally present are the biceps and supinator jerks (C6 segment), the triceps (C7), the knee jerk (L4) and the ankle jerk (S1).

The normal stimulus for the reflex is not, of course, the stretching of muscles by external force but the alterations in length and tension implicit in spontaneous movement. The smooth performance of any movement involves the lengthening and shortening of many muscles and the adjustment of their contraction and of the sensitivity of their spindles, not only to the precise required degree but in precisely correct sequence. It is the stretch reflex that is the basis of this precision. Impulses arising in the spindles reflexly control muscular contraction which in turn modifies the afferent inflow. The stretch reflexes involved in these adjustments are not all of the same type, for in addition to the predominantly monosynaptic phasic reflexes, tonic reflexes also exist that are stimulated by more prolonged stretch and employ more complex central pathways. Evidence is accumulating that the two types of reflex may be served by different receptor organs in the spindles, by separate fusimotor fibres, and possibly even by separate motor units.

As a purely spinal mechanism it is obvious that such reflex activity could neither initiate nor maintain voluntary movement. It is usual to think of voluntary movement as initiated in the motor cortex and stimulating the anterior horn cells through the pyramidal tract. Movement could, however, be initiated by an alteration in the activity of the fusimotor fibres leading to a change in the afferent flow from the spindles and a reflex contraction or relaxation of the muscles. Almost certainly both mechanisms are involved to varying degrees, perhaps depending on the nature of the movement. There are infinite gradations between the extremes of voluntary and automatic movement. However a movement is initiated it must immediately modify the afferent inflow from the spindles, and continued effective movement must depend on the integration of this activity with that derived from all the other sensory receptors.

This integrative action may be illustrated by the control of ocular movement. With binocular vision no useful function can be served by the action of a single cranial nerve on the external ocular muscles. Unless the retinal image falls on the corresponding area of the retina on each side, and especially unless the image at the fixation point is identical, no clear perception is possible. We can direct our eyes voluntarily to focus on any point, and within limits to follow a moving object. A cortical area concerned with such conjugate ocular movements is present in each frontal lobe. The position of the eyes may be signalled by stimuli from the retina, from muscle spindles in the ocular muscles and probably also from the cortical centre that initiates or maintains the movement. These afferent impulses must be integrated with those from other sensory systems, vestibular, auditory and postural. The exact pathways are not fully known, but the cerebellum must play an important role. The coordination of the motor response is effected through important relay stations in the upper part of the midbrain and subsequently by tracts that link the midbrain complex of nuclei (IIIrd and IVth nerves) with the VIth nerve nucleus in the pons. At the same time both the pupil of the eye and the ciliary muscle must be adapted to the intensity of light and the distance of the object viewed. The pupil is to a large extent reflexly controlled, the effective stimulus being the intensity of the light falling on the retina. The afferent fibres run with the optic nerve as far as the midbrain, where they separate to enter the nucleus of the IIIrd nerve, forming synaptic connections with the motor fibres to the constrictor of the pupil. There are, however, many other factors that control the size of the pupil, especially the degree of convergence of the eyes. Convergence is accompanied by constriction of the pupil and by accommodation of the lens, produced by contraction of the ciliary muscle. The nature of the effective stimulus for this apparently reflex constriction is not entirely clear. All these interlinked activities take place with remarkable accuracy and speed, with no conscious awareness apart from our desire to look at something.

THE CEREBELLUM

The cerebellum is an important centre for the integration or coordination of sensory and motor activities. The cerebellar cortex receives fibres, either directly or through intervening nuclei, from all the afferent systems concerned with posture and movement, from the skin, and from the motor and sensory cortex. Fibres from the spinocerebellar tracts convey impulses from the muscle spindles and tendon organs and enter mainly by the inferior cerebellar peduncle on the same side, accompanied by fibres from the vestibular apparatus and nuclei. Fibres from the cerebral cortex relay in nuclei in the pons, and then cross to enter the middle peduncle. The pathways from the visual and auditory systems probably follow the same course after relaying in the superior and inferior colliculi.

Animal experiments yield clear evidence of localization within the cerebellar cortex. It is possible to identify areas in both anterior and posterior lobes in which, for example, afferents from the upper limb are concentrated. Fibres from areas of cerebral cortex concerned with the upper limb are relayed to the same region. This localization is clearly of physiological importance, but has not so far proved to have much clinical significance, except that the vestibular afferents are localized to the flocculo-nodular lobe and the inferior vermis. The former is a small irregular structure almost concealed on the under-surface of the cerebellar hemispheres. The vermis is the central elevation between the two hemispheres.

The afferent fibres terminate on the dendrites of the cells of the deepest layer of the cerebellar cortex. The axons of these cells form an intricate network with the processes of the large Purkinje cells of the middle cortical layer and the granular cells of the superficial layer. This network forms the physical basis of the integration of the impulses originating in the sensory organs with those from the motor and sensory cortex. The outflow from the cerebellar cortex is through the axons of the Purkinje cells and, surprisingly, its function appears to be entirely that of inhibiting, no doubt with great precision, the activity of the dentate and other deep cerebellar nuclei. From these nuclei fibres are relayed through the superior peduncle to the thalamus, the cerebral cortex, the spinal cord and the extrapyramidal motor system. It must be surmised that the interplay of cerebellar cortex and dentate nucleus controls the degree and distribution of excitation over this complex network.

THE EXTRAPYRAMIDAL SYSTEM

This term was introduced in a clinical context and proved most useful in distinguishing the disorders of motor function that could be attributed to disease of the corticospinal (pyramidal) motor pathway from those equally striking disorders that occurred when other motor systems were affected. Anatomically the extrapyramidal system consists of large masses of grey matter in the depths of the cerebral hemispheres (the basal ganglia) and smaller nuclei in the brain stem. Although in most of the classical sections of the brain the corpus striatum appears to consist of several quite distinct anatomical entities it is a single mass of grey matter consisting of the caudate and lentiform nuclei. The elongated caudate nucleus sweeps round the thalamus, at first lying in the floor of the anterior horn of the lateral ventricle but continuing forward as a thin tail in the roof of the temporal horn to terminate in the amygdaloid nucleus deep in the temporal lobe. The lentiform nucleus, fused with the head of the caudate, lies lateral to the thalamus separated from it by the internal capsule. The nucleus is divided into an outer segment, known as the putamen, and an inner segment, the globus pallidus. The lower end of the globus pallidus is continuous with the substantia nigra in the midbrain. The small subthalamic nucleus and the reticular formation of the brain stem are essential components of the system, but the role of the red nucleus, so important in lower animals, is much less certain in man. These nuclei are interlinked by chains of short neurones.

It is not possible to give a comprehensive account of the functions of the basal ganglia because neither their anatomy nor physiology is fully known. The main inflow to the system is to the caudate nucleus and putamen from the motor cortex, and to the globus pallidus from the cerebellum, but many other pathways exist. The main outflow is from the globus pallidus to the thalamus, and from the reticular formation as descending reticulo-spinal fibres. We are much less familiar with the normal physiology than with the effects of disease on the extrapyramidal system. Many of these consist in disturbances of posture or of co-ordinated movement, or in the appearance of abnormal involuntary movements. It is certain that the system is concerned with the maintenance of posture and equilibrium, and there is little doubt that much of this is effected by control of the fusimotor fibres through the reticulo-spinal tracts. It would be absurd to conclude that the prevention of tremor and other involuntary movements are among these functions.

THE CEREBRAL CORTEX

The cerebral cortex is a convoluted layer of grey matter covering the surface of the hemispheres. The useful convention of regarding each hemisphere as consisting of four separate lobes is largely arbitrary. The anatomy of many of the sulci and gyri is inconstant, but certain main landmarks can readily be identified. The central sulcus, dividing the pre- and post-central gyri and forming the boundary between the frontal and parietal lobes, runs downwards and forwards on the lateral surface of the hemisphere. The upper end lies rather posterior to the midcoronal plane, and the lower end almost reaches the Sylvian fissure. This is formed by a deep infolding of the cortex, the insula, and divides the temporal from the frontal lobe. There is no obvious anatomical boundary between the temporal and parietal lobes. Superior, middle and inferior gyri can be recognized in the temporal and frontal lobes. On the medial surface of the hemisphere the calcarine sulcus extends forwards from the occipital pole, and the parieto-occipital fissure forms the anterior boundary of the occipital lobe. In front of this the cingulate gyrus runs parallel to the corpus callosum for most of its length.

Under the microscope the dense masses of cortical neurones can be seen to lie in more or less clearly defined layers. In the motor cortex large cell bodies are present in layer five and in the visual cortex layer four is greatly enlarged. Numerous attempts have been made to divide the remainder of the cortex into specific areas based on the relative density and structure of the cell layers, until recently with only limited success. This is understandable since the complexity of the neuronal structure of the cortex defies description. Within the cortex innumerable radially distributed axons connect the neuronal layers. Short tracts connect neighbouring gyri and long tracts pass from one cortical area to another within the same hemisphere and to corresponding areas in the other hemisphere through the corpus callosum. Afferent and efferent fibres pass between the cortex and many subcortical structures, notably the thalamic nuclei, and in all probability many important connections are still unidentified.

As already described, certain cortical areas are clearly involved in such functions as vision, movement and the appreciation of sensory stimuli. Destruction of these areas produces predictable loss of function. Lesions of comparable size in other areas may produce no consistent loss of function or even no apparent defect at all. This is partly because we have not developed the skills necessary to recognize such defects, but even if a lesion of the right frontal lobe is clinically 'silent' this does not mean that this lobe has no function.

So far we have considered movement and sensation in a largely artificial context of the immediate reaction to stimuli, functions vital indeed but shared with all organisms possessing a nervous system. To an incomparably greater degree than other animals man can learn, predict and plan, can compare one sensation or situation with another; in short, has the power of reason. There can be little doubt that it is the neuronal structure of the cortex that is the physical basis of the sifting of alternatives, the storage of information and the grading of response. There is no *a priori* reason why such functions should be strictly localized, and indeed they would seem to demand a large diffuse organization with alternative pathways. There is evidence that the temporal cortex is concerned with memory and occasional cases are seen where amnesia can be related to focal lesions, but no exclusive 'memory centre' could reasonably be expected. Clinical experience confirms that it is in diffuse disease of the cortex that defects of memory and judgement are most frequently encountered.

SPEECH

The use of words in speech, reading, writing and thought is a highly specialized function acquired with difficulty by the growing child. The full expression of this function is naturally dependent on the visual and auditory systems and on control of the muscles of articulation and of the hand. However, the interpretation and expression of words as meaningful symbols is a function of the cortex of a wide area including the inferior part of the frontal lobe and the temporal and parietal lobes. In contrast to those cortical functions already considered speech is very largely served by one hemisphere, nearly always the left. In less than half of those who are left-handed the right hemisphere is dominant for speech. Most of our information on the physiology of speech is based on observations of its disordered function in patients rendered dysphasic by disease of various cortical areas and the effects of disease can be conveniently described at this point.

It is usual to divide the function of speech into expressive (speaking and writing) and receptive (understanding the spoken and written word). These functions are almost inseparable, and in most dysphasic patients it is easy to demonstrate that both expression and reception are impaired, even if to very different degrees. Nominal aphasia is the commonest form. The patient is unable to name common objects, though he immediately recognizes the name when reminded of it. Nominal aphasia may occur in isolation in lesions of the temporal and frontal lobes and is of little localizing value.

Defects predominantly affecting expression occur in anterior lesions, particularly those involving Broca's area in the third frontal convolution. Spontaneous speech contains mispronounced or misplaced words and is slow and hesitant with little awareness that all is not well. In extreme examples speech is reduced to a few stereotyped and sometimes inappropriate phrases. Writing shows similar defects; words are repeated, omitted or absurdly misspelt. Slight defects may be found only by asking the patient to write to dictation a paragraph containing many polysyllables: deficiencies both in speech and writing are often concealed by circumlocution.

Predominantly receptive dysphasia occurs with lesions in the posterior temporal lobe and adjacent parietal lobe. Simple commands cannot be carried out from lack of comprehension, and written commands are no better understood. Spontaneous conversation is naturally much disturbed, although usually fluent. Even if no mistakes are made in spontaneous speech, repetition of test material is often faulty. Many tests, such as writing to dictation or copying, involve both the motor and sensory aspects of speech. This is shown most dramatically in *jargon aphasia* where the patient emits a continuous stream of incomprehensible words, unable to recognize that he is talking nonsense. The enthusiasm with which apparently 'pure' defects were greeted by an older generation of neurologists was due to their laudable desire to localize each specific function. A more dynamic approach to the physiology of speech has rendered such localization less captivating, though thorough clinical examination of patients with aphasia will reveal some surprisingly specific disabilities. For example, a patient with obvious expressive aphasia may be able to write only in capital letters. To postulate a lesion involving a 'centre' for writing in lower case is absurd, but the explanation of such defects is not obvious.

CONSCIOUSNESS

There is no difficulty in recognizing that a patient is in coma, with no response to stimulation other than simple and often abnormal reflex activity. Such a patient is clearly unconscious of his surroundings. In stupor, often quaintly called semi-coma, where more purposive responses can be obtained, consciousness is still obviously disturbed. After a head injury a patient may appear to respond normally to all stimuli and to answer sensibly, but may later be found to have no recollection at all of these events. In everyday life we are not continuously aware of all external stimuli or even of our own actions; such a state would be intolerable. In sleep we may seem to be oblivious of our surroundings and yet in certain stages of sleep there is electrical evidence of intense activity of some regions of the brain. These different facets of consciousness illustrate the difficulties encountered by those who have sought to hold a single site or system of the brain responsible for the conscious state. Large areas of cortex may be destroyed without effect on consciousness, but quite a moderate blow on the head may instantly result in coma. It now seems probable that consciousness is indeed a function of the cortex but only as activated or alerted by impulses from the reticular formation. Cessation of these impulses causes generalized lapse of cortical function and therefore of consciousness.

THE AUTONOMIC SYSTEM

The autonomic system controls the activity of smooth muscle, cardiac muscle and glandular secretion. It differs from those systems already considered in that all efferent fibres synapse outside the central nervous system and are therefore known as preganglionic fibres. The distinction between the sympathetic and parasympathetic systems is difficult to maintain at all points, but is based both on anatomical and functional differences.

The preganglionic sympathetic fibres originate in the lateral horn of the spinal grey matter from the first dorsal to the second lumbar segments, and leave the cord in the anterior roots, passing to the sympathetic chain as the white rami communicantes. A synaptic connection is formed in one of the ganglia and many of the postganglionic fibres re-enter the anterior roots at the same or a different level as grey rami. Although the sympathetic chain receives fibres from only part of the cord, it extends from the base of the skull to the pelvis. Sympathetic fibres are distributed to the mixed nerves formed by the spinal roots, but they also accompany arteries and form links with parasympathetic plexuses.

The parasympathetic preganglionic fibres originate in the nuclei of the oculomotor, facial, glossopharyngeal and vagus nerves and in the second and third sacral segments of the spinal cord. There are certain well-defined peripheral ganglia such as the ciliary ganglion, but the cell bodies of most parasympathetic postganglionic fibres are close to the viscera.

Preganglionic autonomic fibres are cholinergic; that is to say synaptic transmission is effected by the liberation of acetylcholine. Parasympathetic postganglionic fibres are also cholinergic, while sympathetic fibres liberate noradrenaline, except fibres to sweat glands, which are thought to be cholinergic. The action of noradrenaline on the effector organs appears to depend to some extent on the nature of the receptor mechanism. By examining the selective action of inhibitory drugs it has been possible to recognize two types of receptor, the alpha adrenergic receptor on which noradrenaline has an excitatory effect and a beta receptor where, except for an excitatory action on heart muscle, the effect is inhibitory.

The concepts of sympathetic stimulation as preparing the organism for 'fight or flight' and the parasympathetic as favouring contemplative digestion are too well known to demand repetition. A few aspects frequently encountered in clinical neurology must be considered more fully.

The dilator muscle of the pupil receives a sympathetic supply. This originates in a centre in the midbrain and passes down the tectospinal tract on the same side to the preganglionic cell bodies in the upper two thoracic segments of the spinal cord. Their fibres leave the cord at this level, join the sympathetic chain, pass through the stellate ganglion, and synapse with cells in the superior cervical ganglion. Postganglionic fibres reach the eye through the sympathetic plexus surrounding the internal carotid artery and the short ciliary nerves. The parasympathetic supply to the sphincter pupillae arises in the upper part of the oculomotor nucleus and the postganglionic fibres originate in the ciliary ganglion.

Sweating is under the control of the sympathetic. Central impulses arise in the hypothalamus on both sides, but those destined for one side of the body become localized to that side at the level of the pons. The fibres descend to the cord and stimulate the preganglionic neurones, the axones of which follow the usual course to the sympathetic chain. The postganglionic fibres are distributed mainly through the peripheral nerves but some, especially to the skin of the face, accompany blood vessels.

Loss of control of micturition is a frequent symptom of neurological disease. Like many viscera the bladder receives a dual autonomic innervation, but the sympathetic supply from the first and second lumbar segments of the cord appears to have little clinical significance. The postganglionic fibres from the sympathetic chain form the presacral nerve and then enter the hypogastric plexus from which the muscle of the bladder is supplied. The parasympathetic motor supply originates in the second and third sacral segments and passes through the nervi erigentes to the hypogastric plexus. Afferent sympathetic fibres reach the lumbar cord and the much more important parasympathetic afferents enter the sacral dorsal roots.

Perfectly effective but socially inconvenient emptying of the bladder can occur on a purely reflex basis as in the young child. The bladder distends to a certain pressure which excites afferent impulses that stimulate the parasympathetic action of contracting the detrusor and relaxing the sphincter muscle. Within limits micturition in the adult is under voluntary control. A sensation of bladder fullness is experienced, but emptying can be prevented until a convenient moment. It is even possible voluntarily to pass urine when the level of distension is far below that required for reflex emptying. The cortical centres concerned probably lie on the inferior surface of the frontal lobe and both the ascending and descending tracts are in the lateral columns of the spinal cord. It is obvious that this mechanism can be disturbed in a variety of different ways, ranging from interruption of the reflex arc to loss of cortical control.

The hypothalamus is the chief site of central control of the autonomic nervous system. This group of small nuclei in the walls of the third ventricle controls an astonishing range of vital functions. Certain of the nuclei contain receptor organs sensitive to changes in the circulating blood. Thus the degree of stimulation of thermo-receptors is responsible for the heat-regulating activities of sweating and shivering. Certain aspects of appetite appear to be controlled by hypothalamic receptors sensitive to changes in blood glucose. Receptors sensitive to changes in osmotic pressure control the secretion of antidiuretic hormone in the pre-optic nucleus and the extent to which this passes down the pituitary stalk to the posterior lobe of the pituitary. Other autonomic centres are present in the brain stem, particularly in the floor of the fourth ventricle. Here are the centres concerned with vomiting and with the reflex activity responsible for the alternating activities of inspiration and expiration. In the same region is the vasomotor centre controlling tonic contraction of the smooth muscle of the blood vessels and therefore to a large extent regulating blood pressure. Amongst the many influences that affect this centre are afferent autonomic impulses from receptor organs sensitive to pressure in the carotid sinuses and the aortic arch.

Many of these activities are beyond voluntary control, but this does not imply that the autonomic system functions in isolation. Quite apart from such obvious examples as the voluntary inhibition of micturition, there are close links with those functions of the nervous system concerned with the feeling and expression of emotion. Crying is more than excessive parasympathetic stimulation of the lacrymal glands; it is accompanied by great changes in the facial muscles of expression and normally of course by an emotion of sadness. The cortical and subcortical areas concerned are not fully understood, but probably include the cingulate gyrus and the hippocampus. The autonomic system and its central connections are primitive and mainly concerned with unconscious and uncontrollable activities, but cannot be dismissed as merely 'vegetative'.

BLOOD SUPPLY

The arterial supply to the brain is exceedingly rich, being derived from four large vessels, the internal carotid and vertebral arteries. The right common carotid normally arises from the innominate artery and the left directly from the aorta. Both divide into internal and external branches just below the angle of the jaw. The external carotid supplies the structures of the face and scalp and also the important middle meningeal artery to the dura. The internal carotid gives off no branches in the neck and penetrates the base of the skull through the foramen lacerum. Just above the bifurcation in the neck there is a localized dilatation, the carotid sinus.

The vertebral artery normally arises from the subclavian artery on each side but there is some variation and the left vertebral may arise directly from the aorta. The artery passes up the neck in the foramina of the transverse processes of the vertebrae and enters the spinal canal above the atlas. It then penetrates the spinal dura and enters the skull through the foramen magnum.

Within the skull the first branch of the internal carotid is the ophthalmic artery to the contents of the orbit, followed by the posterior communicating artery which joins the posterior cerebral artery. The carotid then divides into the anterior and middle cerebral arteries. The former passes medially and forward and closely approaches the anterior cerebral of the other side, with which it is connected by the anterior communicating artery. It then sweeps round on the corpus callosum and supplies the medial surface of the hemisphere, apart from the occipital lobe, and a strip of cortex superiorly on the lateral aspect. The middle cerebral artery passes laterally and then posteriorly, lying deep in the Sylvian fissure. It supplies almost the whole of the lateral surface of the hemisphere. Important penetrating branches supplying deep structures arise near the origins of both these arteries.

The vertebral artery gives off the posterior inferior cerebellar artery and other important but unnamed branches to the medulla. The two vertebral arteries then join and pass up in front of the pons and midbrain as the basilar artery. The paired anterior inferior and superior cerebellar arteries arise from the basilar trunk, which then divides into the posterior cerebral arteries. These receive the posterior communicating arteries from the carotid system and then pass posteriorly round the brain stem to supply the occipital lobes and the undersurface of the temporal lobes.

The circle of Willis formed by these communications lies at the base of the cerebrum in the subarachnoid space and is closely related to the cranial nerves passing forward to the orbit, the optic chiasma, and the inferior surface of the frontal and temporal lobes. The conventional pattern of branching is highly variable. The anterior communicating artery may be small or absent and the posterior cerebral on one or both sides may obtain most of its blood flow through the communicating artery from the carotid system. The main cerebral arteries are not end-arteries, as was formerly supposed, but anastomose freely over the surface of the cerebral hemispheres.

The functional significance of these multiple anastomoses is clearly that of safeguarding the oxygen supply to the brain. Provided all the channels are open the blood supply to the brain can be regarded as an integrated system in which any reduction of flow to any part of the brain can be instantly met by increase or even reversal of flow through alternative pathways. The arterial pressure in the cerebral vessels is partially shielded from fluctuations in the systemic blood pressure through reflex mechanisms capable of maintaining an even cerebral blood flow in spite of wide variations in general haemodynamics.

The spinal cord receives its blood supply from arteries that are relatively very small. The anterior spinal artery originates as a branch from each vertebral artery and can be traced the whole length of the spinal cord, but is in reality not a continuous vessel but a series of anastomoses. A variable number of arteries arise from the intercostal and iliac arteries to enter the spinal canal through the intervertebral foramina, and each supplies a length of cord above and below its level of entry. The most constant of these radicular vessels is the arteria magna that is a branch of an intercostal artery at the level of the diaphragm, nearly always on the left side. The posterior spinal arteries are smaller vessels receiving more numerous but also inconstant reinforcements from radicular arteries. Within the spinal cord the anterior spinal artery supplies the anterior and lateral columns and most of the grey matter. Its branches pass alternately to the right and left halves of the cord. The posterior spinal arteries supply the posterior columns of the cord.

The venous drainage of the brain stem accompanies the arteries and needs no special description. The veins of the spinal cord end in the vertebral veins, but also communicate with venous sinuses lying outside the spinal dura. The venous system of the cerebral hemispheres bears little relation to the arterial supply. Blood from the cortex drains either into the superior sagittal sinus, into the transverse and petrosal sinuses or, through the superficial temporal vein, into the cavernous sinus. This also receives the venous drainage from the orbit and is thus connected with the venous circulation outside the cranial cavity. The deep drainage from the hemispheres and from central structures join in the vein of Galen which runs into the straight sinus in the mid-line of the tentorium cerebelli. Posteriorly it is joined by the superior sagittal sinus. The blood then passes forward and laterally in the transverse and sigmoid sinuses to leave the skull in the internal jugular vein through the jugular foramen.

MENINGES

The dura mater is a tough membrane surrounding the entire central nervous system. It is often said to consist of two layers but the outer layer is the periosteum of the overlying bones. The dura forms a deep fold between the cerebral hemispheres, the falx cerebri, which is continuous at its posterior end with a lateral fold, the tentorium cerebelli. This forms the roof of the posterior fossa, the brain stem passing through the tentorial opening anteriorly. The venous sinuses form cavities within the dura. The spinal dura is continuous with that of the cranium and terminates in the sacral canal. The spinal cord is anchored laterally to the dura by the dentate ligaments.

Beneath the dura lies the thin and normally transparent arachnoid membrane. This is closely applied to the convexity of the brain but is not attached to nervous tissue and does not enter the sulci of the brain. Around the base of the brain the subarachnoid space expands to form large cisterns, notably those around the optic chiasma and anterior to the pons, and the cisterna magna lying posterior to the medulla and upper end of the spinal cord. The spinal arachnoid is continuous with that of the brain and extends below the termination of the spinal cord to enclose the cauda equina, ending in the sacral canal.

The pia mater is a fine membrane everywhere adherent to the surface of the brain and cord and loosely attached to the arachnoid by fine trabeculae. The pia dips into all the sulci, and accompanies blood vessels into the nervous tissue for a short distance before fusing with their walls.

THE CEREBROSPINAL FLUID

The subarachnoid space and the ventricles of the brain are filled with cerebrospinal fluid. The essential features of the ventricular system can be seen from Fig. 4. A point of great clinical interest is that the connections between the ventricles, the foramina of Monro and the aqueduct, and also the foramina in the roof of the fourth ventricle, are all narrow passages.

The cerebrospinal fluid is formed by a double process of secretion by the choroid plexuses in the ventricles and filtration from the plasma over the whole surface of the pia-arachnoid and of the ependymal lining of the ventricles, the first process being clinically by far the more important. A choroid plexus is present in each ventricle and consists of an invagination of blood vessels that forms a rich capillary network covered by a layer of thickened ependymal epithelium. Similarly, some absorption takes place over the whole surface, but the predominant site is on the convexity of

FORM AND FUNCTIONS

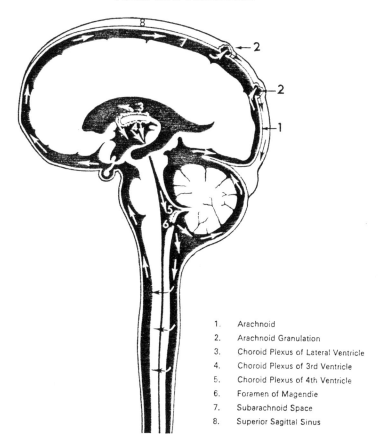

1. Arachnoid
2. Arachnoid Granulation
3. Choroid Plexus of Lateral Ventricle
4. Choroid Plexus of 3rd Ventricle
5. Choroid Plexus of 4th Ventricle
6. Foramen of Magendie
7. Subarachnoid Space
8. Superior Sagittal Sinus

FIG. 4. Circulation of spinal fluid.

the cerebral hemispheres, mostly through the arachnoid villi. These are herniations of arachnoid into the superior sagittal sinus. For practical purposes, therefore, the cerebrospinal fluid is formed in the ventricles, passes through the communicating passages and reaches the subarachnoid space. It diffuses slowly down the spinal canal and upwards around the brain stem to be absorbed over the convexity of the hemispheres.

One function of the cerebrospinal fluid is to maintain the central nervous system in a constant physical and chemical environment, though the factors that control the entry of metabolites into the fluid are obscure. Normal spinal fluid is completely clear and under a pressure of from 50 to

180 mm of water as measured by lumbar puncture with the patient recumbent. Its chemical composition differs in many ways from that of plasma, the protein content in particular being very low. The normal values of those components usually estimated are as follows:

Total protein 0.2 to 0.45 g l^{-1} (20 to 45 mg per 100 ml)
Glucose 2.2–4.0 mmol l^{-1} (40–70 mg per 100 ml)
Cells (lymphocytes) less than 5 per mm^3.

The level of glucose is greatly influenced by the level in the plasma but is always lower in the spinal fluid. Fractionation of the protein is difficult because of its dilution, but is proving to be of increasing clinical importance.

Further reading

Benson D.F. (1977) Neurological correlates of aphasia and apraxia. In *Recent Advances in Clinical Neurology II*, ed. W.B. Matthews and G.H. Glaser. Churchill Livingstone, Edinburgh and London.

Bowsher D. (1979) *Introduction to the Anatomy and Physiology of the Nervous System*, 4th edn. Blackwell Scientific Publications, Oxford.

Brodal A. (1969) *Neurological Anatomy in Relation to Clinical Medicine*, 2nd edn. Clarendon Press, Oxford.

Lance J.W. & Macleod J.G (1981) *A Physiological Approach to Clinical Neurology*, 3rd edn. Butterworth, London.

CHAPTER 2
Examination of the Nervous System

The art and science of neurological examination are based on thorough familiarity with the normal. In practised hands the examination of a cooperative patient does not take long, though detailed assessment of sensory loss or intellectual impairment requires time and patience. Unimaginative routine may lead to the two common errors of conducting tests without positively observing the results, and of failing to pay regard to the patient's actual symptoms. A complaint of difficulty in climbing stairs will not be unravelled by examining the patient lying on a couch. Methods must be adapted to circumstances that range from the hospital environment familiar to the student to the cold ill-lit back room with a confused obese woman lying on the wrong side of a sagging double bed. Detailed tests for aphasia are unnecessary in a patient with an obvious ulnar nerve palsy, but incomplete examination invites disaster, especially when the other systems of the body are ignored.

The scheme of examination outlined can be relied upon to reveal the presence of abnormalities, but their detailed description is left to later chapters.

THE ADULT

Examination begins while taking the history, when defects of speech or memory may already become evident and the patient's attitude to his symptoms and his environment can be noted.

The gait should always be observed, including the ability to turn quickly. Walking heel-to-toe is a good test of balance, but the elderly find it difficult. The normal adult can stand on one leg and does not fall when standing with the feet together and the eyes closed (Romberg's test). The ability to rise from a low chair without help from the arms, to step onto a low stool, or to stand on the toes should be tested if there is any suspicion of weakness of the legs.

THE CRANIAL NERVES

Gross defects in the sense of smell can be detected by blocking each nostril in turn and asking if the patient can smell oil of cloves held to the nose or can distinguish with eyes closed between two commonly encountered smells such as coffee and orange peel. Failure to identify odours by name is normal. If loss of sense of smell is claimed (anosmia) the test should be repeated with ammonia which irritates the nasal mucosa and does not stimulate the olfactory organs. Inability to detect strong ammonia is sometimes claimed in medico-legal cases, and suggests that the patient's statements are unreliable.

The optic fundi should be examined with the room darkened. The disc is inspected for pallor or swelling, the retinal vessels for alteration in calibre, and the retina for exudates, haemorrhages and degenerative changes. Only constant practice engenders confidence in the use of the ophthalmoscope. With the room still darkened the pupils are examined with a bright torch. The normal pupils are equal, round and regular and contract briskly on exposure to light on convergence. In the elderly the pupils are often small and the light reflex more difficult to observe, but a definite decision should be reached on whether the reaction is present or not. It is easy to prevaricate with the description 'sluggish'.

Visual acuity can be tested with Snellen's types read at a distance of six metres. The card should be well-lit and if the patient has glasses he should wear them. In their absence the patient should view the chart through a pinhole. Reading cards for near vision offer a more convenient but less sensitive test of central acuity. Unless it is known that refractive errors have been corrected interpretation may be difficult, but repeated testing under identical conditions will confirm deterioration or improvement.

The peripheral visual fields are tested by confrontation. One eye is covered and the patient fixes on the examiner's eye. A red or white object about five millimetres in diameter is brought in from the periphery in each quadrant of the field and the patient states when the object or the colour is visible. Misleading results can be obtained if the object is brought in on the horizontal or vertical meridian as the stimulus may be inadvertently moved from one half field to the other. The blind spots should also be identified and this will also afford an opportunity to examine for the presence of central or paracentral scotomata. The ability to detect finger movements simultaneously in each temporal field or in both fields is also tested. Confrontation tests are often remarkably accurate, especially since their brevity avoids fatiguing the patient. However, if any abnormality is found or suspected more precise methods must be used (Chapter 4).

The ocular movements are tested in all directions of gaze, and any defect of movement or complaint of diplopia noted. Nystagmus consists of jerking movements of the eyes with failure to maintain fixation. Ill-sustained nystagmus is normal at the extremes of lateral gaze beyond the range of binocular vision, but sustained nystagmus is always abnormal. The analysis of diplopia is described in Chapter 4.

The upper lid normally covers the upper part of the iris but does not encroach on the pupil. Drooping of the lids (ptosis) or lid retraction causing the sclera to show above the iris should be noted.

Facial sensibility is tested in all three divisions of the trigeminal distribution. It is unexpectedly easy to draw blood from dilated veins on the cheeks and care should be taken when testing with a pin. The corneal reflex is best elicited by asking the patient to look up and the cornea is then touched with a wisp of cotton wool. No reflex will be obtained by touching the sclera. The reaction to tickle in the nostril is similarly sensitive.

At this stage also the jaw jerk should be elicited. The mouth is half opened, the examiner's finger placed on the chin and struck with the tendon hammer. In most normal people there is no jerk or only a slight contraction of the masseters. An increased jerk may be found but is an unreliable quantitative sign.

The face and jaws are examined for asymmetry at rest and involuntary movement. The patient is then asked to screw up the eyes, to bare the teeth, and to open and close the jaws. In many normal people the lower jaw may appear to deviate slightly to one side on opening the mouth but this is due to minor abnormalities of the temporomandibular joints.

When hearing is tested, the tympanic membranes should first be inspected to make sure that deafness is not due to wax or to infection or destruction of the sound-conducting mechanism. Intermittent pressure should be exerted over the tragus of the opposite ear, thus producing sufficient noise to block hearing on that side. A quiet whisper or the sound made by rubbing the finger and thumb together should be clearly heard at a distance of a foot. Degrees of deafness can be assessed by repeating numbers in an increasingly loud voice until the patient can repeat them correctly. A list of numbers includes many consonants of high frequency, and inability to repeat correctly such figures as 66 or 77 indicates a high-frequency loss. If hearing is clinically normal there is no need to perform tuning fork tests, but if deafness is detected an attempt can be made to determine whether this is due to damage to the nerve and its receptors or to the conductive mechanism in the middle ear. A high frequency tuning fork (512 cps (C2) or 1024 cps (C3)) is held to the meatus and, when no longer audible, is transferred to the mastoid process. Normally and also in nerve deafness the tuning fork will not be heard, but in middle ear deafness the sound is conducted in the bone past the defect, and the note will still be heard. Some confusion arises from the fact that bone-conducted sound is transmitted across the skull with little loss, so in a unilateral nerve deafness the patient may also apparently have better hearing by bone than air conduction; the sound actually being heard in the good ear. A tuning fork placed on the centre of the forehead will be heard louder in the normal ear in nerve or perceptive deafness, but in the affected ear in conductive deafness.

There is unfortunately no rapid clinical test of vestibular function: a complaint of giddiness on change of posture must always be investigated by observing the effects of such movements, with particular attention to the production of nystagmus.

Sense of taste on the anterior part of each side of the tongue can be tested quickly by applying the terminals of a torch battery, the familiar tingling sensation being a taste and not an ordinary somatic sensation. The classical method is to drop a solution tasting of one of the four true tastes, salt, sweet, acid and bitter, on the protruded tongue and to ask the patient to point to the correct answer on a card. This is time-consuming and less reliable than the electrical method. There is no satisfactory method of testing taste on the back of the tongue.

The movement of the palate is observed on phonation, when the uvula should rise in the mid-line. The uvula is an asymmetrical structure and apparent slight deviations are unlikely to be significant. Sensation on the back of the tongue and pharynx is tested with a spatula and the gag reflex elicited on each side. Any wasting of the tongue or deviation from the mid-line should be observed, and the patient should be asked to move the tongue rapidly from side to side.

Both sterno-mastoid muscles should stand out firmly when the head is flexed against resistance, and can be tested individually when the chin is turned against the examiner's hand. The trapezius muscle can be seen to contract on shrugging the shoulders.

With the patient sitting up, the skull and spine can be palpated and inspected for deformities or tenderness, and active and passive movement of the neck, including lateral flexion, can be tested. This is an appropriate moment to listen for a bruit over the carotid arteries in the neck, over the subclavian arteries in the supraclavicular space, and, if relevant, over the skull and orbits.

THE UPPER LIMBS

Examination of the upper limbs should begin with inspection for deformity, wasting or fasciculation (flickering contraction of muscle bundles) or for involuntary movements in the resting posture. The patient is then asked to hold the arms straight in front of him with the fingers separated and his eyes closed. Tremor or other involuntary movement may become apparent, or one arm may slowly drift down owing either to weakness or loss of postural sense. Each arm is pushed sharply down and should immediately return to its former position without any rebound. First with his eyes open and then closed the patient is asked to touch the tip of his nose with the index finger, when tremor or inaccurate placing may be seen. This test will serve to reveal incoordination due both to cerebellar disease and to loss of proprioceptive sensation, that caused by sensory loss becoming much less pronounced when the eyes are opened. With eyes open he is asked to perform rapid movements such as alternately touching his nose and the examiner's finger, opening and closing the hands or rotating the forearms. Fine finger movements can be tested by rapid tapping with the index finger, or by more functional tests such as doing up buttons.

Tone in the main muscle groups is tested by passive flexion and extension of the wrist and elbow. Power can be tested rapidly by asking the patient to hold both arms abducted, flexed to a right angle at the elbows and with wrists and fingers extended, and to resist any passive movement. Once the patient understands his role an attempt is made to overcome each muscle group in turn. With the exception of abduction of the fingers, which can easily be overcome, a normal adult can maintain the posture of the limb against the degree of force permissible in a clinical examination. The grip of each hand should also be estimated. In special circumstances individual muscles must be examined in more detail, those most commonly overlooked being the spinati and the small muscles of the hands. The action of the former is complex, but can be tested almost in isolation by the resistance to inward rotation of the humerus.

The tendon reflexes normally obtainable in the upper limbs are the biceps, supinator and triceps jerks. Any abnormal spread of the reflex response such as flexion of the fingers on striking the biceps tendon should be noted. When reflex activity is increased a jerk can be obtained from the finger flexors by tapping the palmar surface of the lightly flexed fingers and the response may be repeated several times in the form of a clonic reflex. In many normal subjects the tendon reflexes in the upper limbs are unobtainable but asymmetrical loss is pathological. These reflexes can be reinforced by the patient clenching the teeth or the opposite fist.

Sensation can be tested at this point but is usually best left until the lower limbs have been examined.

The superficial abdominal reflexes are tested by lightly stroking the skin of the abdominal quadrants, the response being a brisk contraction of the underlying muscle. Absent reflexes are not always abnormal or important especially in a lax abdomen, and it is unnecessary to draw blood in an attempt to elicit them. The contraction of the abdominal muscles can be tested by asking the patient to raise the shoulders from the couch. Distension of the bladder should be carefully looked for.

THE LOWER LIMBS

Examination of the lower limbs follows the same principles, beginning with inspection for deformity, wasting or involuntary movement. Coordination is tested by asking the patient to place one heel on the opposite knee and then slowly to slide the heel down the shin. This can normally be performed smoothly and accurately. Slight increases in muscle tone are difficult to detect because many patients are incapable of relaxing, but a gross increase in extensor or flexor tone is easily appreciated on passive movement at the knee.

The muscles of the lower limbs are normally powerful, and marked degrees of weakness may escape detection if the strength of the examiner's arm is the only measure employed. If the limb is held flexed to a right angle at the hip and knee it should not be possible to overcome either the flexor or extensor muscles of these joints. The dorsiflexors and plantar flexors of the feet are also normally very strong, but eversion and inversion at the ankle are less natural movements which the patient may find difficult to sustain. Rapid alternating movements of the toes are always clumsy and irregular. More stringent tests of the strength of the larger muscles may be necessary, including the ability to lift both heels off the couch with the knees straight, to stand on the toes of one foot, or to rise from the floor.

The knee jerks can nearly always be obtained in health, but symmetrical loss of the ankle jerks is common in the elderly. Very brisk reflexes may also be normal when they are symmetrical, but undoubted asymmetry is a significant finding. In many anxious people a few beats of ankle clonus are obtained on sharp dorsiflexion of the foot, but clonus that persists as long as the calf muscles are stretched is abnormal. Clonus at the knee can be produced by sharply depressing the patella and sustaining the pressure. With heightened reflex activity, tendon jerks can be obtained from the adductors and hamstrings.

The plantar reflex is an invaluable physical sign, but is not always easy to elicit or interpret. The area stimulated must be the outer side of the sole, since misleading results may be obtained from the instep. Any blunt point provides a suitable implement, and the stimulus should not be painful. The normal response is flexion of all the toes. The abnormal

EXAMINATION OF NERVOUS SYSTEM 41

extensor response, or Babinski reflex, consists of dorsiflexion of the great toe and fanning of the other toes, often combined with slight contraction of the hamstring muscles. Unfortunately a clear-cut response cannot always be obtained, either because the reflex is genuinely 'equivocal' or because the feet are too sensitive. In doubtful cases the knee should be flexed, and the area to be stimulated rubbed briskly with the hand several times before attempting to obtain the response. Many variants of the Babinski reflex have been described but do not merit enumeration or commitment to memory.

SENSATION

In much of the examination so far described we depend on the co-operation of the patient but with patience this can usually be obtained. Tests of sensation are, however, by definition 'subjective' and provide almost unlimited opportunities for misunderstanding. Vibration sense is tested with a tuning fork (C^0, 124) which should first be applied to the sternum to demonstrate the normal sensation. It can then be applied to bony prominences at the ankle and wrist, and need be explored further only if vibration cannot be felt at these points. Even after careful demonstration many subjects will claim to feel vibration when the tuning fork is still so that if there is any doubt the test should be performed with the patient's eyes closed. Postural sense is normally tested by moving the terminal phalanges of the fingers or toes through a small range and asking the patient to state, without looking, whether the digit is being moved upwards or downwards. The answer 'sideways' after the most careful explanation is one of the unavoidable hazards of neurology. Normally very small movements can be identified with ease. If even large movements of the digits cannot be appreciated, movement at progressively more proximal joints should be tested. In the elderly, vibration sense is often absent in the lower limbs and postural sense less acute.

Sense of light touch is then tested with cotton wool. The patient's eyes are closed, and he is asked to state immediately he feels each touch. Time should be allowed for the response and single stimuli should be applied. Absolute loss or anaesthesia can be readily detected, but slight differences between two areas of skin should be accepted with reserve since they are often inconstant. Superficial pain sensation is tested with a pin, and with a little practice a more or less standardized prick can be given. Here several stimuli within a small area of skin may be necessary as pain-sensitive receptor-organs are not evenly distributed and may be missed by a single pinprick. A hypodermic needle penetrates the skin and is not suitable for sensory testing. Great perseverance may be needed to ensure that the patient genuinely understands what the pin should feel like, and the extent of any area of complete or relative analgesia should be repeatedly confirmed. Needless to say it is not normally necessary to test the entire surface of the body for these forms of sensation, the face and extremities being usually enough, but if loss of sensation is reasonably suspected detailed investigation is essential. An important and often neglected region is the skin of the buttocks and perineum.

Thermal sensation is best tested with metal tubes containing water of known temperature, but perfectly satisfactory results can be obtained with glass test-tubes filled with hot and cold water. If an area of diminished sensation is found during testing any form of superficial sensation, stimulation should proceed from the abnormal to the normally innervated skin, and in this way it is usually possible to map out the areas of altered sensation with some precision. It must not be expected that all such areas will have sharply defined boundaries and some variation must be accepted. It is also possible to become confused by areas of heightened or unpleasant sensation, and particularly by abnormal pain on pinprick—or hyperalgesia. It must be remembered that patients are not accustomed to being tickled with cotton wool or tormented with pins, and a more familiar sensation such as touching the skin with the finger may provide more reliable results.

Deep pain is tested by squeezing the Achilles tendon or first interosseous space with increasing force until pain is experienced.

Two-point discrimination is a useful test. The finger pulps are extremely sensitive and it is normally possible to distinguish two points three millimetres apart from a single point, though there is some variation. One or two points are applied in random sequence, and the proportion of correct answers scored. The distance between the points is progressively increased until a threshold is reached where there are no mistakes. In partial impairment of sensation due to peripheral lesions a threshold can be found, but with loss due to cortical damage occasional mistakes may still be made, however far apart the points are applied.

A refined test is the recognition by touch of objects placed in the hand, or stereognosis. There is no point in investigating this function in an anaesthetic hand since it will certainly be absent, but in disease of the posterior columns of the spinal cord it may be conspicuous when the only other evidence of sensory loss is some impairment of vibration sense and, in the presence of a cortical lesion, astereognosis may furnish the only sensory evidence. The appreciation of bilateral simultaneous stimuli may also be impaired, so that a stimulus is felt on either hand when applied separately but when both sides are stimulated together only that on the normal side is appreciated. This defect is known as sensory inattention or extinction and is a valuable sign of an early lesion of the sensory cortex.

SPEECH

Dysarthria will have been detected while taking the patient's history and may be out of proportion to any defect of the muscles used in articulation found on examination. Weakness of the lips will be emphasized by the repetition of a sentence contining p's or b's and similarly defective movement of the tongue will be revealed by difficulty with r, l and th. Most test sentences, however, merely confirm the presence of dysarthria without throwing any light on its causation. Phonation, the production of the voice sound, is effected by the passage of air through the larynx and is quite distinct from articulation.

The analysis of aphasia can be elaborated almost indefinitely but its detection and broad categorization can be effected by a relatively simple scheme. The patient's spontaneous conversation should be carefully observed, seeking particularly for hesitations and the use of circumlocutions to avoid forgotten words. A series of objects is presented in rapid succession and the patient asked to name them and their use. He should be asked to repeat a number of sentences. The patient's understanding of the spoken and written word is tested by observing the response to increasingly complicated commands such as placing his left hand on his right ear and his right hand on his nose. The patient is asked to write some commonplace dictated sentence, and also to copy from a book. He should read aloud, and be asked to explain what he has read.

When appropriate the patient should also be tested for apraxia. He should be invited to carry out progressively more complex commands. He should also be observed putting on gloves or a pyjama jacket of which one sleeve has been turned inside out. The use of scissors and matches and the folding of a sheet of paper to fit into an envelope should also be tested, and the ability to make symbolic gestures such as shaking the fist or beckoning. Finally the construction of two-dimensional diagrams and drawings and three-dimensional patterns with matches or blocks can be tested. In disease of the parietal lobe such tests often indicate a gross disturbance of the appreciation of spatial relationships.

To the student, uncertain as yet even of the best way to hold a tendon hammer, the experienced neurologist may appear to conduct his physical examination with indecent speed. Familiarity has not, however, bred contempt and such expertise is based entirely on the constant application of the basic techniques outlined above.

INTELLECTUAL FUNCTION

Detailed analysis of defects in reasoning and memory is a skilled and time-consuming task, and the assessment of mental deficiency in the child may demand special expertise. However, it is often necessary to form a rapid preliminary opinion on the integrity or otherwise of intellectual function in the adult. This is not easy, since the recognition of deterioration implies familiarity with the patient's previous level of education and performance. These can seldom be known precisely, but understanding of the general cultural background will go far to avoid serious error.

There are certain tests that an adult capable of earning his living should be able to perform satisfactorily. Tests of common knowledge may be difficult to interpret, but most men can recall the subject of the day's headlines, the results of national sporting events and the fortunes of the local football team. Many normal women appear oblivious of current events. The examination of recent and remote personal memory is far more revealing, but can be effective only if a relative is present who can check the answers. Indeed the independent interrogation of a relative or friend is essential where the patient's mental state is in question.

In order to test memory directly, an imaginary name, address and telephone number are repeated twice and the patient asked to memorize them. He is then asked to subtract seven from 100 and to continue to take away seven from the remainder. A few mistakes in this test are normal, but it is abnormal to get no further than 93 and then to forget the number to be subtracted. The patient is then asked for the name and address he had memorized: he should be able to produce them correctly after an interval of two to five minutes. The Babcock sentence is a useful test of immediate recall and doubtless of other functions. The patient is told he must repeat the sentence as soon as it is finished and then the words, 'The one thing needful to make this country rich and great is a large, secure supply of wood' are clearly enunciated. Failure to repeat correctly after three attempts is abnormal.

By this time it may be obvious that grave defects are present, perhaps altogether concealed in the patient's everyday behaviour, but the investigation can be elaborated by asking for the interpretation of common proverbs or of pictures, and the reckoning of change. Dementia will nearly always be revealed by these rapid tests, but they are undoubtedly open to falsification by those claiming intellectual loss following injury.

STUPOR AND COMA

The neurological examination of the patient who is not fully conscious is naturally somewhat limited in scope. Terminology is sadly imprecise and the distinction between 'semi-coma' and 'semi-consciousness' is obscure. A patient who shows only reflex response to any stimulus is in a coma. A patient who can be roused by painful stimuli to make incoherent noises with withdrawal movements is in stupor. Impaired awareness of the environment accompanied by more purposive movement and speech is the stage of confusion.

An attempt should be made to rouse the patient, the most effective stimulus being painful pressure with the knuckles on the sternum. As well as furnishing a measure of the depth of unconsciousness, this manoeuvre may also uncover the existence of unilateral paralysis. The respiratory rhythm is often disturbed in comatose patients and is an important prognostic sign. The optic fundi and pupils must be examined and any fixed deviation or other abnormal ocular movement noted. The tympanic membranes must be seen. Signs of meningeal irritation may be present, especially neck rigidity. The neck can normally be flexed so that the chin almost touches the sternum. Inflammation or blood in the subarachnoid space causes spasm of the posterior neck muscles limiting flexion to a greater or lesser degree. Similar spasm in the hamstring muscles may prevent full passive extension of the knee when the hip is flexed to a right angle (Kernig's sign).

The state of the tendon reflexes is not likely to be helpful and the plantar reflexes are usually extensor in coma whatever its cause. In deep coma the corneal reflexes are absent. Localized paralysis may be detected by complete loss of muscular tone or unilateral absence of withdrawal from pain. Abnormal postures with rigid extension of the limbs may be present continuously or spasmodically.

Examination on these lines is necessarily brief, but in many circumstances, after head injury for example, careful observation of the changing neurological state, and especially of the patient's level of consciousness, may be of vital importance.

The clinical distinction between deep coma and death has recently assumed great importance. Many patients who would previously have died are now supported by artificial ventilation and the decision to switch off the machinery must be based on the certainty that the brain, evidently the seat of the soul, is dead. The most important criteria are the absence of brain stem reflexes. If the brain is dead, the pupils are in mid-position and do not react to light; the eyes remain fixed on rapid head movement or on slow injection of 20 ml of ice-cold water into the external auditory meatus on each side; the corneal and gag reflexes are absent; the limbs do not adopt rigid extended or flexed postures in response to any stimulus; respiration is absent even when arterial P_{CO_2} is at a level high enough to stimulate the respiratory centre. Spinal reflexes, such as tendon jerks, may, however, still be present. The EEG record will also be silent. It is essential that these observations are repeated after an interval of at least six hours during which the two possible reversible causes of coma of such severity can be excluded: barbiturate intoxication and hypothermia. On many grounds it is essential that the cause of the brain damage, metabolic or structural, be established beyond doubt.

THE INFANT

Neurological examination of the infant is also based on knowledge of the expected normal findings. These change progressively with continued maturation of the nervous system after birth.

The normal newborn child moves all limbs spontaneously and the pupillary reaction to light and the corneal reflex are already present. Other reflexes not seen in the normal adult are also found. The sucking reflex, induced by stimulus near the lips, is of obvious biological importance but the grasp reflex, in which any object placed in the palm is firmly gripped, seems more appropriate to an arboreal life. The Moro reflex consists of rapid abduction of the arms when the child is startled or suddenly moved. Tonic neck reflexes may also be found. If the head is rotated to one side the arm and sometimes the leg on the same side will extend. The absence of these reflexes in the newborn or their persistence after the age of three months is abnormal. The plantar reflex is extensor at birth and a valueless sign until the age of two or three years. Paediatricians have evolved elaborate systems of examination based on the posture adopted by the baby when it is held in different positions, but the interpretation of their findings is obscure and inconclusive.

Apart from obvious abnormalities such as marked loss or increase in muscular tone, or failure to move one or more limbs, examination comprises essentially observation of the development of normal functions. Expression of displeasure is present from birth, but a baby first smiles at about six weeks. Fixation of the eyes on a stationary object can be detected at three to four weeks, but not until 12 weeks is a moving object followed. Some ability to support the head should be apparent by this age, and at 24 weeks sitting with support is possible. By 40 weeks the child should be able to sit unsupported, to crawl and stand with support. The age at which walking unsupported becomes possible is variable between 12 and 18 months and relative delay in an obviously active baby should not cause concern. By this age the faculty of speech should have developed to the expression and understanding of a few words. A child of two should be running about actively and talking freely with a limited vocabulary, and should have normal control of the sphincters in the daytime.

Visual acuity cannot be tested in the small infant beyond the ability to follow a moving object, and the detection of deafness, by judging the response to sudden or meaningful noise, is notoriously difficult.

The circumference of the head may be of great importance and the normal range is as follows:

Birth	13 to 14½ inches	33 to 37.5 cm
3 months	15 to 16½ inches	38 to 43 cm
6 months	16½ to 17½ inches	41 to 46 cm
9 months	17½ to 18½ inches	43 to 48 cm
12 months	18 to 19 inches	44 to 49 cm
18 months	18½ to 19½ inches	45 to 51 cm
24 months	19 to 20 inches	46 to 52 cm

The rate of growth is often more important than the actual size and when necessary this can be plotted on a graph showing the normal range. The anterior fontanelle normally closes between the ages of nine months and two years, but the time of closure is seldom important. The fontanelle should be level with the cranial vault and is abnormal if it is bulging or sunken.

Individual variations in development are common, but gross divergencies are highly suggestive of congenital defect or progressive disease of the nervous system.

LUMBAR PUNCTURE

Lumbar puncture is much dreaded by patients, but with practice and attention to detail it is nearly always a simple and almost painless procedure. The patient lies with the spine fully flexed to separate the lumbar spinous processes. The skin must be carefully cleaned and aseptic precautions maintained to the point of not touching the needle at all except through sterile gauze. The best site of puncture is normally the space between the third and fourth spinous processes, which lies approximately on a line joining the two iliac crests. In the obese the space may not be easy to find, but as the spinal cord terminates at the lower border of the first lumbar vertebra an error of one space in either direction is of no importance. The skin and interspinous ligament should be anaesthetized with a small quantity of 2% procaine. The needle should be straight and sharp and the stylette must fit accurately. The Greenfield needle with a two-way tap is generally manufactured with too wide a bore and is best avoided. Harris's 'trigeminal' needle is excellent. The point is pushed smartly through the skin and then advanced slowly and smoothly through the ligament. If it is aimed correctly it is possible to sense the penetration first of the dura and then of the arachnoid. Difficulties encountered include inserting the needle over the spinous process, when bone will be struck immediately and a new site must be chosen. It is usually easier to find the subarachnoid space if the needle is directed slightly towards the patient's head. A needle inserted too laterally may strike a nerve root and cause a sharp pain down the leg.

Once a flow of cerebrospinal fluid is obtained the pressure must be measured. In the recumbent position this is normally between 80 and 180 millimetres of water, but may be higher if the patient is too tense or too tightly flexed. Queckenstedt's test to demonstrate spinal block is unreliable but before the development of neuroradiology was considered valuable. The jugular veins are compressed, separately and together, by an assistant who should be restrained from obliterating both carotids, light pressure being adequate. The normal response is a rapid rise in cerebrospinal fluid down the spine and up the manometer. Release is followed by a more gradual fall of pressure. Failure to rise may be due to jugular occlusion (rarely), to a block in the flow of fluid down the spinal canal, or to faulty placing of the needle. If no rise occurs, the patient is told to take a deep breath and then bear down, or to cough. This causes distension of the venous system in the spinal canal and a rise in cerebrospinal fluid pressure even in the presence of a block. If the point of the needle is obstructed no rise occurs. A positive Queckenstedt test, implying a spinal block, cannot be accepted unless this full manoeuvre has been carried out.

A cerebrospinal fluid specimen of two millilitres is sufficient for most purposes. If the fluid is blood-stained three separate specimens should be obtained and labelled. If the blood is due to accidental puncture of a vessel the third specimen will contain fewer red cells, while subarachnoid haemorrhage causes uniform mixing of blood and spinal fluid. If the pressure is raised, no more than the contents of the manometer should be removed.

The indications for lumbar puncture will be discussed in later chapters but here it can be urged that the diagnostic help required should be carefully considered before puncture is performed and that the maximum amount of information should be obtained. In particular, the pressure should be *measured* since no reliance can be placed on a mere guess at the rate of flow.

Serious complications occur only if the pressure equilibrium is already distorted by disease. Removal of spinal fluid when the volume of one of the components of the contents of the skull is increased, as with a cerebral tumour, may allow the cerebellar tonsils to descend into the foramen magnum and compress the brain stem. Similarly, the inferior surface of the temporal lobe may be pushed down into the tentorial opening. This 'coning' is the reason for avoiding lumbar puncture as far as possible when the intracranial pressure is known to be raised. Occasionally the signs of spinal cord compression may increase rapidly after lumbar puncture.

The common complication is headache. This is almost certainly due to continued escape of fluid from the hole in the arachnoid and is therefore more common after clumsy or difficult puncture, but it may follow even the most skilful needling. The pain is due to an unduly low pressure and is relieved by lying down. When severe it is distressing and accompanied by vomiting. The accompanying neck stiffness may give rise to fears of meningitis. Prevention can be attempted by enforced recumbency in the prone position for some hours after puncture, but it is not wholly successful. Treatment consists of lying flat and a large fluid intake until the pain subsides.

Cisternal puncture is occasionally necessary when, for example, it is desired to inject therapeutic or diagnostic substances above a spinal block. The technique is easy but is attended by the anxiety naturally induced by the knowledge that the medulla is only a few centimetres from the point of the needle. The hair is shaved on the back of the neck and the site of puncture, the hollow between the highest palpable point of the cervical spine and the base of the skull, is identified. The skin is often very tough and it is distasteful to exert great pressure with the needle pointed directly at the medulla, so the initial puncture is made with the needle deliberately out of line. Once through the skin the point is directed forwards and upwards, aiming at the root of the nose, until it is firmly gripped by the atlanto-occipital ligament. It is then advanced gradually until at a depth of about three to four centimetres it will be felt to penetrate the arachnoid. The point is still a safe three centimetres from the medulla, but cisternal puncture should not be attempted on a struggling patient.

Further reading

Bickerstaff E.R. (1980) *Neurological Examination in Clinical Practice.* 4th edn. Blackwell Scientific Publications, Oxford.

Plum F. & Posner J.B. (1980) *The Diagnosis of Stupor and Coma.* 3rd edn. Davis, Philadelphia.

CHAPTER 3
Neurological Symptoms

Students of neurology often complain that patients do not present with the diseases described in textbooks but with symptoms. This is, of course, true of any branch of medicine, but the symptoms of neurological disease are extremely diverse, in conformity with the multitudinous functions of the nervous system. It is not, however, merely the variety of neurological symptoms that presents the difficulty. Many such symptoms are quite unfamiliar sensations that the patient, however intelligent and willing, is unable to explain in ordinary language. Many do not try to do so but adopt some conventional phrase or word that they hope will convey their meaning to the doctor. A number of these potentially misleading terms will be encountered in this chapter.

HEADACHE

Headache is one of the commonest conditions about which patients consult their doctor and will be encountered as a symptom of many diseases described in subsequent chapters. Although headache is always an unpleasant symptom frequently requiring relief the main point of diagnostic significance is to determine whether it arises from relatively unimportant extracranial causes or from some potentially far more serious lesion within the cranial cavity.

The headache that anyone may experience from fatigue or stress probably arises largely or entirely from the muscles and fascia of the scalp and neck. Medical advice is naturally not sought for this familiar event but chronic headache, apparently of similar origin, is very common. This may occur in children and adults but seldom persists into old age. The pain is described as being present every day on waking in the morning and persisting all day, becoming worse in the evening or with fatigue. The site of the pain is variable but is often bifrontal, bitemporal and in the neck. The character of the pain is seldom described as severe, except for brief periods, and on direct enquiry it may be said that it is 'not really a pain at all' but more a sensation of pressure. The scalp may be tender when the hair is combed. In addition to this diffuse, dull sensation sharp localized stabs of pain are often described. Analgesics are seldom helpful but rest often brings relief and the headache does not prevent sleep. This description has been elaborated to emphasize the significant points of the timing, distribution and character of the pain and of the factors found to aggravate or relieve it. Pain having all the features described would certainly prompt an initial diagnosis of tension headache—unpleasant and difficult to treat but not threatening life, strength or sanity. Naturally this preliminary diagnosis would have to be supported or revised by the results of further enquiry into associated symptoms and of physical examination and, occasionally, investigation. The headache of migraine which also arises from extracranial structures is considered in detail in Chapter 18. Classically this has different characteristics. It is periodic, occurring in definable episodes with intervals of freedom. It may initially be localized to one area of the head and is often severe or even prostrating. Some relief may be obtained from analgesics. The pain of cranial arteritis, although arising from the same structures, has many different features. It is often continuously present but is localized and severe. In both these conditions associated symptoms will provide further evidence but the nature of the headache alone carries considerable diagnostic weight.

The headache caused by intracranial lesions usually differs in many ways from that arising from extracranial causes. The brain itself is insensitive to pain and may be cut or burnt with impunity. The dura and arteries at the base of the brain give rise to painful sensations when stretched. This will occur with raised intracranial pressure. Here the headache is classically intermittent, present and severe on waking, but easing and disappearing within an hour or two. At first it is not present every day. The site of the pain varies to some extent with the site of the expanding lesion, but this correlation is far from exact. In general, a lesion above the tentorium will cause frontal headache, often worse on the side of the lesion. A posterior fossa tumour causes occipital headache. Obstruction of the flow of cerebrospinal fluid with ventricular dilatation may cause intermittent very severe generalized headache. The headache of raised intracranial pressure may be aggravated by straining but this also occurs in other more benign conditions.

The headache of severe arterial hypertension is identical with that of raised intracranial pressure, particularly with early morning predominance. Occasionally hypertension may present with headache resembling migraine. Headache following lumbar puncture is due to lowered intracranial pressure which also results in stretching of the basal meninges and arteries. It is relieved by lying down.

These brief descriptions must not be taken as absolute rules but as important aids to diagnosis. A well-known exception to the intermittent headache from intracranial lesions is that resulting from a pituitary tumour with acromegaly that may cause continuous centrally situated extremely obstinate pain.

NUMBNESS

This is a word used by patients in many different contexts. The doctor may assume that what is meant is loss of cutaneous sensation, but this is by no means always so. Anyone who has had a dental block numbing part of the face will recognize why this should be. The face feels as if it has been paralysed although it moves normally. It is quite difficult to distinguish between loss of feeling and loss of movement, particularly as either may give rise to loss of use. In practice, therefore, a complaint of numbness frequently means weakness and must not be interpreted as necessarily implying sensory loss. The patient with Bell's palsy, an acute lesion of the motor nerve of the face, will often say that the face is numb, which if true would have a quite different clinical meaning implying involvement of the trigeminal nerve as well. There is also often a complaint of numbness on the side of the tongue although here again there is no loss of common sensation but loss of sense of taste. Numbness is also often loosely used to describe impaired function of the limbs, whether from weakness, spasticity or loss of postural sense, but may also, of course, be used in the normally accepted sense of loss of skin sensation.

Other disturbances of sensation are even more difficult for the patient to describe and they may be reluctant to attempt this for fear of being thought neurotic. Great attention should, however, be paid to certain complaints that at first sound bizarre. A sensation as of a tight band round the leg is often experienced when there is a developing lesion of the posterior columns of the spinal cord. A complaint that one hand feels too large or feels 'as if it doesn't belong to me' is nearly always indicative of organic nervous disease. Focal sensory epilepsy may also give rise to totally unfamiliar sensations that can only be imperfectly described or understood but their organic nature is shown by the distribution on one side of the body and by the rapidity of spread.

The commonest abnormal sensation is the familiar 'pins and needles'. This is so easily induced by external pressure on nerve trunks that one would be entitled to assume that no difficulty would be encountered when asking about this symptom. However, many patients seem to confuse pins and needles with cramp, although the two sensations are entirely dissimilar. It is probably more rewarding to enquire about 'tingling' but to be prepared for considerable elaboration on this theme. As already emphasized patients are not deliberately misleading about sensory symptoms—they are simply difficult to describe.

Paraesthesiae may occasionally merge into pain, particularly with lesions of the peripheral nerves. Pain is on the whole far easier for patients to describe than these less familiar sensations and its different characteristics need not be further elaborated in this chapter. The diagnostic significance of paraesthesiae greatly depends on their anatomical and temporal distribution. Thus symmetrical tingling in the extremities would first suggest a generalized peripheral neuropathy. Tingling spreading up from the feet to the waist in the course of days or weeks would most probably indicate a spinal cord lesion. Unilateral paraesthesiae may arise from a variety of peripheral and central causes. Those resulting from a peripheral nerve lesion often seem to be more extensive than the anatomical distribution of the nerve. Paraesthesiae from sensory root involvement are, in contrast, often sharply localizing. Unilateral paraesthesiae involving an expanding area can occur episodically in migraine, in cerebral vascular insufficiency and in epilepsy, the distinction being made by the context and by the rapid spread of the epileptic symptoms. Paraesthesiae around the mouth, quite definitely involving both sides, are common in migraine and in vascular insufficiency of the brain stem, but also occur in hypoglycaemia and following overbreathing where they are accompanied by tingling in the hands and sometimes by tetanic spasm.

DIZZINESS

This word is the prime example of a stereotyped expression used by patients to cover a great variety of different sensations. It is certainly not synonymous with vertigo which implies an element of rotation. In very brief attacks this distinction may be virtually impossible but apart from this patients can usually tell whether their symptoms involve any form of spinning sensation or are episodes of unsteadiness, uncertainty, light-headedness or any of a large number of less well-defined feelings. It is essential to establish this distinction if possible as the diagnostic implications may be very different.

There are other important considerations. It is natural to think of dizziness as something experienced in the head but the word is also used to mean any difficulty in walking, quite unrelated to cranial symptoms. The duration of dizziness must also be determined, as a sensation continuously present during waking hours or always present on walking will have a very different meaning from definitely paroxysmal symptoms. Precipitating factors must also be sought, particularly the effect of change of posture. It must also be realized that many patients use the word dizziness to mean that they feel unwell or a little confused or distressed by the vicissitudes of life.

WEAKNESS

A complaint of weakness is rather less common than might be supposed, patients often preferring to speak of heaviness or of dragging of the leg particularly when this is due to upper motor neurone lesions. In general, lower motor neurone lesions and primary muscle disease are recognized by the patient as causing weakness of the limbs. In contrast, patients with Parkinson's disease may misinterpret their difficulty in rising from a low chair, a common early symptom, as due to weakness rather than to the difficulty in initiating movement seen in this disease. A particular difficulty arises in determining whether a painful limb is also weak as patients may be genuinely unable to decide whether they cannot use the limb because of pain or weakness.

A complaint of generalized fatigue is uncommon in neurological disease but may be encountered in Parkinsonism. A continuous feeling of tiredness may indeed be a symptom of important systemic disorders or of psychiatric disease but the patient with genuine muscular fatigue, the myasthenic, in fact complains of weakness. Rapid increase in disability on exertion is also a common feature in multiple sclerosis but here again the patient does not complain of feeling tired.

CRAMP

Most people have had occasional attacks of cramp in the calf or foot muscles in bed at night and are familiar with the severe pain and obvious muscle spasm. In spite of this the word is used in a very imprecise way to describe many forms of sharp pain, usually in the limbs without, as far as can be determined, any muscular spasm. A complaint of cramp should therefore be followed by an attempt to discover what is meant. Genuine cramp occurs after recovery from sciatica and in motor neurone disease but usually no cause can be found. It should not be confused with the carpo-pedal spasm of tetany.

UNSTEADINESS

A complaint of undue clumsiness is often difficult to interpret and may take many forms. A tendency to bump into doorposts may be due to an ataxic gait but also to defective vision, in particular hemianopia. A common symptom is of a sensation of being drawn to one side while walking. This may sound alarming as it is known that a lesion of one cerebellar hemisphere may indeed cause the patient to veer to that side when walking. However, when this occurs as the result of a cerebellar lesion it can be verified on examination as the patient can be seen to deviate in one direction when walking with eyes open or, a more stringent test, with eyes closed. In the great majority of patients with this complaint no disturbance of gait can be detected and the patients will often admit that their difficulty is not apparent to others and is intermittent. In such patients the symptom remains unexplained but it does not appear to be due to organic nervous disease and otological examination is also normal.

Another complaint that is unexpectedly difficult to understand is that of an increased tendency to drop objects from the hand, usually crockery. This can certainly be the result of the ataxia of cerebellar disease or of loss of postural sense in the hands or simply due to weakness but here again in many patients no abnormality can be found. The complaint appears genuine and may not be volunteered but only brought out on questioning, but in these patients it is an evanescent symptom that remains unexplained. It is certainly not always evidence of organic nervous disease.

DOUBLE VISION

This is another example of a phrase apt to be used unthinkingly by patients and not to be accepted as meaning diplopia without further enquiry. Often enough a complaint of double vision will be found on analysis to mean blurred vision or the uncomfortable sensation of oscillopsia. Some patients with nystagmus find that their field of vision oscillates and this is often described as double vision. In most patients nystagmus does not induce this sensation and what determines its occurrence is unknown. Rather more surprisingly a complaint of double vision may be found to mean just the reverse—hemianopia. This is an alarming and completely unfamiliar disturbance and it is not unnatural that a frightened patient may be unable to provide an adequate description.

A related problem is the difficulty of discovering whether transient symptoms of loss of vision are related to one or to both eyes. Patients will confidently assert that vision of the right eye, for example, was blurred but they are unaware of the anatomy of the visual pathways and believe that the right eye sees to the right and vice versa. Unless the patient has covered each eye in turn during the episode and observed the effect it may be impossible to distinguish between monocular visual loss and hemianopia. The general ignorance of how the eyes work is illustrated by the highly intelligent man who claimed that he knew he had lost his vision in one eye because he could only see one half of his wife.

BLACKOUTS

This word is used by patients in many different contexts, sometimes it seems almost at random. The two common meanings are of loss of vision and of loss of consciousness but the word will be encountered as a description of vertigo, blurred vision, falling, amnesia, speech disturbance such as aphasia, and many ill-defined sensations of the type also often referred to as dizziness. It may be applied to acute episodes of distress and panic, particularly when accompanied by overbreathing. A few pointed questions early in the history taking will at least start the diagnostic enquiry in the right direction.

The characteristic features of the common causes of unconsciousness will be described in subsequent chapters but the general problem of differential diagnosis from other symptoms can be considered. Unconsciousness results either from epilepsy or from failure of oxygen supply to the brain, a very rare cause being lack of cerebral glucose. An additional possibility that must be considered is that of hysterical attacks.

The diagnosis that an attack of unconsciousness was a major epileptic fit will be greatly strengthened by a history of a recognizable epileptic aura, tongue biting and incontinence during the attack and subsequent headache, confusion and drowsiness. In many forms of epilepsy the symptoms that can be recalled by the patient are far less pronounced and in the diagnosis of any form of blackout the description of an eye witness is essential. An account may be obtained of events at the onset of which the patient is unaware, such as turning the head and eyes to one side. Convulsive movements may be confirmed or denied but here the description is often less precise than could be wished. This is due partly to the panic naturally aroused in the inexperienced observer, usually a close relative, but also to popular mythology of what ought to happen in a fit. Stereotyped and unhelpful words such as fighting or struggling are difficult to interpret. A patient in a fit does not 'struggle' but clonic jerking is often loosely described in this way.

A description of colour change in the face is of great value, as in a major fit flushing or cyanosis is the rule while in an anoxic convulsion during a profound syncopal attack the face is ashen. As it is precisely in those patients who have a brief convulsion during their faint that diagnostic confusion arises this point may be of great importance. In other contexts the diagnosis of syncope should not usually present serious difficulty and specific precipitating factors are described in Chapter 17.

The hysterical fit can present serious diagnostic difficulty. The patient is often a young girl who is described as having frequent blackouts, of which the description is not convincingly that of any form of epilepsy. Witnesses are, however, known to be unreliable and there are many variations on the epileptic theme. If the attacks are indeed hysterical the patient usually cannot resist having an attack in front of the doctor when features quite incompatible with genuine unconsciousness can be observed. When those with medical training or patients with genuine epilepsy also have hysterical fits the distinction is impossible.

Hypoglycaemia as a cause of blackouts can be suspected if the attacks occur after starvation and exercise but this is not the cause of the common prevalence of epileptic fits in the period before breakfast.

The fascinating variety of symptoms of neurological disease is almost unlimited and many more will be described in the following chapters. Here an attempt has been made to clarify common difficulties in communication that unless resolved can lead to inappropriate investigation, diagnosis and treatment.

Further reading

Matthews W.B. (1975) *Practical Neurology*, 3rd edn. Blackwell Scientific Publications, Oxford.

CHAPTER 4
The Syndromes of the Cranial Nerves

The specialized functions of the cranial nerves are so frequently disturbed by either localized or diffuse pathology that a knowledge of the effects of cranial nerve palsies is essential to the understanding of a systematic description of nervous disease. In the following account a distinction is drawn as far as possible between lesions of the peripheral nerves and their nuclei, and lesions of central supranuclear structures. Common causes are mentioned but will be elaborated in later chapters and a few conditions in which specific cranial nerves are affected in isolation are described more fully.

THE OLFACTORY NERVE

Unilateral loss of sense of smell causes no symptoms. Bilateral anosmia may also pass unnoticed by those whose food normally tastes of little beyond salt, sugar and vinegar, but the impaired perception of taste that usually accompanies it considerably detracts from the enjoyment of life of those of more discerning palate. Inability to detect escaping gas is a real hazard. Distortion of the sense of smell or parosmia is more unpleasant, since all food may have the same repellent flavour. Most patients eventually adapt to their disability.

The receptor organs may be destroyed by chronic nasal infection, or access to them obstructed by nasal polyps, and the anosmia that accompanies a severe head cold sometimes unaccountably persists. Anosmia may result from damage to the olfactory fibres during their short course from the cribriform plate to the under-surface of the frontal lobe and is an occasional complication of meningitis. A meningioma growing from the dura of the olfactory groove may interrupt the fibres unilaterally. By far the commonest cause of continuing anosmia is head injury, which is thought to disrupt the olfactory fibres by movement of the brain relative to the skull. The severity of the injury is not important and anosmia may follow quite mild concussion. It is nearly always permanent but gradual recovery can occur, sometimes, unfortunately, only to the stage of parosmia.

Refined methods can detect defects in the sense of smell in lesions of a wide area of the cerebral hemispheres, but these are of little clinical relevance.

THE OPTIC NERVE

The term optic atrophy means that loss of fibres in the optic nerve has produced changes in the nerve head visible with an ophthalmoscope, and is therefore a rather confusing mixture of pathology and clinical observation. Important visual loss from disease of the optic nerve may occur without visible atrophy, as in tobacco amblyopia, due to smoking shag, and in vitamin B_{12} deficiency. The normal optic disc is pale pink, and nearly always paler on the temporal side. The white physiological cup is variable in size, but may occupy a large area of the disc. In myopia the disc is large and pale, and in hypermetropia it is small and pink, sometimes with an indistinct nasal edge. This great variation in the appearance of the normal disc naturally causes difficulty in recognizing slight degrees of the pallor found in optic atrophy.

Primary optic atrophy is due to disease of the optic nerve or chiasma, either intrinsic or from external pressure. The disc appears white with sharp edges. Secondary atrophy is due to death of the ganglion cells in the retina that form the optic nerve. Again the disc is pale and sharply defined. Consecutive atrophy may follow papilloedema and the disc is grey with indistinct edges. With the single exception of pallor of the disc following optic neuritis, apparent abnormalities in the colour of the nerve head are unimportant unless there are changes in the acuity or visual fields.

When it is due to infection, toxins, metabolic diseases or genetic disorders of unknown cause, primary atrophy is usually bilateral but may be asymmetrical. Neurosyphilis is now an uncommon cause and easily overlooked. Most drugs that were found to cause optic atrophy have naturally been abandoned and isoniazid is the only common therapeutic agent still occasionally incriminated. Methyl alcohol intoxication is a rare cause. Optic atrophy is a constant feature of cerebro-macular degeneration, a disorder of lipid metabolism in children. A metabolic defect has also been detected in Leber's hereditary optic atrophy (see Chapter 16).

In multiple sclerosis the atrophy as judged by the pallor of the disc may greatly exceed the degree of visual loss, and asymmetry or unilateral affection is common. Tumours of the optic nerve are usually unilateral initially. Ischaemia of the nerve may occur in cranial arteritis.

Primary atrophy due to pressure on the nerve most commonly results from tumours of the pituitary or in the region of the sella turcica, but any expanding lesion, such as an aneurysm of the carotid artery, can have the same effect. Both nerves may be compressed by the floor of the third ventricle when this is distended in hydrocephalus. Severe closed head injury may cause rupture of an optic nerve or injury to the chiasma. Chronic glaucoma exerts pressure on the nerve head and on fibres entering from the retina and is a common cause of atrophy, usually accompanied by marked cupping of the optic disc.

Atrophy secondary to death of the ganglion cells most commonly results from retinal ischaemia due to occlusion of the central retinal artery or its branches. Any severe retinal degeneration must cause optic atrophy, retinitis pigmentosa being a striking example.

Papilloedema

Swelling of the optic nerve head may occur in raised intracranial pressure from any cause. This pressure is transmitted along the sheath of the nerve and causes compression of the veins draining the retina. The appearance of gross papilloedema with the congested disc standing out from the retina, obvious venous engorgement and often retinal haemorrhages, is unmistakable. Lesser degrees are much less easy to recognize, and experts frequently disagree on the slightly pink disc with indistinct edges. Hypermetropia and other congenital anomalies may look very similar. Apart from expanding intracranial lesions, papilloedema may occur in meningitis, subarachnoid haemorrhage and malignant hypertension. Thrombosis of the cavernous sinus blocks the venous drainage with resulting swelling, and retinal venous occlusion has the same effect. Ischaemia of the optic nerve head, usually from cranial arteritis, may initially cause swelling of the disc. Moderate papilloedema due to raised venous pressure may be found in chronic pulmonary emphysema, mediastinal tumour, and polycythaemia vera. An occasional and unexplained finding is papilloedema in acute polyneuritis and in spinal cord tumours.

Papilloedema does not initially cause visual failure, a point of some importance in the distinction from optic neuritis where acuity is usually severely impaired.

With any severe degree of papilloedema there is a risk of consecutive optic atrophy. This may be preceded by obscurations of vision in which vision is totally lost for a brief period, often when the patient bends down, with complete recovery. This is a serious warning symptom of grossly raised intracranial pressure and of blindness that may rapidly become irreversible. More gradual visual loss may also occur in papilloedema, and haemorrhages may obscure the macula.

Optic neuritis

An inflammatory lesion at the nerve head produces appearances very similar to those of papilloedema except that there is less venous engorgement and actual swelling of the disc, although the edges may merge completely with the retina. Haemorrhages are rare but impairment of vision severe. A similar lesion in the nerve but not involving the nerve head produces no changes in the fundus and is known as retrobulbar neuritis. Optic neuritis has been attributed to many diseases but for practical purposes it is either an isolated unexplained episode, or is found to be due to multiple sclerosis and is further described in Chapter 12. It is not due to infected teeth or sinuses, but rare causes are sarcoidosis of the nervous system, post-infective encephalomyelitis and neurosyphilis. Leber's hereditary optic atrophy may present as an acute bilateral retrobulbar neuritis with subsequent atrophy.

The visual fields

The clinical course and characteristic findings of the causes of visual failure listed above will be described in later chapters, but it is necessary to have a clear understanding of the essential diagnostic method, the measurement of the visual fields (Fig. 5). Acuity at the fixation point is enormously greater than that of the rest of the retina and can be measured by the size of letter it is possible to recognize. While it is obvious that large objects can be detected in the peripheral fields, it is possible to read even large letters only within the few degrees surrounding the macula. Acuity in the peripheral field is therefore measured by the size of object it is possible to see at all. This varies with the degree of illumination and the colour of the object, white objects being more easily seen than coloured. If the acuity of the whole retina is reduced, the size of the visual field will be reduced on testing with small objects but may still be full to large or moving objects. However, when there is a localized lesion of the neural apparatus of vision at any point from the retina to the occipital cortex, localized and measurable defects of the visual fields will be found.

The technique of recording the visual fields is time-consuming and not always afforded the care it merits. The peripheral field is measured on the perimeter over which the objective is moved on an arc 330 mm from the eye. The central fields are examined by moving the objective over a black screen one or two metres from the eye. More elaborate perimeters have been developed but have little advantage in practice in patients with neurological disease. With both methods the result is plotted on a chart, and it is vital to state the size and colour of the objectives used and the distance from the eye. Thus the normal field on the perimeter is measured with a two millimetre diameter object and is recorded as 2 mm white/330 and on the screen as 2 mm white/2000. If any abnormality is found it must be examined with objectives of different size and colour. A visual field chart showing that a small white object can only be seen a few degrees from the fixation point is quite useless unless the field for larger objects is also recorded. The central visual acuity must always be noted. The essence of both forms of examination is that the patient must maintain fixation on the central point throughout and this is not always readily achieved. In an inattentive patient simple confrontation testing may be more reliable since it causes less fatigue.

The changes in the visual fields produced by localized lesions can be predicted from a knowledge of anatomy, although in practice this process is naturally reversed. Thus, an area of degeneration in the temporal half of the retina of one eye will cause a nasal field defect in that eye. In papilloedema the swollen nerve head causes expansion of the area of the fundus devoid of receptor organs and therefore enlargement of the normal blind spot, which is not usually noticeable to the patient. Optic neuritis, which may be confused with papilloedema, produces a quite different defect. The maximal impact is nearly always on the fibres from the macula. These make up a large proportion of the total fibres in the nerve, which they enter on the temporal side, reflecting the dense macular concentration of receptor organs and the enormously higher acuity. Damage to these fibres produces disabling loss of central vision, a central scotoma, with relative preservation of the peripheral fields. Retrobulbar neuritis, without visible fundal changes, produces an identical field defect.

In degenerative disease of the optic nerve, as in neurosyphilis, there is often a general reduction of acuity so that the field for small objects is much restricted but remains full when tested with large objectives. External pressure on the nerve may cause selective destruction of fibres. For example, pressure on the lateral side of one optic nerve will damage the fibres from the temporal half of the retina and therefore produce a defect in the nasal field, which may progress to a unilateral nasal hemianopia.

On reaching the chiasma the fibres from the two eyes intermingle, although in an orderly manner (Chapter 1) and a lesion can no longer cause failure of vision in only one eye. At the chiasma the fibres from the nasal halves of the two retinae cross and are especially vulnerable to

THE SYNDROMES OF THE CRANIAL NERVES

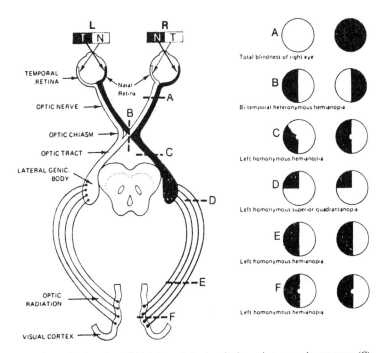

FIG. 5. General points about field defects. 1. Lesions in the optic tract are incongruous (C) as opposed to the congruity of lesions posterior to the lateral geniculate body (D to F). 2. Lesions posterior to the lateral geniculate body often result in quadrantic field defects (e.g. D in which the lesion involves the temporal lobe interfering with Meyer's loop forming the inferior portion of the optic radiation). 3. Lesions involving the visual cortex often spare the macula (F).

pressure from below, typically from a pituitary tumour. The characteristic field defect is therefore loss of both temporal fields or bitemporal hemianopia. When fully developed this is easy to demonstrate, but in the early stages it may be possible to detect only slight indentation of the field in one or both upper temporal quadrants. Chiasmal compression is not always in the mid-line and asymmetrical changes are common.

Behind the chiasma a lesion of the optic pathway must produce changes in the visual field contralateral to the lesion and affecting both eyes. A complete lesion of this kind is called homonymous hemianopia and can result from damage to the optic tract, the radiation in the white matter of the hemisphere, or the occipital cortex. Incomplete defects are common, particularly in lesions of the cerebral hemisphere, and when there has been discrete damage to the occipital cortex the visual field loss is also discrete, sometimes amounting only to a scotoma with full peripheral fields. The scotoma will, of course, also be bilateral and homonymous, that is to say it will affect the temporal field of the contralateral eye and the nasal field on the ipsilateral side.

Visual field defects involving acuity at the fixation point are immediately noticeable to the patient, but gradual loss of the peripheral field is far less obtrusive. The complaint may be of bumping into obstacles on one side, or of difficulty in following a line of print or finding the beginning of the next line. In general, however, defects due to lesions of the optic nerves or chiasma are soon perceived by the patient in terms of visual loss, the scotoma being typically 'positive'—i.e. black. In lesions of the hemisphere, however, there may also be disturbance of the interpretation of visual phenomena and therefore inability to recognize or to interpret quite gross changes correctly. In extreme examples when there has been destruction of the occipital cortex on both sides the patient may even be unaware that he is completely blind and may vigorously deny it.

THE OCULOMOTOR NERVE

A complete lesion of the third nerve causes loss of all movement of the eye except abduction, together with complete ptosis of the upper lid. The pupil is large and unreactive owing to paralysis of its parasympathetic supply. Because of the ptosis there is no complaint of double vision until the lid is elevated. Partial lesions produce lesser degrees of external and internal ophthalmoplegia and may be less easy to identify.

The nerve may be involved in any expanding or destructive lesion behind the orbit, most commonly an internal carotid aneurysm, or by a tumour arising in the ethmoid sinus or nasopharynx or it may be involved in more diffuse disease such as neurosyphilis. An isolated peripheral lesion of the nerve may occur acutely and sometimes painfully in the elderly and also in diabetics, apparently due to occlusion of an artery supplying the nerve. The pupil is not always dilated in these patients. In these cases the prognosis for full recovery is surprisingly and almost uniformly good.

In its central course through the mid-brain the nerve may occasionally be involved in infarction, but a lesion of the nucleus itself does not produce an isolated unilateral palsy owing to the complex grouping of the neurones.

Trochlear nerve

Isolated painless lesions of the fourth nerve sometimes occur in later life and are attributed to arteriosclerosis. Bilateral fourth nerve palsies may occur after comparatively mild head injury resulting in troublesome diplopia on looking down, as in reading or descending stairs, and spontaneous recovery is uncommon.

Abducent nerve

Ths sixth cranial nerve supplies only the lateral rectus muscle which abducts the eye, so that paralysis causes a convergent squint and diplopia. An isolated palsy is common and often recovers spontaneously without any cause being found. Occasionally it is the presenting symptom of a nasopharyngeal or ethmoid cancer. A sixth nerve palsy is also encountered in diffuse disease processes such as neurosyphilis, meningitis or encephalitis. In its long course from the pons to the orbit the nerve is vulnerable to compression from raised intracranial pressure, and unilateral or bilateral palsies may occur without giving any indication of the site of the responsible lesion—a 'false localizing sign'. Nuclear palsy occurs in infarction and other destructive lesions of the pons, though seldom in isolation.

Combined partial or complete ocular palsies on one or both sides may be caused by compression or inflammatory disease behind the orbits where the nerves are close together, a classical but very rare example being cavernous sinus thrombosis. When such lesions develop gradually they may be difficult to distinguish from primary disease of the ocular muscles. An expanding lesion behind one eye may involve these and neighbouring nerves, including the optic nerve and the ophthalmic division of the trigeminal, but often in a selective manner not easily explained on anatomical grounds.

Paralysis of ocular movement also results from lesions of the central pathways. In acute hemiplegia there may be deviation of the eyes towards the side of the cerebral lesion and inability to turn the eyes towards the hemiplegic side, a paralysis of conjugate gaze unaccompanied by double vision. Lesions of the mid-brain may involve supranuclear mechanisms and also cause defects of conjugate gaze, particularly of upward movement. Lower down the brain stem the tracts linking the third and sixth nerve nuclei may be interrupted causing an internuclear palsy. This takes several forms of which the commonest is failure of one eye to adduct on conjugate movement to the side, with normal adduction when the eyes converge. This dissociation shows that the medial rectus muscle is not paralysed but is unable to act in concert with the abductor of the other eye.

Diplopia

Double vision is a common symptom of neurological disease, and the usual cause is deviation of the axes of the two eyes so that fixation cannot be maintained on a single point. This is often due to obvious weakness of the external ocular muscles and may be illustrated by the effects of a right sixth nerve palsy. Abduction is paralysed, and the deviation of the ocular axes and therefore the separation of the two images will be maximal when looking to the right. This is a universal rule: the separation of the images is greatest when looking in the direction of action of the paralysed muscle. On covering either eye, single vision is naturally restored and it is found that the image furthest from the mid-point is that seen by the right eye. This is also a general rule: the false image is displaced in the direction of action of the paralysed muscle. The image seen by the eye affected by ophthalmoplegia is also often somewhat less distinct than that of the normal eye. Such analysis is scarcely necessary when there is an obvious sixth or third nerve palsy, but may be essential when examining slighter degrees of weakness, perhaps involving several muscles. A complaint of seeing more than two objects or of diplopia with one eye closed does not invariably mean that the patient is hysterical. An illusion that objects are moving may be interpreted as multiple vision, and a lesion of the retina or lens can cause monocular diplopia.

Diplopia may also be produced by dislocation of the eyeball secondary to deformation of the bony orbit by injury or tumour.

Nystagmus

Nystagmus is an involuntary oscillation of the eyes. It is a normal phenomenon when gazing out of the window of a moving train when it is not, as might be supposed, due to the voluntary shifting of regard from one object to another, but is reflexly induced. This is optokinetic nystagmus, which may be more conveniently examined by observing ocular movement induced by watching a rotating striped drum or even a tape-measure moved rapidly across the field of vision. Optokinetic nystagmus may be absent to moving objects in one visual field in cases of hemianopia, or in lesions of higher visual centres, but is rarely used as a physical sign.

Ill-sustained nystagmus is also normal at extremes of lateral gaze, when a few jerky movements can be seen. A great exaggeration of this symmetrical gaze nystagmus is seen in alcoholic or barbiturate intoxication.

Congenital nystagmus may be associated with poor central acuity and consequent inability to maintain fixation. This variety is peculiar in that there is no alternation of fast and slow movement, but other forms of congenital nystagmus show rapid jerking in one direction, usually towards the fixation point, and a slower opposing movement typically back to the mid-position. Nystagmus is classified according to the direction of the fast movement but it is in fact the slow component that is abnormal, with a rapid correction.

The complex mechanisms that maintain ocular fixation may be disturbed in many ways and not all forms of nystagmus are fully understood. An acute unilateral destructive lesion of the vestibular apparatus or its immediate connections produces lateral nystagmus with definite localizing features. The rapid movement is directed towards the healthy side and the amplitude of the movement is increased when the eyes are turned towards that side. This is because the eyes are driven towards the opposite side by the unopposed action of the intact labyrinth. Permanent destruction of one labyrinth is compensated for in a few weeks, but nystagmus on looking to the opposite side may remain for as long as several years.

Other forms of nystagmus are not of clear localizing value except that they indicate a lesion either of the cerebellum or of the brain stem: vertical nystagmus always indicates a central brain stem lesion. Nystagmus is not a feature of disease of the cerebral hemispheres. Ataxic nystagmus, in which the movement is much more marked in the abducting eye, is common in multiple sclerosis. Another form seen in this disease is 'jelly nystagmus', clearly evident only on examining the fundus when the eye can be seen to be oscillating rapidly through a small range.

Nystagmus does not usually cause symptoms but some patients in whom it is of recent onset are aware of oscillation of the field of vision and find it highly unpleasant.

The pupils

The size of the pupil and its reaction to stimuli depend on the integrity of the reflex arcs involved. If vision is lost or seriously impaired by a lesion of the optic nerve the afferent fibres concerned with the constriction of the pupil to light will also be destroyed. The pupil will dilate and will be unresponsive to light and as the reflex is interrupted on the afferent side of the arc the consensual constriction of the opposite pupil is also lost. A light shone into the normal eye will cause constriction of both pupils and constriction occurs on convergence even if both eyes are totally blind. A curious phenomenon can sometimes be elicited in cases of optic neuritis. A torch shone into the affected eye causes little pupillary constriction but the consensual reaction from the other eye is normal. If the beam is swung repeatedly from one eye to the other the waning of the consensual reaction causes the pupil of the affected eye to dilate when illuminated. With lesions of the chiasma or optic tract it is sometimes possible to detect a relative failure of the reflex when light is directed to the blind area of the visual field, but this is a very unreliable sign. Even when visual loss due to lesions of the visual pathway behind the lateral geniculate body is total it is not accompanied by any loss of pupillary reflex since the reflex arc remains intact.

As previously noted the pupil dilates if the third nerve is paralysed, and this may be an important sign, even when it is impossible to test ocular movement in a comatose patient. The nerve may be compressed as it crosses the edge of the tentorium if the temporal lobe is pushed into the tentorial opening by an expanding lesion, notably an extradural haematoma resulting from traumatic rupture of a middle meningeal artery.

Horner's syndrome is due to a lesion of the ocular sympathetic pathway, and comprises constriction of the pupil, slight ptosis and, in a complete lesion, loss of sweating on the forehead. The sympathetic pathway may be interrupted in the medulla, as in a medullary infarct; rarely by a lesion such as syringomyelia in the cervical spinal cord; and most commonly as the fibres emerge in the upper thoracic roots or run in the sympathetic chain. This tortuous course means that the syndrome is of little localizing value unless it is accompanied by other signs: an isolated Horner's syndrome often remains unexplained and may recover completely. A severe pain in the shoulder or upper arm accompanied by Horner's syndrome usually implies an invasive tumour at the apex of the lung.

In acute pontine haemorrhage both pupils may be extremely constricted—pin-point pupils—probably due to loss of autonomic control.

The Argyll Robertson pupil is a classical sign of neurosyphilis in all its chronic forms but is occasionally seen after injuries to the orbit. The pupils are small, irregular and unequal, and do not contract on exposure to light but do so on convergence. In congenital syphilis the pupil is sometimes large and unreactive.

The tonic pupil, or Holmes–Adie syndrome, is a condition most frequently seen in young women. It is of unknown cause and usually presents as acute dilatation of one pupil which is completely paralysed, without any weakness of ocular movement. After many months the pupil gradually constricts and then shows the characteristic slow tonic constriction on convergence followed by slow dilatation when gazing in the distance. The reaction to light is usually absent. Eventually both eyes are usually affected. The only symptom due to the pupillary abnormality is discomfort in bright light at the stage when the pupil is large and unreactive. In the later stages there is some danger of confusion with the Argyll Robertson pupil. Accommodation of the lens may also be tonic, and may then cause some difficulty when the focus must be rapidly changed. A curious and almost constant feature is loss of many of the tendon reflexes without any other signs or symptoms in the limbs. The nature of the disturbance of the pupillary reaction and of the loss of phasic stretch reflexes is still controversial. The condition is quite harmless, but often causes alarm.

THE TRIGEMINAL NERVE

The motor fibres of the fifth nerve are seldom involved in disease. A unilateral lesion such as may be seen in paralytic poliomyelitis causes deviation of the jaw towards the paralysed side on opening the mouth and later obvious wasting of the temporalis and masseter muscles. The sensory root and its branches are more frequently affected, particularly the ophthalmic division which may be compressed by an expanding lesion behind the orbit. Tumours in the angle between the cerebellar hemisphere and the pons, of which the commonest is a neurofibroma of the acoustic nerve, frequently compress the trigeminal and facial nerves. Rarely the trigeminal nerve itself may be the site of a similar tumour. A *trigeminal neuropathy* of unknown cause is a rare condition usually affecting women. Progressive sensory loss, eventually bilateral, may be accompanied by mutilation of the nose and danger to the anaesthetic cornea. Equally mysterious is sensory loss on the chin in the distribution of the mental branch of the mandibular division of the nerve as a presenting sign of carcinoma of the breast. In any peripheral lesion pain and paraesthesiae may occur and all forms of cutaneous sensation are impaired. If the ophthalmic division is affected the corneal reflex is diminished or absent.

The long descending sensory nucleus may be involved in infarcts or tumours of the medulla and also in lesions of the cervical spinal cord such as intramedullary tumour or syringomyelia. Pain and thermal sensation will be lost on the face on the side of the lesion, usually accompanied by more widespread signs.

Trigeminal neuralgia is a relatively common and exceedingly distressing condition, occurring predominantly in the second half of life.

There is but a single symptom, pain in the face, often of great severity. It most commonly begins in the area of the mandibular or maxillary division on one side but may spread and is occasionally bilateral. The pain is characteristically brief, lasting no more than a few seconds, during which the face may be involuntarily contorted—the *tic douloureux*. If the paroxysms are frequent, a persistent aching discomfort may also be experienced, but even so the episodic nature of the severe pain can be recognized. The pain may occur spontaneously, but many paroxysms are obviously triggered by touching specific points on the face, as in washing and shaving. Even a cold draught on the face may be a sufficient stimulus, while talking and chewing may become almost impossible. The frequency of paroxysms is highly variable, but in severe relapses the unfortunate patient is virtually incapacitated. Spontaneous remissions, sometimes lasting for many months or years, are common in the early stages.

No consistent pathological lesion has been found in trigeminal neuralgia. There have been numerous theories of causation, varying from compression of the trigeminal ganglion beneath the dura to the effects of hypothetical virus infection, but none have been substantiated. There is of course no reason why the cause of pain originating in the nervous system should be visible under the microscope. The triggering of the pain by peripheral stimulation and the response to treatment certainly suggest an abnormality in the orderly transmission of afferent impulses to the trigeminal nuclei, but no convincing explanation of this functional disorder has been developed.

It might be supposed that such a characteristic, stereotyped and obtrusive symptomatology would be immediately recognized, but in fact the differential diagnosis seems to present unnecessary difficulty. In the initial attack, teeth are often needlessly extracted, and if a natural remission occurs soon afterwards, more teeth are sacrificed when the pain returns, but in vain. Dental neuralgia can certainly occur in paroxysms on eating, but seldom closely resembles tic douloureux. Other pains may be mistaken for neuralgia, particularly the persistent and often unilateral pain that is a common and surprising presenting symptom of depression, particularly in young women. Pain arising in the temporomandibular joint has been dignified by the name of Costen's syndrome. Such pain can certainly arise when the bite is gravely maladjusted in the partially edentulous, but the syndrome has been expanded to include widespread symptoms indistinguishable from those of muscular tension and attributed to mild, or indeed imperceptible, derangements of the joint. Migrainous neuralgia (Chapter 18) is usually initially diagnosed as tic

THE SYNDROMES OF THE CRANIAL NERVES

douloureux, particularly by those members of the medical profession who are themselves its victims.

Pain in all respects identical with trigeminal neuralgia may very rarely result from compression of the nerve or its branches by a tumour or aneurysm, but physical signs can then be detected while in the idiopathic form sensory loss and other signs are never found. Trigeminal neuralgia also occurs as an initial symptom of multiple sclerosis or during the course of the disease, and this possibility must be remembered, particularly in younger patients.

Treatment of trigeminal neuralgia has been revolutionized by the use of carbamazepine (Tegretol). This was introduced as an anticonvulsant and was used in neuralgia because of the temporary beneficial effect of the anticonvulsant drug phenytoin. Both these agents have a stabilizing effect on certain cell membranes but their mode of action is not known in detail. Treatment should begin with 100 mg (half a tablet) thrice daily and should be increased if necessary to a maximum of 200 mg six times a day. On this dose many patients will develop dizziness and ataxia and 600 mg a day is often the limit of tolerance. When this drug is first used, immediate abolition of pain can almost be guaranteed, but this is symptomatic treatment and must be continually adjusted to contain the pain without undue side effects until remission occurs. This treatment is equally effective when neuralgia is a symptom of multiple sclerosis. Unfortunately in some patients carbamazepine loses its effects or proves too toxic and analgesic drugs are quite inadequate.

Alternative treatment consists in interrupting the trigeminal nerve, either a peripheral branch where appropriate or more effectively the sensory root. This is done by injecting absolute alcohol, the insertion of the needle requiring some skill. If successful there is permanent relief, but also permanent loss of sensation over the face. For most patients this is greatly to be preferred to persistent neuralgia, but there is a small group who develop troublesome paraesthesiae, resistant to treatment, in the anaesthetic area. It is possible to make selective lesions of the nerve using a radiofrequency technique that also involves accurate placement of the needle. Light touch can be spared while appreciation of pain is abolished and this is at present the method of choice. Operative treatment is still occasionally necessary, usually partial section of the nerve in the posterior fossa.

Pain of identical character occurs much more rarely in the glossopharyngeal distribution. It is felt in the tonsillar bed and deep in the ear, and is triggered by swallowing. Glossopharyngeal neuralgia responds well to carbamazepine or if necessary to section of the nerve.

THE FACIAL NERVE

The effects of an acute peripheral lesion of the seventh nerve can best be illustrated by a description of the very common condition *Bell's palsy*. This is of unknown cause, although popularly attributed to draughts, and occurs at all ages. The onset of paralysis may be preceded by pain behind the ear for several days or the whole course may be painless. Paralysis develops rapidly or may even appear to be sudden. Often it reaches its full extent within a few hours but progression may sometimes continue for several days. Even in mild examples without complete paralysis, all the muscles on one side of the face are initially affected. In young patients the face may appear symmetrical at rest even when there is complete paralysis, but in older patients such a lesion causes sagging of the lip and lower lid and smoothing of the wrinkles. The eye cannot be closed either deliberately or on blinking, though some lowering of the lid occurs owing to reflex inhibition of the levator. If the lesion is severe the fibres entering the nerve in the chorda tympani will be interrupted with resulting loss of taste on the anterior part of the tongue. The secretion of tears may also be diminished. Similarly the stapedius muscle may be paralysed causing hyperacusis so that noises sound too loud.

The prognosis for full recovery depends on the nature of the damage to the nerve. If this is merely a conduction block, full recovery will take place. In practice, movement detected in all the affected muscles at any time within two weeks from the onset means that recovery will be complete and will occur within about four weeks and often much sooner. This fortunate outcome occurs in at least 60% of cases. However, if the nerve degenerates in whole or in part full recovery does not take place. This does not necessarily mean permanent disfigurement but usually only a barely detectable abnormality of facial movement. Re-innervation of the muscles must be effected by fibres growing again from the point of interruption and this process inevitably takes three months or longer. Moreover, a variable number of fibres will be misdirected, finally innervating muscles other than those they originally supplied. This would be of little moment if it were not for the intricacy of the facial musculature and its use for the public display of emotion. The effect of this faulty re-innervation may be limited to such associated movements as narrowing of the palpebral fissure on pursing the lips, but in severe cases the whole side of the face may contract together on any voluntary movement. This will be accompanied by obvious residual weakness of many muscles. Such misdirection may involve autonomic fibres so that those originally innervating the submandibular salivary gland may supply the lacrymal gland. The eye therefore waters on eating—the 'crocodile tears' syndrome.

It is probable that the outcome is determined within a few hours or at most a few days of the onset. Bad prognostic signs are advanced age, severe pain, loss of taste and complete palsy, but neither singly nor in combination do these features inevitably mean incomplete recovery. Evidence of denervation, and therefore of delayed recovery, can be detected by electromyography after about ten days and delayed conduction in the nerve several days earlier, but probably too late to be of much practical importance in management.

Rational treatment must therefore be directed to the prevention of denervation and must be started immediately if it is to be effective. It has long been supposed that the cause of the paralysis is compression and ischaemia of the nerve in its narrow channel through the temporal bone. In a benign condition a lack of knowledge of the morbid anatomy is inevitable and there is virtually no available information on the state of the extracranial segment of the nerve. Surgical decompression of the nerve has often been advocated but has never convincingly been shown to be effective. Initial hopes that ACTH or steroids would prevent denervation in a high proportion of patients have been over-optimistic, but provided there are no contraindications such as peptic ulceration, infection or pregnancy, the treatment of acute Bell's palsy producing complete paralysis is prednisolone. The dose should be 20 mg four times a day for five days, thereafter reducing rapidly in the succeeding five days. This regime has been claimed to reduce the incidence of denervation if begun within four days of the onset. It has been customary to prescribe galvanism to the paralysed muscles but this is now known to be ineffective and never had any rational basis. The traditional measures of massaging the face and applying splints of sticking plaster may have occasional psychotherapeutic justification, but do not influence the final result.

While it is true to say that the cause is quite unknown in most cases, an identical picture may be the presenting symptom of sarcoidosis of the meninges. Poliomyelitis is a possible cause and there is also an undoubtedly increased incidence of typical Bell's palsy in patients with severe or malignant hypertension, and in diabetics. Recurrent Bell's palsy, on the same or the opposite side, is not uncommon and seems to have no special significance. Likewise, a familial incidence is sometimes encountered.

Facial palsy indistinguishable from idiopathic Bell's palsy may accompany infection with herpes zoster. This used to be attributed to infection of the geniculate ganglion on the sensory root, with resulting oedema and compression of the motor fibres. This may occur, the rash then being in the meatus, but in fact the eruption is often in the trigeminal distribution or in the cervical dermatomes, or even more remote. The facial palsy is probably due to direct infection of the motor nerve. It is usually severe and the prognosis for full recovery is relatively poor.

Other causes of facial palsy due to disease of the nucleus or peripheral nerve are much less common. The nucleus may be involved in infarction and the nerve may be compressed by a tumour in the cerebellopontine angle. It is also exposed to damage from infection in or operation on the middle ear: indeed the diagnosis of Bell's palsy should never be made without examining the ears. Bilateral facial palsy is sometimes overlooked because the face appears symmetrical. It may occur in polyneuritis, sarcoidosis and primary muscle disease, particularly myasthenia gravis.

Supranuclear facial palsy is not often an isolated finding but may occasionally be confused with a peripheral or nuclear lesion. Certainly many patients with Bell's palsy require reassurance that they have not had a stroke. The essential difference is that in a supranuclear lesion the muscles of the upper part of the face are spared owing to their bilateral cortical innervation. As with other supranuclear lesions movements rather than simple muscular contractions are affected so that grinning on demand may be lopsided while spontaneous smiling is symmetrical.

A much less common affection of the seventh nerve is a form of involuntary movement known as *facial hemispasm*. The onset may be at any time in adult life and the first symptom is nearly always spasmodic closure of one eye. This fluctuates from day to day but gradually the movement increases in frequency and spreads to involve all the muscles on one side of the face which contract simultaneously to produce distressing contortions. The condition is painless but a source of great embarrassment. In common with nearly all involuntary movements it is made worse by stress or even by observation and on these grounds is almost invariably misdiagnosed as an hysterical twitch. Close examination, however, will show that the face is abnormal between the spasms as voluntary movement shows features similar to those seen after reinnervation in Bell's palsy described above. A history of a previous facial palsy is hardly ever obtained and the cause remains unknown. Spontaneous recovery is rare and drugs are useless, but partial injection of the facial nerve with alcohol or dilute phenol will produce remission for several months, although the technique is difficult. A more permanent result can be obtained by exposing the nerve in the posterior fossa and surrounding it with foam packing. The effect has been

THE SYNDROMES OF THE CRANIAL NERVES

attributed to fibrosis around the nerve but as cure is often immediate this does not seem entirely plausible. This apparently trivial disorder is so distressing that patients have no hesitation in accepting craniotomy even without an absolute promise of cure.

THE ACOUSTIC NERVE

Nerve deafness results from lesions of the cochlear division of the eighth nerve itself, or from destruction of the receptor end-organs by noise, old age, atherosclerosis, Ménière's syndrome, haemorrhage, and drug intoxication. Nerve deafness may be inherited as an isolated defect, or may form part of more diffuse genetically determined disease such as Friedreich's ataxia. More often congenital deafness is due to intrauterine damage by such agencies as anoxia, jaundice, or rubella. Streptomycin damages the vestibular nerve, but salicylate, neomycin and kanamycin may cause deafness. Another occasional cause is Paget's disease affecting the temporal bones.

Audiometry is essential to differentiate end-organ from nerve deafness. Disease of the receptor organs in the cochlea, as in Ménière's disease, can be recognized by the finding of loudness recruitment. This means that the degree of hearing loss is marked when the intensity of the sound is low, but loud tones are heard normally, and it explains why a hearing-aid is of little value in such cases. The deafness of a nerve lesion is usually evenly distributed throughout the frequency range, and loudness recruitment is characteristically absent. The hearing for pure tones as produced by an audiometer or tuning fork may be surprisingly unimpaired whilst the ability to transmit complex signals like speech is grossly disturbed. This is best tested by speech discrimination audiometry. When the eighth nerve is the seat of disease it is often unusually fatiguable, tested by the tone decay test, in which a pure tone is presented for a minute, and the intensity increased so that the tone remains just audible. In the normal ear, there is no decay, but in the presence of a nerve lesion the decay may be as much as 80 decibels. Using averaging techniques it is now possible to record in astonishing detail the electrical responses evoked in the auditory nerve and brain stem nuclei by a regularly repeated click. This method promises to be of great value in the location of lesions in the auditory pathways.

Lesions of the nerve itself are rare and are caused either by tumours of the nerve, such as acoustic neurofibroma, by meningioma, or by secondary carcinomatosis of the meninges around the nerve. Fracture of the temporal bone may tear the nerve and it may be destroyed by basal meningitis. Disease of the cochlear nuclei produces audiological findings indistinguishable from nerve lesions, but they are often accompanied by other brain stem signs.

Vestibular nerve

The vestibular division of the eighth nerve is functionally distinct from the acoustic, but they are closely related anatomically and often affected together.

The effects of acute loss of vestibular function may be illustrated by the common condition, *Ménière's disease*. This affects both sexes chiefly in middle age. The immediate cause of symptoms is an intermittent increase in the endolymph that fills the labyrinth and cochlea, but the reason for this distension is unknown. The end-organs of both divisions of the eighth nerve are progressively destroyed, and the cardinal symptoms include progressive deafness and tinnitus, at first unilateral and variable, but often eventually affecting both sides. The intermittent symptoms are due to acute temporary total loss of vestibular function on one side. The resulting attacks of acute vertigo are sometimes immediately preceded by an increase in tinnitus and distortion of hearing, but they may be quite abrupt in onset so that the patient falls. Acute labyrinthine vertigo from any cause is a terrifying experience. In addition to the violent sense of rotation and complete inability to stand or even sit, there is often uncontrollable vomiting, prostration and shock, and sometimes loss of sphincter control. Some patients claim to lose consciousness briefly, the mechanism probably being syncopal. In Ménière's disease the severity, frequency and duration of the attacks are very variable but in severe cases they may occur several times a week and last for over an hour. As the receptor organs are progressively destroyed there is naturally less disturbance from acute intermittent loss of remaining functions, and attacks often diminish in severity, unless the opposite side also becomes affected.

No treatment will cut short an attack of vertigo, but vomiting may be mitigated by an intramuscular injection of 50 mg of chlorpromazine. Prevention of attacks is also problematical, though some can be aborted by taking an anti-emetic drug such as dimenhydrinate (Dramamine) or thiethylperazine (Torecan) when increasing tinnitus signals an imminent paroxysm. Vasodilators have also been widely used, betahistone being at present in favour. Many patients with comparatively mild disease fare remarkably well on regular phenobarbitone. There may be prolonged natural remissions as well as a general tendency to slow spontaneous reduction in frequency of vertigo. The deafness is, however, steadily progressive. Attempts at chronic dehydration with salt and water restriction to reduce localized oedema in the inner ear are both useless and unpleasant for the patient.

Surgical treatment is required in no more than 5% of cases. The variety of procedures advocated illustrates the difficulty of curing the vertigo without further injury to hearing. The most promising measure at present is drainage of the saccus endolymphaticus.

Deafness and tinnitus are not influenced by treatment, but the chronic effects of gradual destruction of vestibular function, as opposed to the effects of acute lesions, are remarkably unobtrusive. Chronic complete unilateral loss of function may be entirely asymptomatic.

Epidemic vertigo, sometimes known as *vestibular neuronitis*, is another commonly diagnosed but rather ill-defined disease of the vestibular nerve. It is thought to be due to a virus infection, and although this has not been proven a similar condition may certainly be encountered in mumps. The onset is sudden, with severe vertigo and the usual accompaniments of vomiting and inability to walk steadily, but without other symptoms. Nystagmus of the type due to unilateral vestibular damage is constantly present at the onset but may be seen later only on movement of the head. The course is variable but vertigo is usually severe during the first week followed by a gradual but complete recovery. Brief vertigo on turning the head may be present for many months and is an indication that permanent vestibular nerve damage has been sustained, although this will eventually become fully compensated and asymptomatic. Hearing is not often affected, and treatment, apart from intramuscular chlorpromazine for intractable vomiting, is not effective. In older patients atherosclerosis is a commoner cause of similar syndromes.

Postural dizziness or an unpleasant swimming sensation in the head on rising from a stooping posture is a common complaint, especially during convalescence or after a minor head injury, but is of little importance. It is probably due to a reversible failure in the reflex regulation of blood pressure. A much more distinctive and frequently misdiagnosed condition is *benign postural vertigo*. This may follow trivial head injury but usually there is no discernible cause. The single symptom is of brief but violent vertigo on certain movements. These characteristically involve movement of the head together with the trunk as with lying down in bed, turning over in bed or sitting up or getting out of bed in the morning. The vertigo persists for no more than approximately ten seconds but if it has been induced by standing up the patient may stagger or fall. It is often noticed that lying on one side in bed will induce vertigo while turning to the other side will not. The history is sufficiently distinctive but the diagnosis can often be confirmed on examination. The patient should be sat on a couch and should then rapidly adopt the posture known to induce vertigo. If the test is positive there is a brief pause and the patient then becomes severely distressed. If the eyes can be opened violent rotatory nystagmus can be observed. This reaction is variable and easily fatigued so that repeating the manoeuvre may well prove negative. The condition may last for months or years but eventually remits and most patients come to accept that if they are careful to perform the precipitating movements slowly they will remain free from symptoms. Investigation will not reveal any abnormality of caloric vestibular reactions as the semicircular canals are not involved and the disorder has been attributed to a disturbance in the utricle.

Disease of the vestibular nuclei produces vertigo indistinguishable from that of vestibular neuronitis, but often accompanied by evidence of damage to neighbouring structures. Brain stem infarctions and multiple sclerosis may cause prolonged incapacitating vertigo. In peripheral lesions compensation is established within two or three weeks at the most.

Destruction of both vestibular nerves may result from injudicious treatment with streptomycin, particularly when renal excretion is impaired. It is important to know that this condition may begin some weeks after the drug has been withdrawn, leaving the physician oblivious of the havoc he has wrought. As both nerves are equally affected, vertigo due to acute imbalance of the two sides is not a feature. The almost total loss of vestibular function causes unsteadiness on walking, especially in the dark, to which younger patients may adapt, but which is very intractable in the elderly. A characteristic symptom of bilateral vestibular destruction is an illusion that objects move up and down in time with the head when walking, due to loss of reflex control of eye movement.

The function of the semicircular canals and vestibular nerves are investigated by the caloric tests. The patient lies with the head flexed at 30° so that the lateral semicircular canal is in the vertical plane, and fixes his gaze on a point on the ceiling. Water at 30°C and then at 44°C is run into each ear in turn for 40 seconds. The temperature changes are transmitted to the air in the middle-ear cavity, and then to the fluid in the lateral semicircular canal, inducing a caloric current in the endolymph. This in turn produces ampullar deflection, with a resultant sensation of rotation, which is accompanied by nystagmus, the duration and character of which act as an indirect indicator of vestibular function. The nystagmus normally lasts for about two minutes from the beginning of the irrigation. A common abnormality is canal paresis, when the reaction to both hot and cold water is diminished or absent on

THE SYNDROMES OF THE CRANIAL NERVES

one side. This indicates loss of function on that side and is seen in any peripheral unilateral destructive lesion. Directional preponderance means that the nystagmus to one side is diminished. Normally, cold water causes nystagmus with the rapid phase to the opposite side and this is reversed with warm water. In lesions of the central vestibular connections, either nuclear or in the cerebral hemisphere, the induced nystagmus with the rapid phase to the side opposite to the lesion is reduced. The character of the induced nystagmus is also informative: in peripheral lesions it is regular whilst in lesions affecting the vestibular nuclei or connections it often grossly irregular, phasic or variable in direction. The test is open to much misinterpretation and reliable results are obtained only in expert hands. Electrical recording of the nystagmus does not appear to add much authority to clinical appraisal.

THE GLOSSOPHARYNGEAL NERVE

The ninth cranial nerve is seldom affected in isolation but may be involved together with the other lower cranial nerves in vascular disease of the medulla or in neoplasms in the region of the jugular foramen. The resulting loss of sensation on the pharyngeal wall causes loss of the gag reflex. Glossopharyngeal neuralgia is described on page 75.

THE VAGUS

Although the tenth cranial nerve contains the greater part of the cranial parasympathetic outflow the common clinical effects of a lesion of the nerve are those resulting from interruption of its somatic motor supply to the palate, pharynx and larynx. The motor nucleus may be involved in medullary tumours, in syringobulbia, and in brain stem infarction, and was often affected in epidemic acute poliomyelitis. In its peripheral course the nerve is exposed to damage from any expanding lesion at the base of the skull. The recurrent laryngeal branches, particularly the left which leaves the main trunk in the thorax, may be damaged by tumours in the neck or mediastinum, or at operations on the thyroid.

A unilateral lesion of the vagus causes paralysis of one side of the palate (Fig. 7, following p. 132), which is drawn up to the normal side on phonation, and weakness of the voice and of coughing due to paralysis of the vocal cord. The patient is characteristically unable to sustain the sound 'eee'. Disability from unilateral weakness of the pharyngeal muscles may cause choking or spluttering not encountered in recurrent laryngeal paralysis. Bilateral lesions cause the highly dangerous condition known as bulbar palsy—the bulb being an old name for the medulla. When this is complete the patient cannot swallow. The palate is paralysed so that food secretions may regurgitate down the nose or, much more dangerously, may enter the larynx. Coughing is also paralysed so that there is a serious risk of infection, bronchial obstruction and pulmonary collapse. In its acute form, as in bulbar poliomyelitis, the pulmonary complications are rapidly fatal unless they are prevented or vigorously treated. The chronic form of bulbar paralysis most commonly results from motor neurone disease.

An unexplained and serious feature of bilateral recurrent laryngeal palsy is that the abductor muscles of the vocal cords are paralysed first, causing alarming respiratory obstruction.

Supranuclear lesions of the vagus cause the condition known as pseudo-bulbar palsy. Dysphagia and dysarthria are again prominent, but because of disordered movements rather than paralysis of the pharyngeal muscles. The tongue is also involved and its movements are slow and clumsy. The jaw jerk is exaggerated. Although dysphagia may be prominent during the few days after acute hemiplegia, the common cause of pseudo-bulbar palsy is bilateral cerebral infarction. When fully developed it is accompanied by extreme emotional lability and often some dementia.

THE ACCESSORY NERVE

The eleventh nerve, with its complex origin from both spinal cord and medulla, may be involved in focal lesions of the medulla and at the base of the skull. Paralysis of the trapezius causes drooping of the shoulder and an obvious change in the contour of the neck viewed from behind. The sternomastoid muscle normally stands out strongly on flexing the neck or turning the head to the opposite side and paralysis of this muscle is easily recognized.

THE HYPOGLOSSAL NERVE

The twelfth nerve, the motor nerve of the tongue, is most commonly affected in motor neurone disease, but like other lower cranial nerves, it is sometimes involved in tumours or infarcts of the medulla. Chronic bilateral lesions, characteristically seen in motor neurone disease, cause diffuse wasting, flaccidity, and fasciculation and eventually complete paralysis. In a unilateral lesion the tongue is protruded towards the paralysed side which may also be wasted. As already mentioned, movement of the tongue is severely affected in bilateral supranuclear lesions producing pseudo-bulbar palsy, the palsy being spastic in type.

Further reading

Anon. (1981) Trigeminal neuralgia: treat but do not prolong. *Brit. Med. J.* **282,** 1820.
Brodal A. (1965) *The Cranial Nerves*, 2nd edn. Blackwell Scientific Publications, Oxford.
Dyck P.J., Thomas P.K. & Lambert E.H. (eds.) (1975) *Peripheral Neuropathy*. Saunders, Philadelphia.
Matthews W.B. (1980) Bell's palsy. *Medicine*, 3rd series (Oct.), 1759.

CHAPTER 5
Traumatic Lesions of the Peripheral Nervous System and Spinal Cord

The lower motor neurone

The motor fibres of the peripheral nervous system are derived from the anterior horn cells and the cells of the somatic motor nuclei of the cranial nerves. Destruction of the parent cell bodies, or of all the motor fibres supplying a muscle, causes paralysis with the characteristics of a lower motor neurone lesion. The muscle is flaccid due to loss of the normal stretch reflexes, and tendon jerks are lost. Wasting occurs if the interruption of the motor supply is prolonged. A partial lesion in which some motor neurones are preserved causes weakness rather than paralysis, and tendon reflexes may be reduced in amplitude.

A single anterior root contains fibres destined for many muscles, and most muscles receive fibres from more than one root. A lesion of a single root will therefore cause varying degrees of weakness in several muscles. More peripherally, most muscles are entirely supplied by a single peripheral nerve, so that a complete lesion causes paralysis of all the muscles in the distribution of the nerve.

The lower sensory neurone

The peripheral afferent fibres are derived from the cells of the posterior root ganglia and of the equivalent ganglia of the cranial nerves. There is considerable overlap between the areas supplied by the individual posterior roots, so that a single root lesion may cause no detectable sensory loss. On the other hand, a complete lesion of a peripheral nerve causes loss of all forms of cutaneous sensation within the distribution of the nerve (Fig. 6). There is some overlap with neighbouring nerves, so that the periphery of the area of sensory loss is never sharply defined. Loss of postural sense also occurs, but is much less predictable in its distribution. Partial interruption of the sensory innervation results in blunting of sensation in an area often much smaller than the full distribution of the nerve. Tendon jerks will be absent if the afferent side of the reflex arc is interrupted.

ACUTE TRAUMA OF PERIPHERAL NERVES

When a peripheral nerve is severed, conduction is naturally immediately abolished. For a few days the nerve distal to the site of injury still responds to electrical stimulation, but thereafter the axons are no longer replenished by axoplasm passing down the fibres, and rapidly degenerate. This breaking up of the axis cylinder is known as Wallerian degeneration, and may also follow acute trauma where the nerve remains in continuity. Recovery of motor and sensory function can occur only if the axis cylinders regenerate and establish contact with the motor endplates and receptor organs. This is effected by sprouting of axons from the segment above the injury, which enter the empty neurilemmal sheaths of the distal segment. If the nerve trunk remains in continuity a functionally effective recovery is probable, but even in these favourable circumstances axons or branches of axons enter sheaths other than those they originally occupied. If the nerve is severed misdirection of axons is inevitable, and many axons may not enter the distal portion of the nerve at all, but form a functionless and often painful swelling. Regeneration is not a rapid process and does not appear to begin immediately after the injury.

Conduction may also be completely interrupted without any destruction of axis cylinders. The immediate clinical effect is identical but the implications are quite different. The precise mechanism of this *conduction block* is unknown but the effects are fully reversible. It is a matter of common experience that external pressure on nerve trunks as when sitting with the knees crossed or when lying on an arm in bed will induce rapidly reversible motor and sensory loss. This can clearly be attributed to ischaemia but in pathological states the conduction block may persist for many days or even weeks and is presumably the result of demyelination. If there is no evidence of denervation due to destruction of axons, the prognosis for full recovery is excellent even when paralysis is prolonged.

Many peripheral nerve lesions are incomplete, some axons degenerating while others show conduction block or are unaffected. Prognosis depends on the proportion of destroyed axons, and the detection of partial or complete denervation is therefore important.

About ten days after muscles are denervated, individual muscle fibres begin to contract spontaneously, possibly due to hypersensitivity to circulating acetylcholine. This *fibrillation* is not visible through the skin but can be detected by electromyography. Bipolar needle electrodes are inserted into the muscle and any activity found is amplified and displayed on a cathode ray oscilloscope coupled to a loudspeaker. A normally

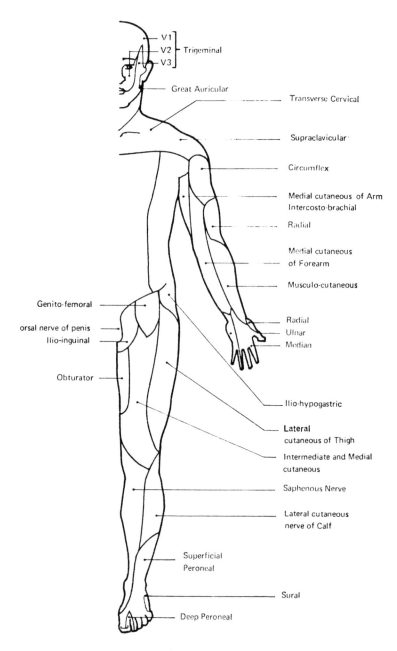

FIG. 6. Cutaneous areas of peripheral innervation. Because of overlap sensory loss following division of a sensory nerve may involve only part of its distribution.

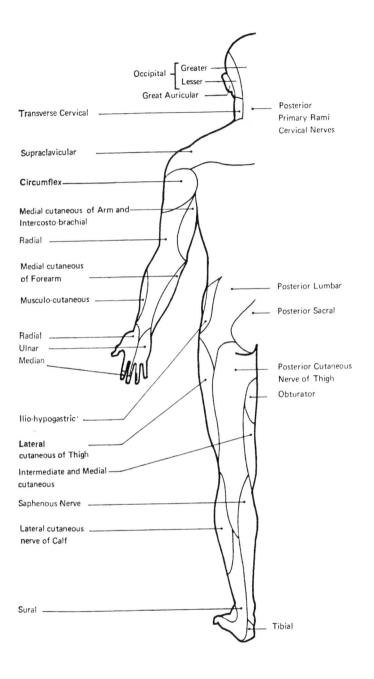

innervated muscle is electrically silent at rest, and abnormal fibrillation potentials are therefore easily seen when many fibres are denervated. The potentials are of low voltage, 100 microvolts, and brief duration. One of the first signs of reinnervation is the diminution or disappearance of fibrillation. Fibrillation does not occur in conduction block.

PRESSURE PALSIES

Certain peripheral nerves are vulnerable to external pressure at points where they lie between the skin and underlying bone. The resulting injury may be due to local ischaemia or to direct pressure on the axons.

Radial nerve

The classical 'Saturday night palsy' is still common but is by no means confined to the weekend. In a drunken stupor the patient sleeps with his arm over the back of a chair so that the radial nerve is compressed against the humerus. On waking the extensors of the fingers and wrist and the brachioradialis are paralysed, and a small area of sensory loss may be detected over the first dorsal interosseous space. The triceps is spared, because the nerve is injured below the branches to this muscle. An acute pressure palsy can occur in less sordid circumstances but nearly always during sleep. Recovery is excellent but may be delayed for many weeks, and is not accelerated by electrical stimulation of the paralysed muscles. A splint for the wrist allows the fingers to function more usefully.

Peroneal nerve

The peroneal nerve is vulnerable to pressure as it crosses the neck of the fibula, and the temporary partial palsy produced by sitting with the legs crossed must be familiar to everyone. This posture is seldom responsible for the prolonged complete palsies, which more often follow kneeling or crouching for long periods, particularly in those unaccustomed to such postures. There is paralysis of dorsiflexion of the foot and toes, and of the peronei which evert the foot. Sensory loss is variable but can usually be detected over the outer side of the foot or shin. The prognosis is again excellent, but recovery is seldom rapid.

Ulnar nerve

The main trunk of the ulnar nerve is relatively protected in its groove at the elbow, and acute pressure palsies are not seen. However, repeated pressure on a hard surface such as a desk may produce a severe palsy in a few days. This may be seen in those who have recently taken up some new occupation involving unaccustomed pressure on the elbow, such as constant use of a telephone handset while sitting at a desk, or in a bedridden patient with a fractured femur who has to lift himself on his elbows. It recovers well with removal of the cause.

An ulnar nerve lesion at the elbow causes weakness or paralysis of the interossei and lumbricals, but spares the muscles of the thenar eminence supplied by the median nerve. In pressure palsies of this type the wasting and deformity encountered in the more chronic lesions described below are not seen. The fingers can still be abducted quite strongly by the action of the extensors, but cannot be adducted. This naturally leads to some clumsiness, but more important is the loss of dexterity of the thumb due to weakness of adduction. Even when the palsy is severe it is often difficult to detect any weakness in the two muscles of the forearm supplied by the ulnar nerve, the flexor carpi ulnaris and the long flexor of the ring and little fingers. Paralysis of the former causes radial deviation of the hand on flexion against resistance. The long flexors act on the terminal interphalangeal joints and weakness can be demonstrated if the proximal joints are fixed. In an incomplete lesion sensory loss may be difficult to find in spite of a convincing subjective complaint of numbness in the ulnar two digits. In complete lesions, loss of cutaneous sensation involves the little finger and usually the ring finger in their palmar and dorsal surfaces and also the ulnar side of the hand, but in contrast with sensory loss from a lesion of the eighth cervical root, it does not extend above the wrist.

Pressure palsies of the ulnar nerve are seldom complete, and usually resolve quickly once the external cause has been removed, with the unfortunate exception of palsies developing during general anaesthesia. Probably because of prolonged pressure during a period of complete immobility the nerve is often severely damaged and recovery is incomplete.

The deep branch of the ulnar nerve in the palm may also be compressed during such activities as weight lifting, lawn mowing, or motor cycling. This branch may also be chronically compressed by a ganglion and the absence of any sensory symptoms may lead to the erroneous diagnosis of motor neurone disease. This branch has no sensory component and does not supply the muscles of the hypothenar eminence, so that there is no sensory loss and abduction of the little finger is spared. The onset is often acute and recovery follows the avoidance of further pressure.

CHAPTER 5

Less common palsies

The other main nerve trunks are not vulnerable to external pressure and isolated lesions are seldom seen except as the result of acute trauma or locally destructive agents. A median nerve lesion in the antecubital fossa causes paralysis of all the flexors of the wrist and digits except those supplied by the ulnar nerve, and of the thenar muscles, the abductor pollicis and the opponens in particular. Sensory loss is confined to the palmar surface of the lateral side of the hand and the lateral three digits, extending on to the dorsal surface of the terminal phalanges. A lesion at the wrist causes similar signs in the hand but the flexor muscles are spared.

The circumflex and musculo-cutaneous nerves may be injured in fractures or dislocations of the humerus. The former supplies the deltoid and a small area of skin over the muscle, the latter the biceps and brachialis and the skin over the radial border of the forearm.

The femoral nerve supplies the quadriceps muscle, which extends the knee and assists in flexion of the hip. Its sensory branches supply the inner side of the thigh and also of the calf to the medial malleolus. The nerve is seldom injured, but may be involved in pelvic malignant disease.

The sciatic nerve supplies the hamstring muscles through branches that leave the main trunk at variable levels, while its two main terminal branches innervate all the muscles below the knee. Its sensory distribution is to the foot and outer side of the calf. A complete lesion is rare except in penetrating wounds, but the nerve may be inadvertently injected with paraldehyde or other destructive agents.

IRRITATIVE AND ENTRAPMENT SYNDROMES

The symptoms and signs of acute traumatic lesions of the peripheral nerves are those of loss of function. Chronic constriction, or entrapment, not only interrupts conduction, but also causes symptoms attributable to irritation of the nerve.

The lateral cutaneous nerve of the thigh:
meralgia paraesthetica

This purely sensory nerve innervates an oval area of skin on the lateral surface of the thigh. It may be subjected to continuous or intermittent constriction in its passage behind the lateral part of the inguinal ligament. This occurs much more commonly in heavily built men, and is frequently bilateral, with unpleasant burning pain in the area supplied by the nerve. As constriction is increased by muscular contraction the pain is aggravated by walking and particularly by prolonged standing, and relieved by rest. Numbness in the same area may be noticed by the patient and sensory blunting is found on examination. Motor signs or loss of reflexes do not occur, and this helps to distinguish the condition from the more proximal nerve root lesion seen in prolapse of a high lumbar intervertebral disc, where sensory loss more anteriorly over the thigh is usually accompanied by a sluggish knee jerk.

The severity of the symptoms of meralgia paraesthetica is difficult to assess, and many patients merely wish to be assured that they have no serious disease. Rational treatment consists in decompressing or dividing the nerve and is effective but seldom necessary. As in other contexts, weight reduction is a counsel of perfection, and injection of the nerve with local anaesthetic at the lateral end of the inguinal ligament is seldom helpful. The symptoms often subside if prolonged standing can be avoided, and natural remission is common.

The median nerve: the carpal tunnel syndrome

The median nerve at the wrist accompanies the flexor tendons in the carpal tunnel beneath the flexor retinaculum. Compression of the nerve in this crowded space is common and produces an unexpectedly complex syndrome. The cause of the compression is seldom obvious, but is probably swelling of the tendon sheaths. An identical syndrome may occur in rheumatoid arthritis where tenosynovitis is a common feature; in myxoedema where there is soft tissue swelling; and in pregnancy where there is fluid retention. The vast majority of those affected are women, and when the characteristic symptoms are encountered in a man the cause of the compression may be unusual, such as a tuberculous palmar ganglion, osteophytes around an old fracture of the carpal bones, gout, or acromegaly.

Symptoms usually begin in middle age, but there is great variation and slight symptoms may have been present for many years before the patient complains. The most distressing symptom is pain which is characteristically nocturnal. It is not present on going to bed but regularly awakens the patient in the early hours of the morning. The pain is not confined to the distribution of the median nerve but may extend the whole length of the arm to the shoulder. It is accompanied by paraesthesiae which are also often of wide distribution. Relief sufficient to allow further sleep is obtained by hanging the arms over the side of the bed or by alternately contracting and relaxing the wrists and fingers. On waking in the morning the hands are stiff and clumsy and feel swollen, but symptoms disappear within a few minutes of use. Paraesthesiae, but seldom pain, may return during any continued use of the fingers, particularly knitting or holding up a book, and now the patient will usually confirm that they are confined to the distribution of the median nerve. Nocturnal pain, clumsiness on waking and diurnal paraesthesiae are present in nearly every case, but they are seldom equally prominent.

Symptoms are often closely related to exercise or unaccustomed use of the hands. The onset may date from injudicious home decorating or gardening, and most patients recognize that the more the hands are used during the day the worst the symptoms the following night. The dominant hand is usually first affected, but all chronic cases are bilateral.

Prolonged entrapment eventually leads to symptoms due to loss of function rather than irritation of the nerve, but these are curiously unobtrusive. Even gross weakness of the thenar muscles that has developed gradually may scarcely be noticed by the patient.

Physical examination may be entirely negative. Slight sensory loss on the terminal phalanges of the thumb, index and middle fingers may be found but is often unconvincing. Weakness always first affects the abductor pollicis brevis, the most lateral muscle of the thenar eminence. The action of this muscle is to move the thumb at a right angle to the plane of the palm and it is tested by putting the thumb in this position and telling the patient to hold it there against resistance. Wasting of the lateral half of the thenar eminence, partial thenar atrophy, may be obvious, but a surprising degree of weakness may be found even when the muscle bulk is normal.

The carpal tunnel syndrome is so common that many women accept it as their natural lot. When they seek advice the diagnosis is unfortunately often missed, mainly because it is difficult to appreciate that a lesion at the wrist can cause such extensive pain. A diagnosis of 'brachial neuritis' is no diagnosis at all, and the carpal tunnel syndrome is much the commonest cause of pain in the arm in women. Often the typical pain and tingling can be provoked on examination by pressure over the carpal ligament, by sustained forcible flexion at the wrist, or by inflating a sphygmomanometer cuff on the upper arm for two minutes at a pressure midway between the patient's systolic and diastolic blood pressures. When such signs are positive they confirm the diagnosis but they may be difficult to elicit even where symptoms are pathognomonic. If doubt exists interference with conduction in the median nerve can be demonstrated objectively in all chronic cases, though the electrical tests may be entirely normal in classical cases with a shorter history: as often, symptomatology remains the most sensitive diagnostic instrument. Longstanding constriction of a nerve causes slowing of conduction in the constricted segment and this can be measured. Recording electrodes are placed over the abductor pollicis brevis and the nerve is stimulated electrically just above the wrist. The muscle normally contracts 5 milliseconds or less after the stimulus, and this can be accurately and simply recorded with standard apparatus. In most cases of the carpal tunnel syndrome the interval between the stimulus and response is prolonged to 7 milliseconds or more. It is also possible to stimulate the digital nerves and to record the resulting action potential in the nerve trunk above the wrist, but the technique is more difficult because of the low amplitude of the potential. If the nerve is constricted, the potential is much reduced or absent, not because the fibres are unable to conduct but because they conduct at different velocities and do not produce a synchronous wave that can be recorded. These tests are of considerable theoretical interest in demonstrating segmental slowing of conduction but they are rarely necessary in the diagnosis of the carpal tunnel syndrome.

It is not easy to account for all the symptoms of the syndrome on the basis of compression of the median nerve, though they are undoubtedly cured by decompressing the carpal tunnel. Efficiently performed operation, with complete division of the flexor retinaculum, produces immediate relief of sensory symptoms, and weakness of the thenar muscles also recovers unless wasting is too far advanced. Operation should always be advised in the presence of either longstanding symptoms or muscular wasting. Conservative treatment is justifiable with a short history of an obvious immediate cause such as pregnancy or recent over-use of the hands. Tight gripping, as in wringing clothes, must be avoided, and a simple splint on the wrist at night often prevents nocturnal pain. Maintained for several weeks, these measures sometimes produce permanent cure in cases of recent onset. Diuretics to reduce local swelling are seldom helpful, and the temporary relief yielded by systemic corticosteroids does not justify their administration in so local a condition. In severe cases complicating pregnancy the local injection of hydrocortisone into the carpal tunnel may provide immediate relief, and the same technique is sometimes helpful in the evaluation of symptoms: temporarily, at any rate, it will obliterate the contribution of median nerve compression to atypical brachial pain in patients where the carpal tunnel syndrome co-exists with significant cervical spondylosis.

The ulnar nerve

In the much less common cubital tunnel syndrome the ulnar nerve is constricted by the fascial band between the two heads of the flexor carpi ulnaris. This occurs more frequently in men, with symptoms of a slowly progressive and usually unilateral ulnar nerve palsy. Sensory symptoms occur first—paraesthesiae and numbness in the ring and little fingers, and pain from the elbow down the inner side of the forearm may be severe but its nocturnal incidence is much less prominent than in the carpal tunnel syndrome. Weakness and wasting of the ulnar muscles of the hand appear later, but it is hardly ever possible to detect weakness of the ulnar flexors in the forearm.

It can usually be demonstrated that the site of the lesion is at the elbow by measuring conduction velocity in the nerve. Recording electrodes are placed over the abductor digiti minimi, the nerve is stimulated at the wrist, elbow, and axilla, and the interval between the stimulus at each site and the response is measured. If the distance between the points of stimulation is known, it is easy to calculate the velocity of conduction in the two segments of nerve, from the axilla to above the elbow and from above the elbow to the wrist. There is some decline in normal velocity with increasing age, and too much importance must not be accorded to slight differences. In the ulnar tunnel syndrome the velocity in the segment including the elbow may be reduced from the normal of 50 to 35 metres a second, with normal conduction in the segment of nerve above the elbow. Like most tests this is not completely reliable but it is a convenient method of convincing orthopaedic surgeons.

Treatment of the ulnar tunnel syndrome consists of decompressing the nerve, a simple and very successful operation.

A chronic progressive ulnar nerve palsy of a rather different type may develop many years after an injury in which the anatomy of the elbow joint is distorted. Here the lesion is due to friction and fibrosis behind the medial condyle of the humerus. Such injuries have not usually involved the joint itself: the commonest cause is a fracture of the humerus that has altered the carrying angle at the elbow. Similar palsies may occur in osteoarthritis of the elbow joint. The clinical features are identical with those of the ulnar tunnel syndrome, except that pain is uncommon and on this account the patient may not present until the ulnar palsy is complete. The paralysis and wasting of the interossei and lumbricals produce the classical 'claw hand' in which the metacarpo-phalangeal joints are hyperextended and the interphalangeal joints flexed. If the palsy has progressed to this stage it is irrecoverable and treatment is pointless. In cases diagnosed earlier, treatment consists in transposing the nerve to the front of the elbow, a less trivial procedure than decompression. The results are not always impressive, but continued deterioration can be prevented and worthwhile improvement may occur.

Causalgia

Causalgia is an uncommon but exceedingly unpleasant manifestation of the incomplete interruption of sensory nerve fibres that may accompany traumatic partial peripheral nerve lesions, especially of the median nerve. The skin in the distribution of the nerve becomes exquisitely sensitive, the slightest touch producing severe burning pain, and the hand is virtually useless. The skin is red, shiny and dry, or may sweat excessively. The cause may be selective loss of large-diameter fibres with relative sparing of small fibres. According to the 'gate' theory, imbalance of this kind would facilitate neuronal systems serving pain within the spinal cord. Relief of causalgic pain has been claimed by restoring the balance by electrical stimulation of surviving large-diameter fibres in the damaged nerve. Sympathetic block is also sometimes successful. This may be tested by a trial procaine block of the stellate ganglion: if this relieves pain, cure is likely to follow alcohol block or excision of the ganglion.

Amputation neuroma

Sprouting axons from the severed nerves in an amputation stump often form painful tender swellings that may prevent the wearing of a prosthesis. Excision may be successful but is often followed by further neuroma formation. It has been claimed that pain and sensitivity can be reduced to a tolerable level by the repeated application of strong pressure to the painful area, usually with a vibratory massage machine. This is not always successful, perhaps because the initial stages of the treatment are so unpleasant that some patients do not persevere with it.

BRACHIAL PLEXUS INJURIES

The brachial plexus is also liable to acute trauma, to pressure palsies and to entrapment. The practical applications of the complex anatomy of the plexus are comparatively limited. Penetrating injuries may cause complete or partial lesions of any of the trunks or cords. The outer cord forms the musculo-cutaneous nerve and part of the median, and may be injured by violent downward movement of the shoulder with resulting paralysis of flexion of the elbow and of the flexors of the wrist and fingers on the radial side of the forearm. The inner cord forms the ulnar nerve and the remainder of the median, and may be injured by forceful abduction at the shoulder. The resulting paralysis involves the intrinsic muscles of the hand and there is sensory loss on the inner side of the forearm.

Injury to the plexus at birth is rare today. The two classical forms correspond approximately to outer and inner cord lesions. They are *Erb's paralysis*, producing paralysis of the deltoid and flexors of the elbow, and *Klumpke's paralysis* in which the hand is paralysed and wasted.

Acute pressure palsies of the plexus are sometimes sustained on the operating table, either from depression of the shoulder or prolonged abduction. The prognosis is relatively good since the nerves remain in continuity.

The plexus may be involved by any locally destructive tumour, particularly at the apex of the lung and in the glands above the clavicle. In addition to progressive paralysis and sensory loss, pain is severe.

CERVICAL RIBS

Chronic compression can occur as the plexus crosses a cervical rib. These structures are usually symptomless, but since it seems that even a normal first rib can occasionally cause a plexus lesion it is hardly surprising that the angulation of the plexus and of the subclavian artery necessary to cross an abnormal rib may sometimes be harmful. Minor paraesthesiae due to such a lesion are not uncommon in middle-aged women, and usually resolve with avoidance of heavy carrying together with exercises designed to overcome drooping of the shoulders. Persistent paraesthesiae and pain may occur in much younger patients and are often aggravated by carrying heavy weights with the arms by the side, though this observation is of limited diagnostic value since it applies in any type of brachial pain. It is the inner cord of the plexus that is affected, and persistent injury results in weakness and wasting of the hand muscles, usually those supplied by the ulnar nerve, and sensory loss on the inner side of the hand and forearm.

Cervical ribs should not be removed unless wasting is present or vascular changes in the hand indicate compression of the artery. However, when such signs are present, relief of compression by removing the rib is essential and should not be delayed. Success is rare following operation for pain alone, or when it is thought that there is a cervical rib or 'costoclavicular compression' syndrome without an abnormal rib visible radiologically. It may be that the plexus can be compressed by fibrous bands or by the scalene muscles, but the poor results of previously fashionable operations for their relief suggests that many symptoms previously attributed to such lesions were in fact due to the carpal tunnel syndrome or other causes.

TRAUMATIC LESIONS

ROOT LESIONS

Severe trauma to the region of the neck and shoulder sometimes avulses cervical nerve roots, resulting in permanent paralysis and sensory loss. The clinical distinction from plexus injury, where partial recovery at any rate is possible, may be difficult. If the lesion is proximal to the entry of the autonomic fibres, axon reflexes through the autonomic system are preserved. Intradermal histamine causes a local flare and pilo-erection, and this reaction is still present if the cervical roots have been avulsed from the cord, but not in a lesion of the brachial plexus.

The nerve roots are also liable to entrapment, and in the lumbar and cervical regions they are frequently subjected to acute, chronic or recurrent compression from disease of the articular structures.

Sciatica

The intervertebral discs in the lumbar spine often fail to withstand the great strains to which they are exposed. The region of angulation at the lumbosacral junction is particularly vulnerable. The annulus fibrosus ruptures, and the comparatively soft tissue in the centre of the disc prolapses, nearly always laterally or posteriorly into the extradural space. Here the prolapsed tissue may compress the roots of the cauda equina, either as they leave the canal in the intervertebral foramina or more centrally as they lie within the canal. A lateral lumbar disc prolapse is by far the commonest cause of sciatica.

The onset may be preceded by recurrent attacks of pain in the lumbar region, often of sufficient severity to produce 'locking' of the back in the flexed position. Pain down the leg may occur acutely following an obvious strain, particularly lifting with the back flexed, or without obvious precipitating cause. The lesion is common enough in the young and athletic, but with advancing age the discs tend to become dry and brittle, and rupture or prolapse may be provoked even by turning over in bed. A more gradual onset over several days or weeks is also common. The site of the pain is in the distribution of the injured root, usually the first sacral or fifth lumbar. The pain is in the buttock, and radiates down the posterior or lateral aspect of the thigh and calf to the heel or toes. It is aggravated by movement, and in the acute stage the patient can find no posture that gives more than momentary relief. The severity varies greatly but may be almost intolerable.

The physical signs are characteristic. The lumbar spine is rigid and there is often scoliosis due to spasm of the lateral spinal muscles. Passive flexion of the leg at the hip with the knee straight is much restricted.

Diffuse muscular tenderness is present in the buttock and thigh. More specific signs of a root lesion are impaired cutaneous sensation over the medial or lateral side of the foot, and loss of the ankle jerk when the first sacral root is involved. Weakness is less common, but it is difficult to assess minor paresis since movement aggravates the pain. If the third or fourth lumbar roots are compressed by a lesion at a higher level the pain is felt anteriorly in the thigh, straight leg raising may be unaffected, and the knee jerk may be reduced or absent. In chronic sciatica the pain is less severe and muscle spasm much less marked, but the signs of root compression may be more obvious. Weakness of dorsiflexion, initially of the great toe, and wasting of the anterior tibial muscles may both be evident.

There are few other causes of acute lumbar or sacral root compression, and these are so rare by comparison that they need not be considered unless aberrant clinical features develop. Lumbar spine X-rays are seldom helpful because disc prolapse often occurs without any narrowing of the disc space, and disc degeneration with gross narrowing is seen without prolapse.

The traditional treatment of acute sciatica is rest in bed on fracture boards for several weeks. This is often effective, but is not easy to achieve, while rest in bed itself is debilitating as well as demoralizing—and may even be dangerous. Immobilization of the lumbar spine in a plaster jacket has much the same therapeutic effect. However, it is more than likely that the natural history of many attacks of acute sciatica is of recovery in six weeks irrespective of treatment. Rapid relief of symptoms has been claimed from a short course of high doses of prednisolone. The doctor working in hospital sees an undue proportion of intractable cases and his view of prognosis is often unduly pessimistic.

The diagnosis and treatment of chronic sciatica is more difficult. When there are neurological signs of a root lesion and pain resists conservative measures, the disc prolapse should be removed by operation. Claims have been made for the effectiveness of manipulation of the lumbar spine, but this should not even be contemplated in the presence of root signs. It is improbable that manipulation can replace a prolapsed disc, but quite certain that it can cause further extensive extrusion. The results of operation are usually excellent, though they depend on careful selection of patients. When physical signs are indefinite and the pain less clearly of root distribution care must be taken to exclude other causes such as pelvic carcinoma with local invasion, secondary deposits and diabetic neuropathy. The most difficult cases are those where chronic pain is accompanied by no evidence of a possible root lesion beyond muscle spasm. Even here operation occasionally reveals a prolapsed disc, but in most no cause for the pain can be found and the patient is unimproved.

A central disc prolapse may extrude large fragments that compress the cauda equina. Even in young adults such a lesion may immediately follow trauma such as a fall from a height on to the buttocks. The effects are serious and retention or incontinence of urine common. The diagnosis is often regrettably missed, since the tell-tale sensory loss is in the lower sacral and coccygeal segments on the buttocks and perineum, where sensation is not always tested. Time may be irrevocably lost, for this is an emergency. The compression must be relieved as soon as possible if sphincter function is to be restored.

Bilateral sciatica is also an urgent indication for full investigation since it suggests cauda equina compression either by central disc prolapse or by tumour.

'Claudication of the cauda equina' is an intriguing variant. Pain and paraesthesiae of sciatic distribution occur on walking and are relieved by standing still. Signs of root compression are usually present at rest, but more conspicuous if the patient is examined after exercise. The pulses in the legs are normal and the syndrome is due to ischaemia of the cauda equina resulting from compression of one or more radicular arteries by disc or osteophytes as they enter through the intervertebral foramina. These symptoms can result from narrowing of the lumbar spinal canal from any cause, notably the overgrowth of bone in Paget's disease.

Cervical root compression

A syndrome similar in many respects to sciatica also occurs in the upper limb. The onset is sudden, with severe pain in the arm down to the hand, accompanied by paraesthesiae usually confined to the digits on the radial side of the hand: the discs in the region of angulation in the lower part of the cervical spine are again specially vulnerable. Although neck pain is a less constant and less conspicuous feature than lumbago in lumbar spine lesions, active and passive movements of the neck are restricted. The commonest signs are those of a seventh cervical root lesion, with weakness of the triceps, loss of the triceps jerk, and impaired pain sensation in the middle digits. It is probable that this syndrome is usually due to an acute lateral disc prolapse in the neck, though opportunity for verification at operation is infrequent. Again the natural history in the large majority of cases is of full recovery in about six weeks. Pain may be severe for the first two weeks and is materially influenced neither by immobilizing the neck nor by traction.

Chronic cervical root lesions are common. The cervical spine is highly mobile and poorly adapted to the upright posture. Chronic disc degeneration and osteoarthritis—referred to in this context as spondylosis—are almost universal with advancing years. Osteophytes and dense fibrous tissue encroach on the intervertebral foramina, compressing the roots. The sixth and seventh are most commonly affected. Symptoms are curiously intermittent, although it is difficult to imagine much change for the better occurring in these narrowed foramina. Few people reach middle age without some symptoms of cervical spondylosis such as aching in the neck and arms with fluctuating paraesthesiae. Unless they persist or are accompanied by undoubted evidence of structural damage to the roots, and not merely symptoms of irritation, they are best treated with analgesics and local heat. Some patients complain of continuous symptoms for years, with physical signs limited to dubious sensory loss and a stiff neck: in these cases operation is to be avoided. Such patients are often treated with a rigid collar which becomes an addiction, worn devotedly for many years. It is difficult to believe that either the symptoms or their relief arise directly from structural change, but many patients seem satisfied with this solution to their problems. Operation to relieve chronic pain should be confined to patients with clear physical signs of root compression. In such patients pain may sometimes be successfully relieved by operations designed to enlarge the intervertebral foramen. Chronic compression of a number of roots by widespread spondylosis occasionally produces extensive muscular wasting in the upper limbs, sometimes with inconspicuous sensory symptoms and without sensory loss, not easy to distinguish from motor neurone disease.

Other causes of root compression are important but far less common, and include neurofibromata growing on nerve roots and indeed any form of tumour involving the spinal canal. Root pain in the limbs must be distinguished from that due to the more peripheral lesions discussed in this chapter, but pain in the distribution of the thoracic roots is often mistaken for that of visceral disease: the motor and reflex changes so helpful in the limbs are absent and even if sensation is tested the results are notoriously unreliable.

THE SPINAL CORD

The spinal cord is well protected by the spinal column, but in these days of high-speed traffic accidents the defences are all too often breached. Before the consequences of spinal cord injury can be discussed the important differences between the effects of peripheral and central lesions on the motor and sensory systems must be understood.

The upper motor neurone

By convention the upper motor neurones comprise the corticospinal fibres in the pyramidal tract, the corticobulbar fibres, and the parent cell bodies in the cortex. Other neuronal systems are involved in motor activity, and it is doubtful whether all the effects classically attributed to an upper motor neurone lesion are due to pyramidal tract dysfunction. However, the concept is undoubtedly useful as a clinical approximation.

The effects of such a lesion are greatly modified by the level of the injury, but they have certain well-defined characteristics. An acute transverse cord lesion, totally interrupting the motor pathways, is immediately followed by flaccid paralysis with loss of all reflex activity. This state of *spinal shock* may persist for hours or days, but is gradually replaced by spastic paraplegia. Spasticity implies an increased resistance to passive movement of the limbs, particularly in the extensor muscles of the lower limb and the flexors of the arm—the antigravity muscles. This increased resistance is due to exaggeration of the normal stretch reflexes. The corticospinal tract appears to exert an inhibitory effect on the excitability of both the alpha motor neurones and the fusimotor neurones. The former are not only rendered more readily excitable, but are exposed to an increased afferent flow from the muscle spindles. In man this increased reflex activity is by no means confined to the antigravity muscles and the comparison with the decerebrate cat is not wholly valid.

The paralysed limbs may be subject to spasms predominantly affecting either extensor or flexor muscles, and these may occur spontaneously as well as in response to passive movement, stimulation of the skin, or distension of the bladder. Severe frequent flexor spasms may herald the onset of the miserable condition, paraplegia in flexion, where the legs are permanently flexed first by continuous spasm and later by persistent shortening with contracture of the hamstrings and flexors of the thigh.

Incomplete lesions permit some voluntary movement in a disordered and inefficient manner. The muscles are weak and no longer contract or relax to precisely the right degree and in precisely the right sequence for any particular movement. All the muscles of the limb contract together, producing a limited range of stereotyped movements, and reciprocal innervation of agonists and antagonists is lost. Movement is therefore not only weak but slow and inaccurate. In walking, a spastic leg is rigidly extended at the knee and the foot is plantar flexed so that the toe scrapes the ground.

In any upper motor neurone lesion the tendon jerks are increased, sometimes to the extent that a single stretch causes repetitive contraction of the muscle, or clonus. Tendon jerks may be elicited in muscles where they are not normally found, such as the hamstrings, the adductors of the thigh and the flexors of the fingers. The spread of reflex hyperexcitability may be such that muscles quite remote from that stretched by the tendon hammer may contract.

The cutaneous reflexes are also disturbed. The plantar reflex that normally causes flexion of the toes on stroking the outer side of the sole becomes extensor. The toes fan and the big toe is dorsiflexed—the Babinski response. The superficial abdominal reflexes and the cremasteric reflex are often lost.

The sensory tracts

A complete lesion of the sensory pathways in the spinal cord causes total sensory loss with a distinct though not absolutely abrupt upper level corresponding to the segment involved. The effect of partial lesions depends on the tracts affected. Postural sense is lost and light touch impaired if the posterior columns are involved. Vibration sense is also lost, although the situation and course of the fibres concerned is not entirely clear. Injury to the lateral and anterior columns containing the spinothalamic tracts, on the other hand, causes loss of pain and thermal sense and also some change in the subjective sensation of light touch. In partial lesions sensation may be no more than blunted, and this may not extend over the whole area below the lesion, while the upper level of the sensory change may be hard to define.

THE BROWN–SÉQUARD SYNDROME

Hemisection of the cord produces a characteristic clinical picture, the Brown–Séquard syndrome. There is spastic paralysis and loss of postural sense on the side of the lesion and loss of pain and thermal sense on the opposite side. The spinothalamic fibres ascend on the side of entry for a few segments before crossing, so that the sensory level is well below the level of the lesion and there may also be a band of spinothalamic loss on the side of the lesion. A complete Brown–Séquard lesion of this type is hardly ever seen, but elements of the syndrome are common. One leg may be weaker and more spastic than the other in which pain and thermal sense are lost, but the upper level may bear little relation to the known site of the lesion.

THE SPHINCTERS

In spinal shock both voluntary and reflex emptying of the bladder are impossible. Retention of urine occurs, eventually with overflow incontinence. As reflex activity returns so reflex voiding becomes possible, but after a severe cord lesion this is often difficult to establish and retention may persist for many weeks. Reflex emptying is never complete, and the residual urine is a source of infection. In paraplegia, voiding may be induced on provoking the mass reflex of withdrawal of the legs by stimuli such as stroking the sole of the foot.

Incomplete lesions may cause heightened reflex activity of the bladder, with frequency and precipitancy of micturition. Incontinence of urine with a small hyperactive bladder is a common and distressing symptom which may be accompanied by episodes of retention.

The spinal tracts concerned with control of the bladder are in close association with the lateral spinothalamic tracts.

Constipation is common in all forms of spinal cord lesion and spontaneous evacuation of the bowel may cease altogether, but rectal incontinence is distinctly uncommon.

TRAUMA TO THE CORD

Apart from penetrating wounds, trauma to the spinal cord results from violent distortion of the vertebral column in industrial and traffic accidents. The spine may be fractured at any level by direct injury, and bone fragments may be driven into the spinal canal. A crush fracture resulting from a fall from a height in a standing or sitting posture is usually less harmful but many also narrow the canal. The great mobility of the cervical spine is a source of danger, since rapid deceleration causes acute flexion followed by extension. This is seen in the so-called 'whiplash' injury, often postulated in traffic accident claims on account of subjective complaints that are difficult to disprove, authenticate, or evaluate. However, there can be no doubt that the most transient dislocation with rupture of the anterior ligament, spontaneously and immediately reduced, imperils the spinal cord.

Even when no fracture or dislocation has occurred severe trauma of this kind can cause *concussion* of the spinal cord. There is no immediate means of distinguishing this temporary functional failure of conducton from more serious irreversible damage. The lesion may appear to be complete and its comparatively benign nature manifest only in rapid recovery. It is possibly comparable to peripheral nerve conduction block without destruction of axons, but it is briefer.

A severe lesion that improves within a few days with some residual disability is usually attributed to *contusion* of the cord, although opportunities for verifying the supposed bruises are necessarily few.

Laceration or transection of the cord inevitably causes permanent disability because divided axones in the central nervous system do not effectively regenerate. It is difficult to determine how much of the damage is due to direct impact of bone fragments or pressure of the angulation of the dislocated spine, and how much to the secondary effects of haemorrhage or loss of blood supply.

Cervical cord injury may produce a neurological syndrome indicating a centrally situated lesion destroying the spinothalamic fibres as they cross the pyramidal tracts in the lateral columns. This has been traditionally attributed to a central haemorrhage or *haematomyelia*, but is in fact probably due to infarction in the distribution of the anterior spinal artery. It is seen most characteristically after flexion injuries such as may be sustained by diving into shallow water.

A complete permanent lesion of the high cervical cord is scarcely compatible with life. The innervation of the diaphragm is mainly from the fourth cervical segment, and a transverse lesion at or above this level causes total quadriplegia with paralysis of respiration.

A common site of injury is at the seventh cervical segment. Although the intercostal muscles are paralysed diaphragmatic breathing continues. Loss of the anterior horn cells causes flaccid paralysis of the triceps and of the extensors of the wrist and fingers. Below this level spastic paralysis develops. Movement at the shoulder and flexion of the elbow are retained, but there is little useful movement of the fingers. Although their central connections are a segment higher than the lesion the biceps and supinator jerks may be increased, perhaps because of some interference with the blood supply of the upper cervical cord. The sensory level extends along the inner border of the arms.

Dorsal cord transection causes motor and sensory loss at the appropriate level. Since the cord is shorter than the vertebral column the vertebral and segmental levels do not correspond. A lesion at the eighth dorsal vertebra, for example, will produce a motor and sensory level at the eleventh dorsal segment.

The conus medullaris lies at the level of the first lumbar vertebra. Although the motor and sensory loss resulting from a lesion may be comparatively slight there is a grave risk of destruction of the reflex arcs controlling micturition, the action of the bowels and sexual activity in the male. These functions are, of course, impaired or lost in any complete cord lesion at a higher level, but reflex micturition may still be established. This can never be achieved if the reflex arcs are permanently destroyed.

Below the first lumbar vertebra the spinal canal contains the cauda equina, which may be injured by severe trauma to the lumbar spine.

TRAUMATIC LESIONS

Such lesions are seldom complete, and the disability from motor and sensory impairment in the lower lumbar and sacral segments may be relatively mild but accompanied by permanent loss of sphincter control and by impotence.

MANAGEMENT

It is unfortunately true that the effects of an acute severe spinal cord lesion are sometimes misdiagnosed as hysteria. This almost incredible blunder is due to failure to appreciate the significance of the initial flaccid paralysis. If a man who has been injured says that he cannot move his legs he is probably telling the truth. In most cases, however, it is immediately obvious that a potential disaster has occurred. Avoiding movement of the spine as far as possible, X-rays of the appropriate area should be obtained. Unfortunately the failure to visualize conspicuous bone lesions does not exclude serious cord injury. A tell-tale finding in cervical injuries is a small flake of bone pulled off the anterior aspect of one vertebra where the anterior longitudinal ligament has been torn away. Lumbar puncture should be done to see if there is a spinal block. Opinion is still divided on the value of operative exploration and some authorities think it has hardly any place. Spinal block confirmed and localized by myelography, or progressive paraplegia, are fairly widely accepted indications for surgery. Even here the only hopeful finding is the rather uncommon one of cord compression by a haematoma that can be evacuated. Removal of bone fragments from the spinal canal is valueless since the cord damage has occurred at the moment of impact.

If the cause is irreparable every effort must be made to mitigate its effects. Retention of urine must be relieved by a fine indwelling catheter, preferably released every few hours rather than draining continuously. Urinary infection is almost inevitable in the bacteria-ridden atmosphere of a hospital ward, and prophylactic antiseptics should be used provided urinary output is adequate. A paralysed patient soon develops bedsores if he is not turned every two hours, but to move him at all may be dangerous if there is an unstable lesion of the spine. A specially devised turning frame is essential for the best results.

As soon as possible the patient should be transferred to a special unit for the treatment of paraplegia. The principles of management consist of early mobilization, training in the use of surviving muscular power, and vigorous treatment of any urinary infection or bedsores that may have developed. The latter are treated by the avoidance of all pressure on the area, the clearing of infection by local and systemic antibiotics, and the replacement of the heavy protein loss in the exudate by means of a high protein diet. Anaemia is common but does not always respond well to oral iron, and blood transfusion may be needed for its prompt correction. The paraplegic gravely handicapped but usefuly employed, and with the freedom of the wheelchair, is in happy contrast with the demoralized emaciated wreck that is the end-result of inexpert management.

The care of the bladder and urinary tract in chronic neurological disease is of great importance as neglect can lead to persistent infection and eventually to fatal renal damage. As reflex activity returns to the legs, following an acute cord lesion, reflex bladder emptying becomes possible. This can be assisted by suprapubic pressure and is best done at progressively longer timed intervals. In partial cord lesions, such as in multiple sclerosis, different problems may arise. Reflex emptying of the bladder may become over-sensitive and voluntary inhibition is inadequate. Frequency and urgency of micturition result and at this stage occasional incontinence occurs. As the disease progresses, incontinence becomes an increasing problem, sometimes punctuated by recurring episodes of retention. Management is difficult as, although urgency can sometimes be helped by ephedrine, 15 to 30 mg twice or thrice daily, or by anticholinergic drugs, incontinence scarcely ever improves on such treatment. Timed deliberate micturition, at first at frequent intervals, sometimes leads to reasonable retraining of the bladder. In most male patients a rubber urinal provides a tolerable solution, but no effective urinal for the female has been invented. The choice lies between absorbent padding, a catheter, or diverting the flow of urine. Padding and waterproof pants offer the safest method and have become far more comfortable since the invention of fabric that allows urine to pass in one direction only so that the skin can remain dry and the soaked padding conveniently removed. An indwelling catheter nearly always leads to chronic cystitis and pyelonephritis, but modern plastic catheters are far less irritating than the rubber catheters previously in use. The formation of an artificial bladder from a loop of ileum discharging into a bag on the abdominal wall has proved disappointing as management is difficult and complications are frequent. Despite much ingenuity, it is undeniable that chronic urinary incontinence, particularly in the female, is one of the most miserable consequences of disease of the nervous system.

In chronic spinal cord disease, retention is less frequently a problem and is usually a passing phase, although sometimes recurrent. Catheterization is needed and should be maintained for a few days. Voluntary micturition then usually returns and may be assisted by carbachol 2 mg twice daily by mouth, but this drug should not be given by injection. In unusually persistent retention, resection of the bladder neck has been recommended but there is a risk of permanent incontinence.

A common diagnostic problem is whether disturbance of micturition as an isolated symptom is due to disease of the nervous system. This is certainly rare in the complete absence of other signs of nervous disease, but if there is genuine doubt, a cystometrogram can be used to elucidate the bladder function. Sterile saline is run into the bladder 50 ml at a time and the intravesical pressure can be measured by leading off to a manometer through a Y-tube. Pressure is plotted against volume. Normally the presssure rises steadily with increasing volume, until at about 300 ml reflex bladder contractions occur. If the reflex arcs are interrupted, pressure rises very little and no contractions are induced, even by a large volume of fluid. In the hyperactive bladder of chronic spinal cord disease, pressure mounts steeply and uncontrollable contractions may be induced by 50 or 100 ml. The micturating cystogram and other radiological refinements have not greatly added to the ease of diagnosis of the neurogenic bladder.

MYELOPATHY DUE TO SPONDYLOSIS

The cervical and much more rarely the dorsal cord may be injured by chronic trauma in a manner comparable with the entrapment syndromes of the peripheral nervous system. Degenerative disease of the cervical intervertebral discs with osteophyte formation on the posterior aspect of the vertebral bodies is found on X-ray examination of the large majority of middle-aged and elderly subjects who have no symptoms whatever (Fig. 10, following p. 152). Nevertheless central disc protrusions encroach on the cervical canal and are a potential source of spinal cord injury (Fig. 11, following p. 152). Chronic cord compression is especially likely if the antero-posterior diameter of the canal was already below average. Chronic arthritis of this kind is accompanied by ligamentous thickening, and the ligamentum flavum posterior to the cord may be thrown into deep folds that further narrow the canal especially on extension of the neck. These bony and ligamentous changes of cervical spondylosis are now recognized as a common cause of cervical myelopathy. A disc protrusion with accompanying osteophytes may similarly encroach on the canal in the dorsal region, but it rarely induces myelopathy.

The precise causation of the myelopathy is uncertain. Actual indentation or flattening of the cord certainly occurs and could itself possibly cause neuronal degeneration. However, compression of venous drainage and especially of a marginally adequate arterial blood supply are almost certainly more important factors.

The clinical syndrome is variable, but is most commonly a slowly progressive spastic paraparesis beginning in middle age. Stiffness of the gait or dragging of one leg increase almost imperceptibly until walking becomes continuously difficult. Sensory symptoms in the lower limbs are uncommon, and sensory loss is usually confined to loss of vibration sense and some impairment of postural sense in the toes. The occasionally unilateral impact of the disease on the spinal cord may produce a partial Brown–Séquard syndrome: pain of central origin is accompanied by loss of pain and thermal sense in one leg which the other is clearly spastic. Sometimes the upper level of cutaneous sensory change is thoracic and does not immediately suggest a cervical lesion. The abdominal responses are often retained.

Pain in the upper limbs due to root compression is uncommon, the protrusions being central rather than lateral, but some abnormality in the arms is nearly always present. There is usually some alteration in the tendon jerks, especially loss of the triceps jerk with increased biceps and supinator jerks, or a generalized but asymmetrical reflex overactivity. Wasting due to root compression or more probably to anterior horn cell damage is occasionally extensive. A curious variant is a condition of severe disablement from loss of postural sense in the fingers.

The course of spondylotic myelopathy is not invariably chronic and in some patients disability advances in the course of a few weeks: in a patient with previously mild symptoms an apparently trivial fall or jerk may immediately precipitate a severe cervical cord lesion.

The signs of cord compression due to prolapsed dorsal disc are of course indistinguishable from those of any other progressive spinal cord lesion in this region.

The diagnosis of cervical myelopathy may often be suspected on clinical grounds but cannot be regarded as definitive without investigation. Multiple sclerosis often produces a closely similar clinical syndrome and should be suspected especially if control of the bladder is impaired at an early stage of the disease: a pale optic disc, sustained nystagmus or intention tremor may clinch the diagnosis. Subacute combined degeneration must always be excluded in any progressive spinal cord syndrome of this type, particularly when the signs are limited to loss of vibration sense and spasticity: the ankle jerks are usually absent and the calves tender. In any case of progressive paralysis a spinal cord tumour must be considered as a possible cause. Radiological evidence of cervical spondylosis is so common that in itself it is of little help except that spondylotic myelopathy is very unlikely with a cervical spine that is completely normal on X-ray. Narrowed disc spaces are unimportant and the only significant finding is encroachment on the spinal canal. If the clinical course is slow, X-ray changes marked, and the diagnosis highly probable initial investigation should be limited to lumbar puncture. If there is no evidence of block and the fluid is normal, other causes of cord compression are unlikely though not impossible. The patient must be re-examined at regular intervals. If at any stage deterioration is rapid, if any unexpected or inappropriate clinical findings appear, or if the cerebrospinal fluid protein is raised a myelogram should always be carried out. In spondylosis the contrast medium may be held up at several levels (Fig. 12), and complete block may develop when the canal is further narrowed on extending the head.

Treatment must be based on knowledge of the natural history. In most patients disability progresses only slowly over many years and never becomes very severe. It is unusual to find a patient bed-ridden or unable to walk from cervical myelopathy. However, all such patients are at risk from the effects of quite minor trauma and when the onset is acute the condition may rapidly become disabling. It has been customary to treat the chronic form of the disease with a rigid collar, the rationale being to prevent the repeated narrowing of the canal every time the neck is extended. The effectiveness of this treatment is doubtful and difficult to assess against the background of a comparatively benign natural progression. Enthusiasts counter any doubts by extolling the superiority of their own particular type of collar.

Surgical treatment of cervical myelopathy is often highly beneficial but the results can never be accurately predicted. Certainly if the condition is rapidly deteriorating despite attempts at treatment with a collar, decompression of the cervical canal should be undertaken. This will usually involve laminectomy of most of the cervical vertebrae thus allowing ample space for the spinal cord. Earlier attempts included vigorous efforts to remove the protruding osteophytes on the anterior aspect of the cord with frequently disastrous results. Multiple laminectomy naturally does not leave a normal neck and a collar is advisable for several months after operation. In favourable cases there is rapid improvement in walking and in the use of the hands. An anterior approach by drilling through the disc space has been used in patients in whom the cord is compressed at only one or two sites.

Further reading

Guttman L. (1976) *Spinal Cord Injuries*, 2nd edn. Blackwell Scientific Publications, Oxford.

Koppel H.P. & Thompson W.A.L. (1963) *Peripheral Entrapment Neuropathies*. Williams and Wilkins, Baltimore.

Nurick S. (1972) The natural history and the results of surgical treatment of the spinal cord disorders associated with cervical spondylosis. *Brain* 95, 101.

Seddon H. (1972) *Surgical Disorders of the Peripheral Nerves*. Churchill Livingstone, Edinburgh and London.

CHAPTER 6
Peripheral Neuropathy

Disease of the peripheral nervous system may be diffuse, causing multiple symmetrical peripheral neuropathy, otherwise known as polyneuritis, or may affect individual nerves, either singly or in combination: mononeuritis multiplex. In neither form does the suffix -itis imply an inflammatory disorder and these traditional terms have the merit of brevity.

In polyneuritis the clinical picture always contains elements of a syndrome comprising bilateral lower motor neurone weakness, distal sensory loss and absent tendon reflexes. Despite great variation in extent and severity and in the relative loss of motor and sensory functions, within wide limits the symptoms and signs are characteristic. Sensory symptoms are commonly the presenting feature even when sensory loss is found to be slight. Paraesthesiae, variously described as pins and needles, tingling, burning or even pain, are experienced in the extremities, usually at first in the toes and feet and later in the fingers. A change or loss of feeling on putting the foot to the ground is a later symptom. At the onset symptoms may be asymmetrical or even unilateral, a cause of diagnostic confusion. Cutaneous sensory loss or blunting may not be detectable but when present affects distal segments of the limbs in the so-called glove and stocking distribution. This pattern is also seen in hysteria but the distinction is not difficult. In organic disease the upper limits of sensory impairment are not sharply defined and, as a result, are apt to vary between different examiners and with the fatigue of the patient. In hysteria the upper limit is sharp and can be made to vary by adjusting the patient's clothing, the level rising and falling according to the length of the sleeve. Postural sense may be impaired, sometimes profoundly, and always to a greater extent at distal joints. Vibration sense is commonly lost.

Weakness predominantly affects distal muscles in most chronic cases of polyneuritis, but in acute forms may be proximal. Wasting and, more rarely, fasciculation, occurs if weakness persists for long. Muscles supplied by cranial nerves may also be affected.

Tendon reflexes are lost because of delayed or blocked conduction in a proportion of fast-conducting axons in the afferent side of the reflex arc. This prevents a synchronous burst of impulses reaching the spinal cord and firing the monosynaptic stretch reflex. The reflexes may therefore be lost even when weakness is minimal or absent, and may not return even after apparent full clinical recovery. The plantar reflexes, of course, are flexor or absent.

The clinical features of mononeuritis multiplex are those of lesions of the individual nerves affected, for example, bilateral peroneal nerve palsies, when there would be foot drop but retained ankle jerks. The two forms of neuropathy may, however, coexist, leading to complex clinical presentations.

PATHOGENESIS

We are accustomed to think of polyneuritis as a disease of peripheral nerve fibres. It is, however, important to remember that these motor and sensory fibres are in fact the long protoplasmic processes of lower motor neurones in the anterior horns of the spinal cord and of the sensory neurones of the posterior root ganglia. Furthermore, these cell processes that subserve movement and sensation in the toes from cells in the lumbosacral region may be three feet in length. The cells are by far the largest in the body, and their axons are dependent for their health and nutrition on at least three separate factors. The first of these is the intact function of the parent cell. The second is the maintenance of the myelin sheath by healthy Schwann cells, and the third the blood supply furnished to the nerve trunk along its course by the small entering vasa nervorum. The vulnerability of a lengthy structure of this kind is evident, and the observations outlined above imply three fairly well-defined pathological patterns, though they more often operate in combination than in isolation. They consist first in poisoning of the nerve cells of the motor and sensory neurones by toxic substances; secondly in demyelination, most typically affecting the proximal nerve roots and often associated with oedema and inflammation; and thirdly in a group of lesions of the supporting tissues and vasculature of the peripheral nerves that damage nerve trunks along their course.

The first effects of neuronal poisoning are seen and felt at the distal end of the neuronal process, where interference with the nutrition of the cell first becomes evident, and this is the basis of the peripheral onset of symptoms. This pattern of polyneuritis due to poisoning of the neurone is characteristic of intoxication with many drugs, diabetes and alcohol. It is seen in deficiency diseases such as beriberi, pellagra and intestinal malabsorption: it is also an endotoxic effect of acute intermittent porphyria.

Demyelination of some degree is found in most severe cases of polyneuritis, but selective massive proximal demyelination, involving especially the dorsal nerve roots and ganglia, is characteristic of the Guillain–Barré syndrome (infective polyneuritis), where it is accompanied by lymsphocytic infiltration of nerve roots. It is probably allergic in origin, analogous to experimental polyneuritis induced in animals by auto-immunity to peripheral myelin.

Segmental demyelination is commonly found in many forms of chronic polyneuritis, especially those of unknown cause, and appears to be a primary lesion that affects the Schwann cells. Each cell maintains the myelin sheath between two nodes of Ranvier, and since the disease process rarely affects the entire tissue the effect is loss of myelin over many segments of each fibre, some segments retaining the normal sheath. Segmental demyelination is characterized by marked slowing of conduction in the axons, measured by stimulating the nerve and recording the muscular contraction. Conduction velocity in the fastest fibres may be reduced from about 60 metres per second to 20 metres per second or even less. Some axonal degeneration almost invariably accompanies chronic segmental demyelination, but where polyneuropathy primarily affects the axons the effect on nerve conduction is much less conspicuous. Even when weakness is severe motor nerve conduction may be normal, because those axons that are conducting at all do so at normal velocity, even though their number may be much reduced. Demyelination of nerve roots does not reduce conduction velocity in peripheral segments of the nerve.

Polyneuritis due to lesions of the supporting and vascular structures of the nerve trunk is epitomized by polyarteritis nodosa, where the arteritic lesion causes multiple infarctions along its course. It occurs also in such conditions as leprosy, sarcoidosis, and xanthomatosis, where the nerves are involved by the gross structural lesions of the causative process.

There are a multitude of causes of polyneuritis but these fall naturally into defined groups.

EXTERNAL TOXINS

Alcohol

Alcoholic addiction may be a symptom of several psychiatric disorders, amongst which depression is conspicuous. In many cases, however, it occurs in the absence of any other evidence of mental illness or abnormality. Furthermore, some robust individuals are capable of consuming inordinate amounts of alcohol over periods of many years without apparent ill-effect. Nevertheless, chronic alcoholism remains one of the commonest causes of peripheral neuropathy in the hospitals of the Western world. It presents an excellent example of polyneuritis caused by neuronal poisoning, with peripheral ascending axonal degeneration. Secondary nutritional deficiency plays a larger part in its genesis than a specific toxic effect of ethyl alcohol. Vitamin B_1 (thiamine) is certainly involved, and sometimes indeed the alcoholic syndrome approximates closely to classical beriberi. However, the condition resembles all such disorders in that the deficiency is nearly always multiple and deficiency of protein as well as of the other components of the Vitamin B complex is also concerned.

The typical patient with alcoholic polyneuritis is a middle-aged male, past his prime, and with a long history of excessive consumption. Earlier obesity has often given place to loss of weight and sometimes to emaciation, years of morning nausea to dyspeptic anorexia. The facial appearance is ravaged: there are dilated venules in the skin of the face, the tongue is furred, there is a coarse tremor of the outstretched fingers and enlargement or later shrinking of the liver.

Asymptomatic absence of the ankle jerks and some calf tenderness is almost invariable in such circumstances. However, the established disease is essentially painful, and it usually begins with painful muscular cramps and unpleasant paraesthesiae in the feet and calves, a feeling as though walking on cotton wool, and unsteadiness of gait, especially in the dark. Examination reveals blunter knee jerks as well as absent ankle jerks, and the deep reflexes of the upper limbs are also often difficult to elicit. All forms of sensation are impaired in a stocking distribution. Despite the impairment of superficial sensation the calves are acutely tender to pressure. If alcoholic indulgence continues, unsteadiness when the eyes are closed (Romberg's sign) progresses to inability to walk or stand at all, and the patient is confined to his bed or chair. Flaccid weakness of the upper limbs may progress to wrist drop, but the cranial nerves are spared and if sphincter control is impaired it is only by mental clouding in a drinking bout.

Wernicke's encephalopathy

Alcoholism is also the commonest cause of Wernicke's encephalopathy which is certainly due to thiamine deficiency. It can occasionally occur in other forms of malnutrition, particularly those associated with carcinoma. The onset is usually abrupt with ataxia, nystagmus, ocular palsies and confusion. Retinal haemorrhages may be present. Evidence of polyneuritis can usually be detected even if no more than absent ankle-jerks. The initial lesion appears to be biochemical because all symptoms can be rapidly cured in most patients by the administration of thiamine. Only minute doses are needed but there is no point in being niggardly and 30 mg by intramuscular injection should be given. If the diagnosis is missed the condition may be fatal when multiple haemorrhages are found in the midbrain.

In some patients the encephalopathy is accompanied by Korsakow's psychosis or this may occur independently in alcoholics. This is a profoundly amnesic state with complete loss of immediate recall so that events even of the previous few seconds may not be remembered. A few patients confabulate in an apparent attempt to conceal their disability. A patient who has been ill in hospital for weeks will describe extensive travels undertaken and people encountered during the past few days and his account may be so lively and circumstantial that the unwary student is entirely deceived.

Unfortunately Korsakow's psychosis responds far less well to thiamine and in the majority of patients serious defects persist.

Alcoholic polyneuritis itself is completely recoverable, but improvement is slow and all too often nullified by renewed drinking. The management of alcoholism is a discouraging business and the small proportion of patients who recover often do so spontaneously, for no apparent reason, and after the doctor has abandoned treatment. The polyneuritic alcoholic should be treated in hospital with total abstinence, a liberal diet, and a multivitamin preparation containing thiamine. Pain and muscle tenderness improve rapidly but improvement in motor and sensory function is very slow.

Drugs

There are few classes of drug that have not been incriminated as a cause of polyneuritis but with the great majority this is so uncommon as not to interfere with their use in practice. Examples are sulphonamides, anticonvulsants, tricyclic antidepressants and non-steroid anti-inflammatory drugs. Some drugs are more neurotoxic, for example, thalidomide, nitrofarantoin and perhexilene and have been abandoned or used only with due care. Most drugs cause axonal degeneration rather than demyelination and recovery is often very slow when the drug is withdrawn.

A few drugs are retained because essential, vincristine for leukaemia and isoniazide for tuberculosis. INH commonly induces a largely sensory neuropathy. In part it is a function of dosage, though it affects less than half even of those treated with massive amounts of the drug. This is a pyridine derivative related to pyridoxine, and the concurrent administration of this vitamin protects against the development of the neurological complication.

The particular interest of isoniazid neuropathy is that it has been shown to develop only in subjects in whom metabolic inactivation of the drug is slow. The condition resembles the polyneuritis that sometimes complicates the treatment with nitrofurantoin of patients with impaired renal function due to pyelonephritis, in that it depends on a high circulating level of the drug. But in the case of isoniazid the high circulating level is due to the constitutional quirk of slow inactivation; fast inactivation shows a dominant heredity. It may be that other forms of idiosyncrasy and familial susceptibility have a similar explanation.

OTHER FORMS OF POLYNEURITIS

Heavy metals

Lead neuropathy is now a rarity because of improved industrial hygiene, and is more often seen in accumulator-breakers than in lead-workers, painters or plumbers. Lead damages especially the motor fibres of the nerves supplying muscles that are repeatedly and continually contracting. The lesion is entirely motor and comprises demyelination, though anterior horn cell degeneration in the spinal cord has also been described. Bilateral wrist drop and finger drop is characteristic. The shoulder girdles may be involved, sometimes with extensive wasting, but the lower limbs usually escape. Constipation, nausea, abdominal pain and anaemia usually accompany lead neuritis, but the typical severe colic is less common. Treatment comprises withdrawal from exposure and attempts to speed the excretion of lead by the use of chelating agents such as penicillamine. In contrast, arsenic and gold produce typical multiple symmetrical neuropathy, the former accompanied by hyperkeratosis of the soles and increased pigmentation.

Industrial hazards

Although a great many potentially harmful compounds are used in industry the risk to workers of developing polyneuritis is not great. The organophosphorus compound triorthocresyl phosphate has caused outbreaks of severe neuropathy when it has contaminated food. Organic solvents must be regarded with suspicion but there have been few reports of neuropathy.

NUTRITIONAL CAUSES

In the experimental animal polyneuritis can be produced by pure deficiencies of thiamine, nicotinamide or pantothenic acid in the presence of an adequate carbohydrate intake. The discovery that tropical beriberi was due to thiamine deficiency was important in the prevention and treatment of this condition but did not, as was hoped, throw much light on the pathogenesis of other forms of neuropathy. It is still common practice to prescribe compound vitamin pills for 'neuritis' of any kind, but this is entirely without foundation. Thiamine-deficient neuropathy from nutritional causes is now rare even where malnutrition is prevalent.

Subacute combined degeneration of the spinal cord due to vitamin B_{12} deficiency is preceded by symptoms and signs of peripheral neuropathy. Paraesthesiae, sometimes extremely unpleasant, nearly always begin in the feet but occasionally in the hands. At this stage typical signs of polyneuritis may be found: distal sensory loss and absent ankle jerks, but little evidence of weakness. As the lateral columns of the spinal cord become involved the plantar reflexes become extensor and the knee jerks exaggerated, but the ankle jerks usually remain absent.

INTRINSIC DISEASE

Diabetes

The classification of diabetic peripheral neuritis is difficult because it almost certainly comprises several different conditions. It is common in poorly controlled though not necessarily severe diabetes of long duration. Even in the absence of relevant symptoms, many elderly diabetics show loss of ankle jerks and peripheral impairment of vibration sense as well as diminished electrical conductivity in the peripheral nerves.

One rather uncommon form of diabetic neuritis is mononeuritis multiplex due to the atherosclerosis and the endarteritis of smaller vessels that often accompany the metabolic disorder. This may for example present as a painful unilateral or bilateral sciatica. The same type of ischaemic lesion is also responsible for the usually painless double vision that often arises from a motor cranial nerve lesion in the elderly diabetic.

Much the commonest variety of diabetic neuropathy is a painful, symmetrical, mostly sensory neuropathy affecting particularly the lower limbs. Burning and shooting pains are particularly conspicuous at night, motor weakness slight or even undetectable. In one variant of this condition profound loss of vibration and postural sense accompanied by impairment of the pupillary reaction to light closely simulates tabes dorsalis. The pupillary changes indicate a peculiar tendency of diabetic neuropathy to affect the peripheral autonomic nervous system, sometimes with troublesome intermittent and often nocturnal diarrhoea, postural hypotension, impotence, and trophic changes in the form of penetrating ulcers and Charcot-type arthropathies in the lower limbs.

In a minority of cases asymmetrical painful weakness of the lower limbs (so-called diabetic amyotrophy) may be accompanied by an increased protein content in the spinal fluid. The quadriceps muscles are often affected and the primary lesion is in the spinal nerve roots. An occasional extensor plantar response is probably due to coincident cervical spondylosis.

Many clinical cases of diabetic neuropathy include components of several of the above clinicopathological syndromes. Since polyneuritis complicates neglected diabetes it is rarely a presenting symptom of the disorder, nor are minor changes of glucose tolerance likely to have any causal significance in cases of severe chronic polyneuritis.

The intrinsic cause of diabetic polyneuritis is unknown. Atherosclerosis is not invariable, and evidence of vitamin deficiency is as unconvincing as evidence of any benefit from vitamin treatment. The apparent response of many cases to improved diabetic control and the occasional appearance of acute polyneuritis during the stabilization of a diabetic patient (so-called 'insulin neuritis') support some specific disturbance of nerve cell metabolism, but its nature remains obscure.

Carcinoma

Asymptomatic cancer is today one of the commonest causes of subacute polyneuritis. Although occasional cases arise as a complication of pelvic or even gastrointestinal carcinoma, there can be little doubt that the wider recognition of carcinomatous polyneuropathy reflects a genuinely increased incidence due to the current epidemic of bronchogenic cancer. This is the cause of most cases encountered at the present time, and it is important to appreciate that the neurological complication may antedate the symptomatic onset or radiological signs of neoplasm by months or even years.

Polyneuritis is one facet of a complex of non-metastatic neurological complications of cancer which affect every level of the nervous system from cerebral cortex to skeletal muscle, and that may be evident in intermittent confusional and atypically depressive states; cerebellar ataxia; a group of polyneuritic syndromes; and muscle disorders that may amount to polymyositis or dermatomyositis and may also simulate myasthenia gravis. These syndromes often occur in mixed forms. Their nature is uncertain except that they are unconnected with dissemination of the growth and can probably best be regarded as toxic in the broad sense. The finding of complement-fixing antibodies to brain tissue in some cases of carcinomatous sensory neuropathy suggests that autoimmune mechanisms may be involved. Improvement sometimes follows surgical removal of the growth, but the neurological signs often wax and wane spontaneously quite independently of its progression.

The neurological syndrome most pathognomonic of cancer is a rare exclusively sensory neuropathy characterized by peripheral pains and paraesthesiae followed by a progressive loss of all forms of sensation ultimately involving the face and trunk as well as the limbs. The pathological basis of this uniquely selective condition is a fall-out of sensory neurones in the posterior root ganglia, followed by secondary degeneration of the peripheral nerves and the posterior columns of the spinal cord: involvement of the sensory nuclei of the cranial nerves usually ensues. This syndrome sometimes responds in some degree to steroid treatment.

Much commoner is a very chronic non-specific sensorimotor polyneuritis beginning with ill-defined pains in the lower limbs, frequently remittent, and sometimes followed or accompanied by myopathy, slowly progressive dementia, and diffuse degeneration of the cerebellum characterized by increasing ataxia and dysarthria.

It is clear that cancer and especially bronchogenic neoplasm must be suspected in any atypical neurological disorder of middle or later life. In many cases the erythrocyte sedimentation rate (ESR) and X-rays remain normal at successive examinations. Sometimes sputum cytology gives an earlier clue, but it may be as long as four years before the diagnosis can be clinched. Response to steroid or other therapy is unimpressive.

Collagen-vascular diseases

Polyarteritis nodosa presents the classical form of polyneuritis due to multiple ischaemic lesions of nerve trunks secondary to disease of the nutrient arteries. The condition is characteristically a painful *mononeuritis multiplex*, with successive and often asymmetrical involvement of nerve trunks. In a typical case the right ulnar and the left sciatic nerves might be successively involved. Sometimes this condition develops into a generalized symmetrical sensorimotor polyneuritis, and indeed sometimes it takes this form from the outset. Whether this less specific variety of polyneuritis as it occurs in polyarteritis nodosa is also due to multiple ischaemic lesions or to some undefined toxic cause is uncertain, but the frequency with which microscopic vascular lesions are found in the peripheral nerves in this disease lends some support to the former view. Mononeuritis multiplex is so characteristic of polyarteritis nodosa that if leprosy and diabetes are excluded this is almost the only cause. The polyneuritis usually develops in the context of a subacute febrile illness with polymorphonuclear leucocytosis and usually myalgic and arthralgic symptoms and abdominal pain. It may present a picture resembling acute or subacute rheumatic fever complicated by visceral and neurological involvement, or as pyrexia of unknown origin with vascular hypertension of renal origin in a young patient. Polyarteritis is one of several disorders such as Addison's disease, myxoedema, and porphyria that is easily diagnosed if its existence is remembered. Like the other syndromes of polyarteritis, polyneuritis often shows some response to treatment with steroid hormones though the illness remains serious and often fatal.

The non-specific mild sensorimotor polyneuritis that occasionally complicates systemic lupus erythematosus is probably of a similar nature, and the same consideration applies to the more severe subacute polyneuritis that sometimes complicates advanced rheumatoid arthritis.

Amyloidosis

Systemic generalized 'primary' amyloidosis must be distinguished from the traditional amyloid disease that complicates protracted sepsis. It occurs both in a familial form and in association with multiple myelomatosis, and causes a very chronic painful sensorimotor polyneuropathy with thickening of the palpable nerves. Diagnosis depends on microscopic examination of the sural or some other accessible peripheral nerve, by which the irregular deposits of glycoprotein amyloid material in and around the affected nerves can easily be distinguished from the lamellar onion-like thickening seen in the familial hypertrophic polyneuritis mentioned above. Autonomic neuropathy is often severe and the presentation may be with postural fainting due to hypotension.

Metabolic diseases

The prolonged survival of many patients with chronic renal failure now achieved with modern treatment has revealed severe polyneuritis as part of the syndrome of uraemia. The precise metabolic defect responsible has not been identified but appears to be related to poor renal function rather than to any effect of dialysis. To a lesser extent polyneuritis is also being recognized as a complication of chronic hepatic failure.

Porphyria

Acute intermittent porphyria is an inborn metabolic error inherited as a dominant trait, symptomatically commoner in the female and usually beginning in early adult life. The severity of the condition is highly variable, and its commonest clinical manifestations are intense abdominal pain (with flaccid abdomen), leucocytosis, low fever, constipation, tachycardia, and transient hypertension. Such episodes are intermittent, as are the very miscellaneous psychiatric disturbances that often precede recognition of the true nature of the disorder; these may be of 'hysterical' type, but are sometimes toxic-confusional, manic, or even convulsive. Needless to say such a history may lead to the abdominal episodes being wrongly regarded as psychogenic, and most of these patients are initially diagnosed as psychoneurotic. Attacks of acute porphyria are often provoked by barbiturates administered to control the earlier psychiatric symptoms or prior to laparotomy for abdominal pain.

Polyneuritis is often acute and severe, usually though not always accompanying the abdominal episodes. Pathologically it is characterized by both patchy demyelination and anterior horn cell damage: initially it is an acute biochemical lesion in which electrical conductivity may be normal in the presence of severe paralysis—an interesting limitation of electrodiagnosis. Pain in the limbs is followed by a rapidly developing almost exclusive motor polyneuritis which may begin focally but often progresses to profound flaccid quadriplegia, with or without proximal and cranial nerve involvement. Respiratory paralysis is often fatal. Recovery is protracted, but often surprisingly complete in view of the wasting and contractures that may characterize severe cases. There is some tendency to improve with age, and the patients learn to avoid the many drugs (including sulphonamides and oestrogens as well as barbiturates) that are known to precipitate attacks.

The clue to diagnosis is the conversion of the colourless porphobilinogen present in the patient's urine during an attack to a red pigment by Ehrlich aldehyde in HCl, not extractable with chloroform after neutralization.

GENETICALLY DETERMINED NEUROPATHY

Paroneal muscular atrophy and hypertrophic polyneuritis are described in Chapter 16.

Although the nature of the defects involved is entirely speculative it seems very likely that these and similar disorders arise on the basis of some metabolic anomaly. This suspicion is strengthened by a consideration of the recessively inherited Refsum's syndrome of chronic sensori-motor polyneuritis with cerebellar ataxia and retinitis pigmentosa. This is much more than a medical curiosity. The finding of an increased serum content of fatty acid has led to the identification of an abnormal metabolite (phytanic acid) present in striking excess in these patients' tissues. The relation between the biochemical abnormality and the neurological syndrome seems to be consistent. Phytanic acid is largely derived from dietary constituents, and the door has been opened to the possible control of a bizarre genetic abnormality by dietary measures.

THE GUILLAIN-BARRÉ SYNDROME

First described a century ago as Landry's acute ascending paralysis, this condition occurred in epidemic form in the First World War as 'acute infective polyneuritis'. It has also been described as 'polyneuritis cranialis' (because of a tendency to cranial nerve and especially bilateral facial nerve involvement) and more recently 'polyradiculitis', because oedema and subsequent demyelination are especially prominent in the spinal nerve roots. The key to its understanding is probably its frequent relation to antecedent infection, either banal in the form of a sore throat or even a head cold, or more specific as in the case of hepatitis or mononucleosis: it may also follow various inoculations and vaccinations. Although acute infective polyneuritis is often loosely attributed to virus infection there is no direct evidence of this and it is probably an auto-immune reaction to peripheral myelin induced by virus infection. Sometimes persistent infection with cytomegalovirus can be detected during the attack of polyneuritis, but even here the neuropathy is not directly due to infection. In fatal cases the nerve roots contain a heavy lymphocytic infiltration, again suggestive of a disturbance of immune mechanisms.

The syndrome may occur at any age. The onset is frequently with mild tingling of the extremities rapidly followed by advancing weakness of the legs. Pain in the back is often prominent at this stage, particularly in children, and this may obscure the diagnosis. The paralysis reaches its height in about ten days when, in a severe case, there will be profound weakness of all limbs most marked in proximal muscles. Sensory loss is usually difficult to detect but sometimes postural sense is severely affected. Cranial nerves are often involved, particularly the facial nerve, and occasionally bilateral facial palsy is the main feature of the disease. Complications commonly include temporary retention of urine and rarely, a curious finding, papilloedema, unconvincingly attributed to the high cerebrospinal fluid protein.

In all patients there is a risk of respiratory and bulbar paralysis. Respiratory function must be monitored at frequent intervals, the vital capacity being the most useful measurement. This may be difficult because facial palsy may prevent the application of the lips to the mouthpiece but with ingenuity this can be overcome. If the vital capacity falls to one litre preparations should be made for a tracheostomy and assisted respiration.

Investigation will nearly always show that the cerebrospinal protein is raised to around 100 mg/100 ml (1 g l^{-1}) but it is occasionally normal early in the disease. There is no increase in cells. It is usual to do the lumbar puncture but when the diagnosis is obvious it is scarcely necessary.

The prognosis in the Guillain–Barré syndrome is good provided that respiratory function is maintained. Full recovery can be confidently expected in young patients but in those of more advanced age some persistent disability may remain. It has never been adequately decided whether ACTH or corticosteroids improve the prognosis in the sense of speeding recovery. In most patients no dramatic effect is seen and certainly there are strong reasons for not persisting with ineffective and potentially harmful treatment. In occasional patients there is rapid recovery on treatment and relapse if the dose is reduced too quickly, so that there is good reason also for a trial of steroids which should, however, be abandoned if there is no immediate response. Recent reports suggest that both very high doses of steroids and plasmapheresis can lead to rapid recovery. Spontaneous recovery is never rapid and may not be full for six to twelve months. If postural sense is lost this may prove the most obstinate disability. At the height of the illness patients do not believe that recovery is possible and it is not easy to maintain morale.

Relapse or recurrence are rare but both are well recognized.

In a smaller number of cases a less acute syndrome otherwise identical with the Guillain–Barré disorder begins much more insidiously and may recur several times over a period of years. This uncommon condition is sometimes strikingly responsive to treatment with steroids, but the response is unpredictable.

Post-diphtheritic polyneuritis is probably a variant of the Guillain–Barré syndrome, and where the initiating infection has escaped notice an onset with palatal weakness causing nasal speech and regurgitation, together with paralysis of accommodation, may reveal the cause of the polyneuritis. Again the spinal fluid protein is raised without any increase in its cell content. In this instance the risk of myocarditis is added to the potential danger of respiratory paralysis. However, the large majority of patients recover uneventfully.

NEURALGIC AMYOTROPHY

This condition is relatively common and gives rise to diagnostic difficulty. Preceding infection is uncommon but in a significant proportion of patients the onset is while they are in hospital with some unrelated condition. An identical condition can follow injection of foreign serum and an allergic cause must be probable. Pain in both shoulders develops acutely and is extremely severe for up to a week. Weakness probably develops simultaneously and affects the muscles of the shoulder girdle in a scattered and asymmetrical way so that, for example, the spinati and deltoid are paralysed on one side and the deltoid on the other. Sensory symptoms apart from pain are insignificant but in the acute stages it is usually possible to detect an area of cutaneous sensory loss over one deltoid. The affected muscles waste rapidly—the amyotrophy of the title—but the prognosis for full recovery is relatively good although often delayed for up to two years. It is not known whether steroids at the onset would avert paralysis.

Sudden isolated unilateral paralysis of the serratus anterior causing winging of the scapula is probably a related condition but is painless (Fig. 8, p. 152). In some families a tendency to recurrent neuralgic amyotrophy may be transmitted by dominant inheritance.

POLYNEURITIS OF UNKNOWN CAUSE

In spite of a formidable list of known causes in the majority of cases of chronic polyneuritis no cause can be found on intensive investigation or even sometimes at autopsy. There is no particular reason why such a cause should be present; we do not, for example, look for a cause of rheumatoid arthritis but accept the diagnosis. Some of these cryptogenic forms of polyneuritis are found many years after the onset to be associated with, and presumably due to, myeloma or some less obviously pathological disturbance of the serum proteins. The clinical picture is naturally varied but in general weakness is mainly distal and sensory loss is present but is not profound. Cranial nerves are seldom affected. Hypertrophy of the nerves may become obvious, particularly if the condition has remitted and relapsed. The natural course is unpredictable but in many there are marked fluctuations or even complete remission, sometimes from a state of grave paralysis. The response to steroids, usually given in desperation, is also unpredictable. Some patients respond and do not relapse when treatment is stopped but others become steroid dependent, requiring ever larger doses to maintain even partial remission. However, chronic polyneuritis of unknown cause progressive to a fatal outcome is rare.

RESTLESS LEGS

The strange condition variously known as restless legs or Ekbom's syndrome is sometimes mistaken for polyneuritis, although there are no abnormal physical signs unless the syndrome accompanies organic disease, in particular multiple sclerosis. The essential symptom is of an intensely distressing creeping sensation or pain in the legs and occasionally in the arms, occurring only at rest and relieved by exercise. In some patients there is also involuntary jerking of the legs. In the daytime this is tolerable, though prolonged sitting may be impossible, but in bed at night sleep may be almost entirely prevented. The sensation can be momentarily interrupted by moving the legs but can be stopped only by walking. Mild intermittent symptoms of this kind are common, but the severe form is incapacitating, since a mere two hours of drugged sleep are an inadequate basis for an active life. This is a well-recognized symptom of iron deficiency and when this is present, even mildly, the symptoms can be cured by oral iron therapy. In other patients iron is ineffective and the condition difficult to treat. Clonazepam 0.5 mg an hour before retiring to bed often affords complete relief and has recently proved unexpectedly successful in some obstinate cases.

Further reading

Ashbury A.K., Arnason B.G. & Adams R.D. (1969) The inflammatory lesion in idiopathic polyneuritis. *Medicine (Baltimore)* **48**, 173.

Becker D.M. & Kramer S. (1977) The neurological manifestations of porphyria. *Medicine (Baltimore)* **56**, 411.

Bradley W.G. (1974) *Disorders of Peripheral Nerves*. Blackwell Scientific Publications, Oxford.

Dyck P.J., Thomas P.K. & Lambert E.H. (eds.) (1975) *Peripheral Neuropathy*. Saunders, Philadelphia.

Stein J.A. & Tschady D.P. (1970) Acute intermittent porphyria. *Medicine (Baltimore)* **49**, 1.

Tsairis P., Dyck P.J. & Malder D.W. (1972) Natural history of brachial plexus neuropathy. *Archs Neurol.* **27**, 109.

Victor M., Adams R.D. & Collins G.H. (1971) *The Wernicke–Korsakoff Syndrome*. F.A. Davis, Philadelphia.

CHAPTER 7
Diseases of Voluntary Muscle

Skeletal muscle forms about 45% of the weight of an adult male, but until recently it has been remarkably neglected as a tissue, particularly by pathologists, whose routine post-mortem sections seldom include even a single specimen of muscle. These deficiencies are now being made good, and both primary muscle disease and muscle disorders secondary to systemic diseases are recognized with increasing frequency.

PROGRESSIVE MUSCULAR DYSTROPHY

This is a group of uncommon genetically determined diseases in which the primary fault has long been thought to be in the contractile tissue of voluntary muscle. While histochemistry and the electron microscope have revealed the structure and function of the muscle fibre to an almost molecular level, the defect in muscular dystrophy has proved elusive and there is increasing evidence that part at least of the pathology may not be primarily muscular but involve the nerve supply. Although there are many forms distinguishable by age of onset, mode of inheritance, distribution of muscle involvement and rate of progress, the identifiable lesion in all is similar. In an actively affected muscle there is great variation in size of fibres. Some are abnormally large and others small, and they may show necrotic changes. The sarcolemmal nuclei may be centrally placed in the large fibres or apparently present in excessive numbers when atrophy is pronounced. Phagocytosis of necrotic fibres is seen and there is some evidence of regeneration. The amount of fat between the fibres is increased and in the final state the contractile tissue is entirely replaced by fat and fibrosis (Fig. 9, p. 152).

The clinical description of muscular dystrophy is confused by the existence of small groups, members sometimes of only a single family, that defy classification. The broad categories are, however, sufficiently distinctive and of these the *Duchenne* type is probably the most stereotyped. This is nearly always inherited by sex-linked recessive transmission, which means that the full clinical syndrome is confined to males.

The symptoms begin before the age of ten and usually at three or four years. Weakness develops first in muscles of the trunk and proximal segments of the limbs. The gait becomes waddling and running impossible because of lack of control over the pelvic girdle, and the lumbar lordosis is increased. Extension at the hips and knees, as in standing up, is affected early and the characteristic mode of standing known as 'climbing up the legs' results. To assist in extension at both these joints and to support the weight of the trunk when assuming the upright posture the hands are placed on the knees, pushing them backwards at the same time as raising the trunk. The spinati and upper limbs are also soon affected, but the deltoid is often relatively spared.

The curious condition of pseudo-hypertrophy is often a very early physical sign and is seen most commonly in the calf muscles. The affected muscles are enlarged and may be weak. In such cases the contrast between the bulk of the calves and their profound weakness is immediately impressive.

The disease is progressive and eventually severe paralysis leads to helpless disability, although the distal muscles often remain relatively strong. Acute infections and especially confinement to bed lead to rapid deterioration, and deformities due to fibrous contracture in the destroyed muscles are common. The great majority of these boys do not reach adult life, some dying from cardiomyopathy.

The transmitted biochemical abnormality underlying the disease has not been elucidated but there are recent indications of a generalized defect of cell membranes. The dying muscle fibres liberate certain enzymes into the blood-stream, aldolase and creatine kinase in particular, and in this form of dystrophy where destruction is comparatively rapid the serum levels are greatly increased in the early stages of the disease. Diagnosis can be made at birth by examination of blood from the umbilical cord and indeed the highest levels are found at about the age of 12 months, in the pre-clinical phase of the disease. The electromyogram shows features characteristic of any disease in which muscle fibres are primarily affected. There is no electrical activity at rest and the number of motor units recorded during voluntary activity is not reduced, but the amplitude and duration of the action potentials are much diminished. This is clearly because each unit contains fewer contractile fibres, and when the changes are well developed the contrast with the effects of denervation (Chapter 5) is unmistakable. Treatment is wholly ineffective. From time to time claims are made that irrational treatments increase muscle power, even if they do not actually cure the disease. To disprove such claims has involved much work and the disappointing of falsely raised hopes.

Known carriers of this disease are women with a positive family history who have had an affected son. Many of these show minor electromyographic abnormalities and rather more than 50% can be recognized by quantitative serum enzyme (creatine kinase) estimation. Occasionally there are clinical signs such as slight weakness or unduly bulky calf muscles. The application of these tests to potential carriers—young girls with affected brothers—is clearly important and it is the doctor's social responsibility to inform the family about the risks involved in having children. There is a one-in-four chance that any pregnancy will result either in a carrier or an affected child.

The prognosis in other forms of muscular dystrophy is rather better, since although these are all progressive diseases for which there is no effective treatment, and all of which often lead to severe disability, their course is much more protracted. It is usual to recognize a *limb-girdle* type beginning a decade or more later than the Duchenne form and usually transmitted by autosomal recessive inheritance, both sexes therefore being affected. The weakness and wasting are usually closely confined to the proximal muscles of the limbs and trunk. Life expectancy is reduced as disability eventually becomes severe, but useful mobility may be retained for many years. Because this is a less acute process the serum enzyme levels may not be raised. The intensive current investigation of muscle pathology has clearly revealed that many cases which would formerly have been diagnosed as suffering from limb-girdle dystrophy are in fact instances of spinal muscular atrophy (Chapter 16), and this finding may in part account for the favourable reputation of the muscle disease in the matter of prognosis.

Facio-scapulo-humeral dystrophy may not be easy to distinguish from the limb-girdle type since both the age of onset and the distribution of the weakness are similar. However, as the name implies the facial muscles are also affected and the detection of even slight facial weakness is of considerable prognostic importance. There is much variation, but some patients survive to old age with little disability. Inheritance is almost always dominant.

The distal limb muscles can be involved in any form of dystrophy; for example, foot drop is common in some families with the facio-scapulo-humeral form. Onset with weakness and wasting confined to the distal muscles is extremely rare, although a distal form described by Gowers is part of our traditional heritage from the era when accurate clinical observation was virtually the only instrument of diagnosis. This form is relatively common in Sweden, very uncommon in Britain.

The curious and still controversial condition known as *ocular muscular dystrophy* presents with ptosis and weakness of external eye movements, but diplopia is rare since the muscles are symmetrically involved to a precisely similar degree on the two sides. Argument continues as to how far this is primarily a muscle disease and how far a system degeneration of the nervous system; the specificity of the myopathic changes described in the extra-ocular muscles is dubious. The difficult differential diagnosis will be discussed below. What is clear is that in some such cases weakness extends to the limb muscles, particularly those of the limb girdle, and that there is a further small group in which the pharynx is involved, causing dysphagia.

The commonest form of muscular dystrophy encountered in adult patients is *dystrophia myotonica*. This is transmitted by dominant inheritance and is a complex disorder by no means confined to skeletal muscle. The dystrophic element consists of diffuse weakness and wasting of the limbs and also particularly the sterno-mastoid and facial muscles. Ptosis is almost invariable and ocular palsies may also occur. The weakness may present at any age from infancy to the seventh decade, but most commonly in early adult life. It is only slowly progressive and severe disability may not occur for many years.

The curious phenomenon of myotonia consists of a failure of rapid muscular relaxation after voluntary contraction. This is nearly always best demonstrated by asking the patient to open his hand to command after gripping the examiner's, and indeed this is often the only evidence of myotonia. If an affected muscle is struck a sharp blow with a tendon hammer a local contraction is excited, producing a lump or a dimple that subsides over a period of several seconds. Myotonia is nearly always worse in cold weather but can usually be abolished by repeated contraction of the affected muscles. It is a much more striking feature in *myotonia congenita* or Thomsen's disease. This is exceedingly rare and is also transmitted by dominant inheritance in nearly all affected families. Myotonia is the most prominent and often the only symptom. It affects the entire musculature to varying degrees. Opening the eyes may be difficult after firm closure, the smile is oddly lingering, and an injudicious bite may be followed by difficulty in opening the mouth. The patients are often athletic but can excel only in long-distance races in which they have time to 'work off' the myotonia.

When it is very troublesome myotonia can be partially controlled by quinine sulphate 300 mg t.d.s. or procaine amide 250 mg q.i.d. and also in acute exacerbations by corticotrophin. Phenytoin is probably more effective than any of these.

Some have thought that Thomsen's disease is no more than a variant of the dystrophic form, but there is a striking difference between the appearances of the two groups of patients. The fully developed dystrophic syndrome includes frontal baldness and testicular atrophy in the male, cataract, and an often extremely difficult personality leading eventually to dementia. In some families there is a history of cataracts or frontal baldness for several generations before muscular disease becomes evident. Incidental findings are a small bridged pituitary fossa on the skull X-ray, and cardiac arrhythmias. Many patients ultimately succumb to cardiomyopathy, others to respiratory paralysis. The thin face, drooping eyelids, wasted neck and premature baldness present an unmistakable appearance, recognizable as the patient enters the room. Diagnosis may however be difficult in the young child, when hypotonia may be the only sign. Dysphagia is often prominent in the terminal stages and may cause death from the inhalation of food.

POLYMYOSITIS

This is a rare disease in which weakness is also due to muscle fibre degeneration, but it lacks any genetic element and as its name implies there is some evidence of an inflammatory reaction. It occurs at any age, and in about half of those affected is associated either with carcinoma or with one or other of the collagen disorders. The relation to cancer is especially prominent in male patients over the age of fifty. Beyond this the cause is not known. The clinical features are extremely diverse, varying from an acute illness with severe systemic symptoms to a mild indolent weakness of selected muscle groups. In the more acute forms weakness is widespread, often involving respiratory and bulbar muscles, and is accompanied by pain and tenderness. Oedema of the face and extremities and a violaceous erythema are common, and this association has long been recognized as acute dermatomyositis. There may be a high fever and prostration with a raised erythrocyte sedimentation rate but without any characteristic change in the white blood count. There is an immediate threat to life from respiratory paralysis or from involvement of cardiac muscle. The diagnosis should present no difficulty, the only possible confusion being with acute polyneuritis, or with infestation with *Trichina spiralis* where this is endemic, since it can also produce diffuse muscle pain and weakness with oedema of the face.

In more chronic forms involvement of the skin is less common. When it is present it takes the form of scleroderma of the face and limbs, with shiny skin adherent to underlying structures. Raynaud's phenomenon, polyarthritis and other evidence of collagen disease may be present. Perhaps the most characteristic clinical presentation of the chronic form is that of slowly progressive weakness of the neck muscles and the proximal muscles of the limbs, without symptoms of systemic disease.

Weakness is seldom completely symmetrical and is often unduly severe in comparison with the relatively slight degree of wasting. Muscular pain may sometimes point to an inflammatory cause, but the possibilities of diagnostic confusion with limb girdle muscular dystrophy and with other forms of neuromuscular disease are obvious.

A positive diagnosis can nearly always be established by the combined use of muscle biopsy, serum creatine kinase estimation, and electromyography. The disease process is commonly patchy and the biopsy may miss an affected area. Another source of error arises from the examination of a fragment of muscle into which an EMG needle has been thrust a few days earlier, inevitably producing an inflammatory reaction. This difficulty can be simply averted by undertaking routine electromyography on one side of the body and biopsy on the other. A positive biopsy shows necrosis of muscle fibres and infiltration with mononuclear inflammatory cells, characteristically grouped round small blood vessels. Muscle regeneration can also be seen. The serum creatine kinase can be normal in the more indolent forms but even here it is often raised. The EMG shows an unexpected finding. In addition to the reduction in amplitude and duration of the action potentials on voluntary action that is characteristic of primary muscle disease, fibrillation and positive sharp waves ('sawtooth' potentials) are also present. In other contexts this is taken as indisputable evidence of denervation, and indeed in polymyositis it is possible that the lesion involves the terminal motor neurones.

Although complete recovery has occurred in a few untreated cases the prognosis in polymyositis is generally bad. Remission can be induced in about half of all cases by full doses of corticosteroids, and a favourable response is more easily obtained in the acute and subacute forms. Relapse is unfortunately common and complete cure can seldom be claimed. Even if improvement in strength is slight, relief of pain may justify prolonged treatment. An initial response is obtained in polymyositis associated with carcinoma but seldom lasts for more than a few months. Treatment with the immunosuppressant drug azathioprine may occasionally be successful when steroids have failed.

In polyarteritis nodosa arterial lesions can often be seen in muscle biopsies, but weakness due to inflammatory change in the muscle is less common and the picture is often complicated by coincidental polyneuritis. In sarcoidosis muscle biopsy is positive in about 50% of cases, but in spite of the extraordinary profusion of sarcoid nodules there is usually no effect on function. Occasionally chronic progressive proximal weakness occurs, though the biopsy may show little obvious loss of muscle fibres. The condition responds unpredictably to corticosteroids.

DISEASES OF VOLUNTARY MUSCLE

Polymyalgia rheumatica is a disease of the elderly and middle-aged and is closely related to cranial or giant-cell arteritis. Severe pain around the shoulders and neck restricts movement of the arms but probably there is no real weakness. Certainly muscle biopsy and EMG are normal. The erythrocyte sedimentation rate is grossly raised, and even in the complete absence of headache biopsy of a temporal artery may show arteritis. The cause of the muscular symptoms remains obscure but they respond immediately to an initial dose of 60 mg of prednisolone a day, which can be gradually reduced to a maintenance level of 10 to 15 mg daily.

MYASTHENIA GRAVIS

The cardinal symptom of this uncommon but important disease is excessive muscular fatigue and weakness on sustained or repeated contraction, with recovery at rest. It may occur at any age but the onset is most commonly in the third decade and women are more frequently affected. The mode of onset may be protracted, rapid or even sudden, but although there is much variation certain patterns can be distinguished.

The muscles supplied by the cranial nerves are usually those first affected so that diplopia, ptosis, weakness of the voice, and difficulty in chewing, swallowing and holding up the head are characteristic early symptoms. Fatiguability is often evident from the history in that diplopia is only present at the end of the day, only the first few mouthfuls of a meal can be masticated, or the voice is lost only after prolonged gossiping. Weakness of ocular muscles alone or combined with slight facial weakness is common.

Muscles of the limbs and trunk may be involved at the same time or later, but in one form of the disease these muscles may be involved alone for many months or years. In most patients diagnosis is long delayed, usually until there is persistent weakness of some muscle groups, irrespective of fatigue. Muscular wasting is exceptional. The severity of the disease varies greatly. At one extreme it presents with mild intermittent unilateral ptosis and at the other with incapacitating generalized muscular weakness threatening life from bulbar and respiratory paralysis.

Weakness is due to failure of normal neuro-muscular transmission. Acetylcholine liberated by the terminal motor axons normally excites the receptor mechanisms of the muscle end-plates, and is then rapidly destroyed by cholinesterase. Recent evidence indicates that the defect in myasthenia gravis is due to blocking of the acetylcholine receptor sites on the muscle fibres by antibodies that can also be detected in the serum. Myasthenia is therefore an autoimmune reaction to acetylcholine receptor sites. The classical effect of fatigue is due to the loss of the normal reserve capacity of the muscle resulting from blocked receptor sites. This conclusion is in agreement with many facets of the disease that have suggested an autoimmune cause. There is a definite association with other such diseases, in particular rheumatoid arthritis, disseminated lupus and thyroid disease. The muscles contain collections of lymphocytes, presumably immunologically active. The association of myasthenia with thymoma and with active germinal centres in the non-tumorous thymus was known before the role of the thymus in immunity was recognized. Opinion has changed so frequently that it is unlikely that the present hypothesis will go long unchallenged.

Clinical diagnosis can be difficult and there are several sources of confusion. A complaint of 'feeling tired all the time' is in no way suggestive of myasthenia, but of depression or some grave systemic disease. Purely ocular weakness may be difficult or impossible to distinguish from ocular muscular dystrophy, but this is seldom of much clinical importance. Myasthenic bulbar palsy may be mistaken for motor neurone disease. Misdiagnosis is commonest when weakness is confined to the limbs and trunk and this presentation is often regarded as hysterical. Fortunately the diagnosis can be confirmed in most cases by the intravenous injection of the rapidly acting anticholinesterase edrophonium chloride (Tensilon). One milligram should be given, followed by the remainder of the 10 mg ampoule if there is no untoward reaction after a minute. In myasthenia the effect is astounding. Persistent weakness vanishes within a minute or two, and it is then obvious that many muscles not thought to be involved have also responded, shown particularly by the patient's vivid smile at the almost instantaneous cure. Diplopia may not be fully corrected and especially in very long-standing myasthenia other muscles may also be unresponsive, but there is seldom much doubt about a positive test, except occasionally in minimal cases. The effect wears off in a few minutes and the patient should be warned to expect this. In a non-myasthenic subject edrophonium produces brief flushing of the face and fasciculation of facial muscles.

For many years the standard symptomatic treatment has been with anticholinesterase drugs by mouth in carefully supervised dosage. Neostigmine and pyridostigmine are the only two agents in common use, 15 mg of the former being equivalent to 60 mg of the latter. Neostigmine acts more quickly but its effect is also less prolonged. It is sometimes difficult to parallel the effect of edrophonium by oral therapy, but most patients gain useful benefit and some are almost relieved of symptoms on 60 mg or more of pyridostigmine every three to four hours when awake. In severe cases a subcutaneous injection of 1 mg of neostigmine may be necessary before meals to allow mastication and swallowing. Abdominal discomfort and colic may prove limiting factors in dosage but can usually be controlled by 0.5 mg of atropine thrice daily.

While many myasthenics can be maintained in reasonable health for many years by these measures and some even go into complete remission, others are less fortunate. Bulbar palsy, which is particularly common in the presence of a thymoma, often responds poorly to treatment. Following infections, undue exertion, unwise sedation or for no apparent reason a myasthenic crisis may occur. Profound generalized weakness is accompanied by respiratory paralysis requiring assisted respiration. If this is efficiently maintained there is no immediate danger and treatment with intramuscular neostigmine can be judiciously pursued. The utmost skill and experience are needed to distinguish this emergency from the equally grave cholinergic crisis due to overdosage with anticholinsterase drugs, for this also causes respiratory paralysis from the neuromuscular blocking effect of excess acetylcholine. Sweating, bradycardia and constriction of the pupil are important confirmatory signs. If doubt exists edrophonium may be used to make the distinction between the two forms of crisis, but no more than 2 mg should be injected and assisted respiration should be immediately available: in cholinergic crisis this minute dose may cause immediate further deterioration or even apnoea. Treatment of the cholinergic crisis otherwise consists of 2 mg of atropine by intravenous injection every hour until the pupil dilates and the mouth is dry, as it is important to counteract possible cardiac complications. The usual causes of such a crisis are over-enthusiastic treatment in a vain attempt to produce complete reversal of symptoms, or the unwise prescription of barbiturates.

The difficulties and dangers of anticholinesterase treatment have prompted the search for more effective means. Almost as soon as steroids were available their effect was naturally tried on this mysterious disease. The effect was alarming; most patients became much worse. It is only recently that further attempts at steroid treatment have been made and, if the initial deterioration can be overcome, the results are often remarkable. The patient must be in hospital because of the possible adverse effect. Different regimes have been advocated but high dose, 100 mg, alternate day treatment will induce remission in many patients. Further management cannot be stereotyped but the aim is to stop anticholinesterase treatment and then, if all remains well, to attempt to reduce and eventually stop the steroids. It is not yet known how successful this will prove.

The surgical treatment of myasthenia gravis was initially based on its association with tumours of the thymus, and has subsequently gained an insubstantial theoretical justification from the link between the thymus and immune reactions. Removal of a thymoma was found to be hazardous but was undoubtedly sometimes followed by remission, and this led to the removal of the macroscopically normal gland. In young women with generalized myasthenia who have not had the disease for more than three years, the chances of a substantial remission are undoubtedly increased by thymectomy, but a beneficial result can never be guaranteed. The operation should not be confined to this group of patients and should be considered in any disabled myasthenic whose symptoms cannot be effectively controlled by drugs. It is never indicated when weakness is confined to the ocular muscles. The operation is within the scope of any thoracic surgeon, but in the post-operative stage the balance between myasthenic and cholinergic crisis swings rapidly and requires the most expert management. The failures may be due to the permanent structural changes that occur in the muscles.

There are still many mysterious aspects of this disease, not least the tendency to sudden death, particularly following an enema. Pregnancy can usually be managed successfully, but severe relapse is common in the puerperium. The presence of some circulating factor, now known to be antibodies to receptor sites, is shown by the myasthenia sometimes present in newborn babies of myasthenic mothers, requiring appropriate treatment but resolving completely within a few days.

THE NON-DYSTROPHIC MYOPATHIES

This vague title covers a variety of quite unrelated conditions in some of which the muscle lesion is apparently primary while in others it is clearly secondary to established disease. The acceptance of 'myopathy' as a complete diagnosis is never justified even though the cause may never be found.

Congenital myopathy and the floppy baby

The syndrome of the weak and floppy baby has many causes. There may be initial difficulty in feeding and the normal activities of early infancy are delayed. The muscles of the limbs, trunk and neck are hypotonic in that there is little resistance to passive movement and the baby can be placed in postures involving an abnormal degree of mobility at the proximal and distal joints. The cause may declare itself as cretinism, primary amentia, progressive spinal muscular atrophy (Chapter 16) or cerebral palsy due to birth injury or congenital malformation. Of the muscular dystrophies only the Duchenne type is sometimes seen at this age. There remains a small group where, although development is delayed, it may progress relatively favourably. *Amyotonia congenita* has long been recognized as a benign condition without discernible pathology in the muscles or elsewhere. It is now often known as benign congenital hypotonia in order to emphasize that these children learn to walk and that many eventually become normal: some diffuse lack of muscular development may persist. More clearly identifiable as myopathies are a group of cases with similar clinical features but distinguishable by the pathognomonic appearance of the muscle biopsy. Central core disease, nemaline myopathy and a number of distinct varieties of morphological changes in the mitochondria are interesting but very rare conditions, in some of which a genetic cause is established. Definitive clinical diagnosis is impossible and since most forms are not progressive it may not be established until adult life.

Metabolic myopathies

The metabolism of glycogen is disordered in a number of rare inborn errors of metabolism. As the energy for muscular contraction is largely derived from the breakdown of stored glycogen to glucose, disorders of muscle function naturally occur in some of these diseases. Deficiency in acid maltase results in one form of glycogen storage disease affecting mainly cardiac and skeletal muscle. Presenting in infancy the prognosis is poor but in more benign forms there may be little disability until adult life. The symptoms in *McArdle's disease*, or muscle phosphorylase deficiency, are distinctive. There is a lifelong tendency to incapacitating muscular pain and weakness on exertion. Glycogen cannot be broken down to lactic acid, so that contraction must depend on circulating glucose. Exercising the hand while the arterial supply is cut off by a sphygmomanometer cuff therefore rapidly produces pain, and the venous blood from the forearm shows no rise in lactic acid. The disease is relatively benign, but in some patients progressive permanent weakness develops, with episodes of myoglobinuria from muscle breakdown. Glucose cannot be utilized but treatment with oral fructose though rational is ineffective.

Periodic paralysis is described in Chapter 14.

Endocrine myopathies

All patients severely affected by *thyrotoxicosis* have weakness of the trunk, neck and proximal limb muscles, but the resulting symptoms are seldom obtrusive and although there may be wasting there are no recognizable pathological changes in the muscles. Less often the disease presents with weakness and wasting of similar distribution but with scant evidence of thyroid disease, and diagnosis can then be difficult, particularly as fasciculation is sometimes present. The acute forms are cured by treatment of the thyrotoxicosis, but in occasional cases where diagnosis is long delayed weakness may be permanent. Myasthenia gravis may accompany thyrotoxicosis and it is sometimes difficult to determine whether the fatiguability that naturally accompanies any form of general weakness is truly myasthenic or not.

Ophthalmoplegia, usually causing diplopia, is one of the more distressing eye signs of Graves' disease. It is usually associated with exophthalmos, bulging of the eyelids, conjunctival oedema and lid retraction. When eye signs occur in the absence of hyperthyroidism, the condition is best referred to as ophthalmic Graves' disease. Eye signs in such patients are commonly asymmetrical or unilateral and may give rise to fears of an orbital tumour, though the presence of a small, firm goitre or a family history of thyroid disease or pernicious anaemia may give a clue to the diagnosis. Thyroid abnormalities can be revealed by triiodothyronine suppression tests in about half of these patients and circulating thyroid antibodies are present in a similar proportion. Ophthalmoplegia first limits upward gaze and only later are lateral movements affected. In some instances limitation of upward gaze may be due not to weakness of the superior rectus but to tethering and adhesions between the inferior rectus and inferior oblique where they cross in the lower part of the orbit. The muscles and other contents of the orbits are initially swollen and oedematous with an increase in fat and a cellular infiltration of lymphocytes and plasma cells; later atrophy and fibrosis supervene. Ophthalmoplegia tends to improve slowly in the majority of patients, and the diplopia can be helped by covering one eye and sometimes by prismatic lenses. When the condition has been static for at least a year muscle recession can be carried out. If the symptoms in the eye become acute with pain and swelling and failure of visual acuity, high doses of prednisone are needed, and if this does not cause rapid improvement it may be necessary to resort to surgical decompression of the orbits.

Muscle weakness is common in *myxoedema,* and aching and stiffness of the muscles may also be a prominent feature. Perceptibly delayed relaxation of the tendon jerks is a characteristic and helpful sign and one that remits rapidly with therapy. Lethargy and general muscular weakness and fatiguability are common in Addison's disease and cortisol deficiency from other causes, responding dramatically to corticosteroid treatment. Proximal limb weakness is an invariable accompaniment of Cushing's syndrome or steroid therapy beyond physiological requirements. Triamcinolone is more likely to cause myopathy than equivalent doses of other steroids. Reduction of circulating steroid levels is followed by improvement of muscle power. Patients with acromegaly not infrequently complain of muscle weakness and fatiguability, and electromyographic and histological studies reveal evidence of a patchy myopathy.

Disorders of calcium metabolism are now being recognized with increasing frequency as a cause of chronic weakness, again mainly of proximal muscles. *Osteomalacia,* such as may occur many years after gastrectomy, in renal disease, or from malnutrition, may be accompanied by a low blood serum calcium, while in hyperparathyroidism the serum calcium is raised. The symptoms and signs of muscle disease are, however, very similar in all such instances and clearly do not depend on the blood levels of calcium, phosphate or phosphatase. Pain is common but not invariable, and the tendon jerks may be unexpectedly brisk. The weakness of osteomalacia, which may be profound, can be reversed provided the dose of vitamin D is adequate.

Toxic myopathy

Alcoholic myopathy is rarely seen in Great Britain. The commonest form is chronic weakness punctuated by exacerbations due to excesses. The antimalarial drug chloroquine, used in the treatment of collagenoses, may cause myopathy as well as retinal degeneration if given for a prolonged period.

Carcinoma

The frequent association of polymyositis with remote carcinoma has already been described, and a closely similar or possibly identical condition sometimes presents as a proximal myopathy without distinctive histological features. Far more characteristic, however, is a syndrome resembling myasthenia gravis. The complaint of fatiguability may be out of proportion to any weakness that can actually be demonstrated after exertion. The carcinoma is nearly always bronchial and since it may be very elusive these patients are sometimes regarded as hysterical. The muscles supplied by the cranial nerves are seldom affected and the complaint is of difficulty in walking or climbing stairs or in holding up the arms. There is no wasting, but the tendon jerks may be lost, whereas they are retained in myasthenia gravis. Improvement following edrophonium is occasionally dramatic, but the more hopeful diagnosis of myasthenia is belied by the paradoxical failure of any worthwhile response to anticholinesterase drugs by mouth. Guanidine 20–50 mg/kg body weight may produce symptomatic relief.

In a high proportion of the diseases described in this chapter the initial symptoms are those of weakness of the pelvic girdle. These normally powerful muscles cannot be adequately tested against the strength of the examiner's arm, and if gross diagnostic errors are to be avoided the ability to perform more exacting tasks must be observed. Rising from the floor or from a low chair, or stepping on to a chair seat all involve supporting the entire weight of the body, the natural function of these muscles. The ability to perform these and other stringent exercises with the speed and ease conformable with the patient's age should always be tested if there is any suspicion of proximal myopathy. Failure to do so may lead to a treatable condition being falsely diagnosed as hysteria for a decade or longer.

Further reading

Brooke M.H. (1977) *A Clinician's View of Neuromuscular Disease*. Williams and Wilkins, Baltimore.
Rowland L.P. (1978) Myasthenia gravis. In *Recent Advances in Clinical Neurology II*, ed. W.B. Matthews and G.H. Glaser. Churchill Livingstone, Edinburgh and London.
Walton J.N. (ed.) (1981) *Disorders of Voluntary Muscle*, 4th edn. Churchill Livingstone, Edinburgh and London.

CHAPTER 8
Head Injury

A rising incidence of head injury is one price of an increasingly mechanized society, and there are few doctors who are not concerned with such cases. The crucial problem of initial assessment is usually in the hands of the casualty officer, while the evaluation of late complications often concerns both the neurologist and the psychiatrist, and their management the general practitioner. The neurosurgeon is involved only in the small minority of patients who require operative interference either for such immediate results of cranial trauma as a compound or depressed skull fracture, or on account of an early complication such as intracranial bleeding.

Head injuries are conventionally divided into the open or closed varieties. The open head injury is the typical war casualty where it results from gunshot or shrapnel wounds, but it is also seen amongst such industrial injuries as those resulting from a heavy tool being dropped from a height on the patient's head, or after the violent trauma of a motor-cycle accident. In open head injury there is compound fracture of the skull where both scalp and skull are breached and there is some exposure of cranial contents. These are severe injuries that come immediately within the scope of the neurosurgeon.

Under peace-time conditions the closed head injury is very much commoner. It accounts for most industrial head injuries and for many deaths sustained in car accidents. In closed head injury there may be scalp lacerations and either linear or depressed fracture of the skull, but there is no compound fracture in the literal sense and indeed there may be no fracture whatever even in fatal cases. This chapter is mainly concerned with this commoner type of injury.

Closed head injury may be of any severity, from a moderate blow on the head with momentary dazing to cerebral damage severe enough to render the patient unconscious for many months. In all except trivial cases there is some impairment of consciousness. The transient loss of consciousness following head injury is known as concussion and is probably directly due to reversible neuronal injury to the reticular substance of the brain stem interrupting afferent inflow and producing a syndrome in many ways similar to normal sleep. The pathological changes following closed head injury vary considerably. In immediately fatal cases it may be difficult to find evidence of any abnormality, but especially where the patient survives for a day or two contusion or laceration may be found both at the site of the injury and at the opposite pole of the brain (contrecoup). The mechanism of the closed head injury is either rapid acceleration of the head, in which the brain floating within it is bruised by the impact against the rigid skull posteriorly and torn from its moorings anteriorly, or more often rapid deceleration of the head, in which case the brain comes forward and sustains bruising at the point of impact and traction injury at the opposite pole. Small subarachnoid haemorrhages are therefore especially common at the contrecoup area, though in very severe cases they may be massive and more generalized. In fatal cases brain stem haemorrhage is a striking feature and is of the same order as that caused by distortion of the brain stem in the presence of severely raised intracranial pressure from cerebral tumour.

Amnesia is a more reliable measure of the severity of a closed head injury than obvious unconsciousness, and retrograde is less significant than post-traumatic amnesia. Retrograde amnesia (RA) is loss of memory for the period preceding the injury. Except sometimes after extremely severe injury, or where exaggeration serves some purpose to the patient, it is rarely prolonged. In the typical running-down case the patient's recollection is clear until a few seconds before actual impact, when he may remember the vehicle approaching a hundred yards away.

The duration of post-traumatic amnesia (PTA) is much more important, and its duration is measured from the time of injury until *the restoration of continuous awareness*. This qualification is important because PTA may be interrupted by 'islets of consciousness', brief periods of recollection as on admission to hospital or the visit of a relative, without sustained restoration of memory.

Measurement of PTA depends on the patient's cooperation, but it is rarely the subject of exaggeration and is more liable to underestimation. The injured footballer may play on automatically after the blow, sometimes becoming more obviously 'unconscious' after a period of minutes, and a patient may be described as conscious in the hospital casualty officer's notes even though he has no subsequent recollection of being examined: more searching interrogation at the time would almost certainly have revealed confusion or disorientation. Another interesting feature of PTA is that it often tends to 'shrink' during the months that follow restoration of clear consciousness, some vague and fragmentary but genuine impressions of the period appearing in the patient's memory.

Other things being equal, the duration of PTA is the most reliable measurement of the severity of brain damage sustained by closed head injury. It is of little value in relation to open injury, where the patient whose brain has been traversed by a high-velocity missile may walk into the casualty clearing station in a state of clear awareness.

In minor concussion, unconsciousness and amnesia last only for minutes, but in more severe closed injuries there may be profound coma, and death may ensue within a few hours or days when compression of the medulla arrests the vital functions of respiration and the heartbeat. If signs of returning consciousness appear within a week there is reasonable prospect of good recovery, but only a few survive when coma persists for many weeks. Improvement from traumatic coma is signalized by response to powerful stimuli, increasing restlessness, and a phase of noisy delirium. At this stage signs of focal damage to the brain may emerge from the general picture of generally flaccid paralysis and depressed reflex activity. Delirium gives place to a variable confusional state, with unsteady gait, vertigo and headache, but in recovering cases improvement is usually progressive even if slow.

Management of the acute head injury comprises management of the unconscious patient with strict attention to maintaining an adequate airway; to avoiding dehydration and the electrolyte disturbances that often complicate prolonged coma; and especially in the early stages constant vigilance for the deepening unconsciousness, pupillary changes or increasing hemiparesis that may betoken cerebral compression by haemorrhage. Restlessness indicates recovery but may become so violent as to require sedation, chlorpromazine 50 mg by injection, repeated as necessary, being the drug of choice. Of necessity many patients with serious head injury must be cared for in centres where CT scanning is not available. Its use has shown an unexpected frequency of intracerebral haemorrhage in such patients and has also confirmed the importance of cerebral swelling as a dangerous and potentially lethal factor. Unfortunately the agents so useful in reducing oedema in relation to brain tumours are far less effective in head injury.

Although the vast majority of closed head injuries are of little importance and leave no disability whatever, the complication of extradural haemorrhage from a torn middle meningeal artery is so serious and so unpredictable that all patients who have sustained such an injury sufficient to cause loss of consciousness should be kept under close medical supervision for 48 hours and all should have a skull X-ray. That this is a sensible medico-legal precaution is less important than that it may show an entirely unsuspected fracture. Admittedly only the depressed fracture requires surgical treatment, but a fissured fracture crossing the middle meningeal groove greatly increases the risk of haemorrhage from the artery that lies within it.

EXTRADURAL HAEMATOMA

The most important early complication of closed head injury is extradural haemorrhage, in which blood usually from a torn middle meningeal artery collects progressively between the skull and dura over a period of hours, causing cerebral compression, raised intracranial pressure and very often death. This is the lesion that accounts for the boxer found dead or comatose in bed the morning after a knock-out, and for the onset of drowsiness in a patient sent home from the casualty department after what appeared to be a minor injury. It is the casualty officer's nightmare.

In the classical case consciousness has been briefly lost and rapidly regained after a fairly minor injury. During the interval the patient may retire to bed and to sleep, no concern being felt until he is found unrousable in the morning. In other cases the classical lucid interval gives place to insidious drowsiness, with constriction and then dilatation of the ipsilateral pupil due to successive irritation and paralysis of the intrinsic fibres of the third cranial nerve, and insidious but progressive hemiparesis on the opposite side from hemisphere compression. If available the CT scan will reliably confirm or exclude the haematoma, but otherwise the diagnosis must be made on clinical grounds. Neglected, a fatal outcome is almost inevitable. The case is so urgent and simple surgical treatment so dramatically effective that operation cannot await transfer to a distant neurosurgical centre and must be in the repertoire of the general surgeon responsible for emergency work. Unless exposure and control of the artery has been delayed recovery is excellent. The time factor is crucial and determines the issue between complete recovery and death.

CHRONIC SUBDURAL HAEMATOMA

Extradural bleeding is the characteristic early and acute complication of closed head injury, subdural bleeding its late and chronic analogue. At one time chronic subdural haematoma was regarded as a disease of mental hospitals and of chronic alcoholics. It is in fact an occasional asymptomatic finding wherever large numbers of elderly patients come to autopsy. The elderly psychotic is more than averagely likely to sustain unobserved head injury, but although the shrunken brain of the dement may render the subdural venous system more vulnerable the pathological relationship is not specific. The important points about subdural haematoma are that the syndrome is insidious, that the patient is usually elderly, and that the head injury may have been no more than a jolt, or even so inconspicuous as to attract no attention whatever (Fig. 25, following p. 152).

Chronic subdural haematoma is an encapsulated collection of venous blood overlying the cerebral cortex, originating in oozing from damaged subdural veins, swelling and shrinking over a period of weeks in relation to osmotic influences. In many cases hemiparesis on the side of the haematoma is caused by pressure of the opposite crus cerebri against the edge of the tentorium, impairing corticospinal tract function above the pyramidal decussation. In others the haematoma is bilateral, lying asymmetrically over the vertex on either side of the sagittal sinus. Its clinical signature is fluctuation both in symptoms and signs. The elderly patient is observed to be intermittently confused or drowsy and it may therefore be particularly difficult to elicit any history of minor trauma. Anxiety felt in the evening may be dissipated by the patient's alert behaviour next morning, a left extensor plantar response may no longer be elicited—or may even be found on the opposite side.

If chronic subdural haematoma is kept in mind it will not be missed. On the other hand it will often be sought in vain when the correct diagnosis is cerebral infarction or glioma with a misleading story of minor injury. The CT scan will not always detect a subdural haematoma, particularly when bilateral and therefore causing no shift of mid-line structures. Often, however, the haematoma is seen as a high density lesion. If not available other investigations may be useful or diagnostic. Sometimes a localized depression of alpha rhythm on the EEG may give a clue, more often an avascular clear area overlying the cortex seen in the antero-posterior projection on angiography, remembering that any hemiparesis may be on the *same* side as the haematoma. Lumbar puncture should not form part of the routine investigation but if performed the spinal fluid may be yellowish, but curiously its pressure is often reduced rather than increased. In emergency or where ancillary investigations involve serious delay, burr-holes will give the answer. The recovery of consciousness that follows immediately on evacuation of a large haematoma is so gratifying that it excuses a considerable number of negative explorations. The outcome is not always so fortunate and coma persists in those patients in whom the brain fails to re-expand following aspiration of the blood.

Acute subdural haematoma is of much less clinical importance. Always associated with serious brain damage, it results from tearing of the major dural sinuses. Even when the subdural blood is evacuated at operation, survival is exceptional.

CHAPTER 8

SEQUELAE OF HEAD INJURY

Apart from the anatomical differentiation between open and closed injury the most significant distinction is between minor and major cases. The minor closed head injury with brief unconsciousness is usually made too much of, causes disproportionate loss of work, and attracts excessive compensation in courts of law. Exactly the opposite is true of severe cases, where subjective complaints are few and may indeed be entirely lacking because of lack of insight, where unfitness for skilled employment may be genuine and prolonged but inapparent, and where expert assessment may be the victim's only protection against the risk of serious injustice in the matter of compensation.

The post-concussional syndrome of headache, postural dizziness, irritability, impotence and failure of concentration is one of the curiosities of medicine, and argument persists as to whether it is the result of subtle brain damage, or largely artifact. The symptoms are certainly most persistent and by no means always subside when litigation has been settled. Headache may be migrainous and vertigo may be of the postural type described on p. 77 but the giddiness complained of is usually far less specific in character. Depression and anxiety are often evident. Extreme views have been adopted, one school maintaining, somewhat illogically, both that the symptoms are due to neuronal loss, and that they can be cured. At the other extreme is the claim that the symptoms are fabricated for motives of greed. There is probably no all-embracing truth. It has long been recognized that indistinguishable symptoms can arise from an accident in which no physical injury was sustained, even an accident merely witnessed. Opportunities for neuronal loss in such circumstances are slight. On the other hand it would be absurd to deny dogmatically that a blow sufficient to cause amnesia for several hours might well result in some permanent damage even in the absence of classical neurological signs. It seems probable that the sequelae of slight or moderately severe closed head injury result largely from mental depression and disturbance of peripheral vestibular mechanisms. Such an approach at least affords hope of treatment and recovery. The recognition of, at one end of the scale, slight cerebral damage and, at the other, malingering, both of which occur, is sometimes difficult.

Unlike many patients who have had trivial injuries, the victim of severe head injury often makes little of his residual disability, which may consequently be ignored or underestimated. In these cases subjective complaints are few, headache and dizziness being rarely mentioned. Emotional and intellectual impairment may remain undetected at routine clinical examination, and even the severity of local disability may be disguised by euphoria. The patient's family often furnish the most reliable evidence as to his incapacity.

In more than half of all head injuries admitted to hospital, medico-legal assessment of disability is required at some time or other. The average period between injury and settlement of a compensation claim in Britain is two years. This period is too long for the minor cases, where it is often a factor in prolonging subjective disability. It is much too short for the equitable assessments of severely head-injured patients, where follow-up studies show that slow and almost imperceptible improvement may continue for nearly a decade.

Young patients stand head injury much better than the elderly, and children recover best of all. To deal with physical disabilities first, hemiparesis usually recovers well except where there has been gross laceration of brain substance, and this of course usually implies severe bony injury. The same considerations apply to aphasia. In childhood especially, severe aphasia often shows excellent recovery over a period of months or a few years. In the elderly patient recovery of speech, as with other complicated physical functions, is usually less complete.

The cranial nerves are frequently damaged in severe head injury. Anosmia is a classical complication of fracture of the anterior fossa of the skull where the olfactory apparatus may be actually torn across. However, it is commoner in closed head injury without fracture, and is usually regarded as an indication that the injury has been material. Anosmia following head injury is nearly always permanent.

Failure or impairment of ocular movement after head injury is sometimes due to haematoma in the orbit directly affecting or disturbing the muscles that move the eyeball. This variety rapidly recovers. More often muscular weakness or paralysis is due to a lesion of one or other of the cranial nerves and will show the characteristics of third, fourth or sixth nerve paralysis. Again such lesions may complicate simple closed head injury, but in general their prognosis is good, and any question of surgical interference to achieve mechanical relief of double vision should be deferred for at least a year and preferably longer. In fact it is not often required. The fifth nerve is rarely affected as a whole, but pronounced tingling in the distribution of its infraorbital branch often complicates injury that has involved the face. It causes discomfort rather than disability and since it is usually due to bruising of the nerve it clears up within six to twelve months.

Facial nerve paralysis after head injury has a good prognosis and this applies not only where the paralysis is sustained at the time of injury, but in the rather curious cases in which it appears without warning about a week later, presumably due to nerve involvement by organized scar tissue. The only exception to this good prognosis is where the nerve has been torn across by an extensive fracture of the temporal bone, and such cases are rare.

A complaint of deafness following head injury is more often due to a traumatic exacerbation of pre-existing middle ear disease, which may be denied by or even unknown to the patient, than to nerve damage. In some instances there can be no doubt that the injury drew attention to deafness already present, but it can also permanently aggravate pre-existing damage to the delicate conducting mechanism of the middle ear. Post-traumatic nerve deafness usually shows little improvement, and indeed for practical purposes deafness resulting from head injury must be regarded as irrecoverable.

It is difficult to assess the significance of mental symptoms following minor closed head injury. It is undeniable that if monetary compensation is being claimed symptoms may be exaggerated and on occasions even fabricated. Standard psychological tests show no abnormality but these do not necessarily examine the appropriate aspects. Adequate tests for concentration, which is the main subject of complaint, have not been developed.

In severe head injury the problem is different. The patient may have little or no insight into his mental handicap, and if he has insight he often makes every attempt to disguise his disability. However, his impairment of memory is evident in an account of errands unfulfilled, objects mislaid, names and places forgotten, and unreliable performance of simple duties and obligations. Evidence of this nature is more convincing than that yielded by psychological testing, though such simple tests as remembering a name and address given at the beginning of a consultation, repeating a complicated sentence after the examiner has read it aloud two or three times, or serially deducting seven from 100 may confirm the slowness and inadequacy of the patient's mental processes in the more outspoken cases. In more difficult clinical situations, especially where there is complicating emotional disturbance, skilled psychometric testing may be of great value. Expertly carried out it may enable the examiner to make some assessment as to how far the patient's poor intellectual performance is inherent and constitutional, how far it is due to reversible emotional disturbance, and how far it is genuinely due to brain damage; in the latter instance the patchiness of the test results is characteristic. In very severe cases the patient may remain severely demented and such dementia may be complicated by disorientation and dysphasia due to superadded focal brain damage.

Even two years after a severe head injury the patient's poor memory, easy flustering, and air of rather dazed confusion may lead the examiner to the view that he will never work again, even with simple closed head injury. There are some patients to whom this certainly applies, but for the most part these are instances where there has been gross focal brain destruction: in other words this situation arises much more often after open than closed head injury. However, even after open injury, and more so after closed injury, the brain has an enormous capacity for functional recovery except after middle age. A minority of these patients are left with some degree of permanent intellectual impairment that may be evident on testing even ten years later. However, this may not be incompatible with steady and continued occupation, except in the most highly skilled and intellectual pursuits. A few patients remain unemployable, either because of epilepsy (which is discussed below); because of serious and persisting changes in personality and temperament, usually dependent on severe damage to the temporal or frontal lobes of the major hemisphere; from persistent hemiplegia as a result of open injury; and from more severe dementia. There is incidentally no evidence that progressive dementia results from head injury.

TRAUMATIC EPILEPSY

Traumatic epilepsy is a complication of severe head injury. It is seen most often after open head injury, and especially following the wartime gunshot or shrapnel wound where cortical scarring complicates severe damage to scalp, skull and dura mater. Some such patients develop fits within hours or days of the injury. Most of those who will develop traumatic epilepsy do so within two years of the injury, but there is a minority in which the onset is delayed for several further years. The focal onset of the fit may disclose its site of origin, but most often traumatic epilepsy presents as a major convulsion without local signature. Some of these patients show a tendency to status epilepticus, but in many the condition can be controlled by the usual anti-convulsant measures and especially by some combination of phenobarbitone and phenytoin. In some the fits tend to cease spontaneously. The difficulties of employment for the epileptic are well known, but contrary to expectation most of our patients suffering from traumatic epilepsy have returned to work.

Traumatic epilepsy after closed head injury is very much less frequent and is indeed a rarity. The fact that it is so often claimed in children probably reflects the tendency of primary generalized epilepsy to begin about the time of puberty rather than any genuine predilection of the younger patient for the traumatic condition. Except where there is a depressed fracture with probable underlying cortical damage, where there has been intracerebral or intracranial bleeding of some degree, or where there has been very prolonged unconsciousness for at least several days, the claim that fits have resulted from closed head injuries should be scrutinized with great care. In some instances it will be found that the injury itself occurred in the course of an epileptic fit. Since the interseizure EEG even in authentic traumatic epilepsy is often normal, diagnosis is a matter of opinion. However, it must be based on statistical probabilities. The fact that fits have followed a head injury does not mean that they are due to it. Except for surgical elevation of a depressed fracture, treatment is the same for other forms of epilepsy.

TRAUMATIC CEREBROSPINAL RHINORRHOEA AND OTORRHOEA

Cerebrospinal rhinorrhoea due to anterior fossa fracture involving the paranasal air sinuses is much commoner than leakage of spinal fluid from a petrous temporal fracture passing through the ear. Otorrhoea practically always clears up within about a week, and rhinorrhoea usually does so. In either case the patient should be nursed in a sitting position, protected as far as possible from respiratory infection, and given antibiotic cover. Because of the risk of recurrent meningitis the occasional case of persistent rhinorrhoea requires surgical repair.

Further reading

Gurdjian E.S. & Gurdjian, Edwins (1978) Acute head injuries. *Surg. Gynaec. Obst.* **146**, 805.

Northfield D.W.C. (1973) *The Surgery of the Central Nervous System.* Blackwell Scientific Publications, Oxford.

Potter J.M. (1974) *The Practical Management of Head Injuries*, 3rd edn. Lloyd-Luke, London.

CHAPTER 9
Vascular Disease of the Nervous System

The brain receives a rich blood supply from four large arteries connected by an extensive anastomosis. Nevertheless, cerebrovascular disease is one of the commonest causes of death and disability. In contrast, although the spinal cord is supplied by small arteries with little effective anastomosis it is seldom affected by clinically significant vascular disease. The explanation lies in the differential incidence of atherosclerosis, which is a disease of large and medium sized arteries. Some degree of thickening of the arterial wall and loss of elasticity is inevitable with advancing years, but atheroma is not simply the result of ageing. Until its causes and their prevention are discovered cerebrovascular disease will continue to be common and largely intractable.

Knowledge of cerebrovascular disease has, nevertheless, enormously expanded in the last decade and, as a result, much of what was previously accepted without question has been shown to be wrong. The arterial supply of the brain must be regarded as a dynamic system capable of adjustment to meet varying demands in health and disease. Cerebral blood flow is within wide limits protected from the effects of fluctuations in systemic blood pressure by variation of the calibre of the cerebral arteries. Thus, if one or more of the main vessels in the neck is stenosed or occluded, the blood supply of the brain can be maintained through the remaining arteries and the anastomosis of the circle of Willis. Such a supply is precarious since the reserve is not inexhaustible. Occlusion or stenosis of an anastomotic vessel, transient disturbance of flow due to the passage of an embolus, or even mild anoxia during a general anaesthetic may impoverish the blood flow to some part of the brain sufficiently to cause infarction. Investigation may then reveal the stenosed or occluded vessels in the neck—an essential but far from immediate cause of the infarction. The view that the arteries that arise from the circle of Willis are end-arteries is no longer tenable. There is a further possibility of collateral circulation over the surface of the brain, where dilated arteries may carry blood to ischaemic areas outside their normal distributions. Thrombosis may therefore occur in the extracranial or cerebral arteries without infarction, and infarction in the territory of any artery may result from remote causes. It remains true, of course, that occlusion of the main trunk of the middle cerebral artery will cause massive infarction if there is no effective collateral circulation. Similarly the circle of Willis is often incomplete, and occlusion of an internal carotid artery may cause infarction even if the remaining arteries are healthy.

ISCHAEMIC VASCULAR DISEASE

Pathology

Atheroma may occur in any of the main arteries and their larger branches, but it has a predilection for the common carotid and vertebral arteries at their origins, the internal carotid just above its bifurcation in the neck and in the siphon, the basilar artery just before its division into the posterior cerebral arteries, and the main trunk of the middle cerebral artery. The lumen may be further narrowed by collections of fibrin and platelets on the diseased intima, or by actual blood clot that may occlude the artery. Fragments of clot, clumps of platelets, or cholesterol crystals may break away to traverse or lodge in distal arteries. Although the intimal lesion is the most important, thickening of the media is an additional cause of arterial narrowing, especially where the blood-pressure is raised and particularly in smaller vessels where atheroma is uncommon.

An infarcted area of brain becomes soft and necrotic, and may be surrounded by extensive oedema. Haemorrhage from capillary rupture is common. If the patient survives, the area becomes shrunken and scarred (Fig. 13, following p. 000) or the necrotic tissue may break down to form a cyst. At autopsy it is usual to find evidence of several infarcts of different ages. Some of these can be clearly related to the distribution of main cerebral arteries, most commonly the middle cerebral. The artery supplying the infarcted area may be occluded but infarction of the middle cerebral artery territory is commonly seen in internal carotid artery occlusion. Fatal infarction is usually accompanied by severe swelling of the hemisphere with herniation of the uncus of the temporal lobe through the tentorial opening and distortion of the brain stem which is sometimes the site of secondary haemorrhage. Other infarcts are related to the 'watersheds' at the margins of the distribution of the main vessels, areas that are theoretically and in practice vulnerable if blood supply is precarious. Perhaps the commonest pathological evidence of infarction, particularly in hypertensive subjects, is the presence of 'lacunae'. These are cysts a few millimetres in diameter and are found most frequently in the brain stem, basal ganglia and other central structures.

Pathogenesis

The incidence of cerebrovascular disease rises sharply in the sixth decade, but no age group is exempt. Evidence of diffuse atherosclerosis may be prominent in the elderly but absent in younger patients. Coronary artery disease is common, and may be a source of emboli or a cause of ischaemia due to relative failure of flow through narrowed cerebral vessels in a period of hypotensive shock following cardiac infarction. The incidence of diabetes is higher than in the general population. Hypertension of the order of 180/90 is common in patients with extensive arteriosclerosis but is a sign of the disease and not a cause of cerebral infarction. The association between hypertension and cerebral haemorrhage is well known but hypertension is also the main risk factor in ischaemic brain disease. Recently attention has been redirected to the possible harmful effects of a moderately raised haematocrit slowing blood flow and increasing the risk of infarction.

Oral contraceptives undoubtedly contribute to occlusive cerebrovascular disease in young women. Although only a minute proportion of those who take these agents are affected, their use is so common that the number of women involved is not insignificant. The cause is a defect in clotting mechanisms, the arteries remaining normal. In fatal cases the vascular occlusion appears to result from embolism but the source of the emboli may not be found.

In younger patients mitral stenosis is still an important cause of cerebral embolism. In children disastrous cerebral infarction is a rare complication of tissue infections around the carotid in the neck.

Arterial disease other than atherosclerosis occasionally causes infarction. Syphilitic arteritis is a rarity but the cerebral vessels may be involved in giant-cell arteritis and in the rare arteritis of the aorta and its branches that occurs in young women (Takayashu's disease; pulseless disease).

Chronic anaemia is well tolerated by the brain and is hardly ever a contributory factor in infarction. Polycythaemia vera often presents with cerebral symptoms apparently because the increased viscosity of the blood impedes its passage through a previously adequate arterial tree.

Transient cerebral ischaemia

There is an important clinical distinction between transient episodes followed by full recovery, and strokes that leave persistent evidence of brain damage. The former are considered to be due to ischaemia causing reversible loss of function, and the latter to infarction with inevitable permanent neuronal loss. Transient cerebral ischaemia is usually defined as a neurological deficit of vascular cause with full recovery within 24 hours. This figure is entirely arbitrary and full recovery is relatively uncommon if symptoms have lasted for more than a few hours and most such attacks are much more brief. As any part of the brain may be affected the clinical features are naturally varied, but may be divided into those due to involvement of the carotid and of the vertebrobasilar territories.

Recognizable symptoms of ischaemia in the carotid territory are transient hemiparesis, hemisensory symptoms and aphasia. The onset is abrupt and loss of function is often slight. Weakness may be confined to the face or to one limb and sensory symptoms, paraesthesiae, numbness, or sensory ataxia may be similarly restricted. Aphasia may take any form, most commonly that of mispronouncing words, or there may be sudden inability to comprehend the printed page or to write coherently. Resolution of the symptoms is less rapid than the onset, but the duration of most attacks is half an hour or less. Headache may be severe but is inconstant.

The carotid also supplies the eye through its first branch, the ophthalmic artery, and attacks of unilateral loss of vision, *amaurosis fugax*, are common. These are often described as being like a black curtain being drawn rapidly over the eye and vision may be totally lost or small peripheral islands retained. Such attacks are usually brief, and last for less than five minutes.

The symptoms of ischaemia in the vertebrobasilar distribution are more complex and less easy to recognize for what they are. Transient hemianopia or less severe defects such as shimmering in one half-field result from ischaemia of one occipital lobe. If both posterior cerebral artery territories are involved simultaneously there may be alarming attacks of total blindness. In the brain stem, ischaemia of the cranial nerve nuclei may cause diplopia, tingling on one side of the face, or facial weakness. Vertigo is common and may be recognizable as due to ischaemia only if it is accompanied by other symptoms. Hemisensory symptoms may occur from involvement of the spinothalamic tract. The cause of 'drop attacks', when these are due to cerebral ischaemia, in which the patient suddenly falls to the ground without loss of consciousness or vertigo, is more speculative, but may be ischaemia of the reticular formation causing sudden loss of tone in the limbs.

The strange condition known as *transient global amnesia* has been attributed to ischaemia of the temporal lobes. This occurs in middle-aged people and consists of the sudden onset of confusion and amnesia which may stretch back many years into the past. During the episode, which lasts for up to an hour, the patient frequently asks where he is and what is going on, but is capable of voluntary activity. On recovery there is complete amnesia for the period of confusion but the retrograde amnesia recovers. There are many points resembling temporal lobe epilepsy but recurrent attacks are rare. One strange precipitating factor that can be identified in some patients is sea bathing.

A recently recognized cause of transient ischaemia of the brain stem is the *subclavian steal syndrome*. If the subclavian artery is occluded or severely stenosed proximal to the origin of the vertebral artery the flow in the latter may be intermittently reversed, resulting in vertigo and other symptoms of brain stem ischaemia, particularly when exercise of the relatively ischaemic arm causes an increased demand for blood. The subclavian block is revealed by a significant lowering of the brachial blood pressure compared with the other side.

There are two recognized causes of cerebral ischaemia induced by turning the head; the carotid sinus syndrome, and narrowing of a vertebral artery by osteophytes in the neck. The former results from hypersensitivity of the carotid sinus, and can be detected by gross bradycardia or asystole on massaging the sinus on one or other side. The latter can be diagnosed only by elaborate angiographic studies of the vertebral arteries. Both conditions are potentially curable, by denervating the carotid sinus or removing the offending osteophytes respectively, but both are rare. In most patients with typical symptoms no such abnormality can be found.

Transient ischaemic attacks may be single or repetitive. Multiple attacks are usually stereotyped, but in some patients two or three different forms of attack occur independently. The frequency varies greatly, but in a few dramatic examples attacks of aphasia or hemiparesis occur many times every day.

Transient ischaemic attacks may be confused with other forms of temporary loss of cerebral function. The distinction between ischaemia of the sensory cortex and a focal sensory fit may be a matter for conjecture, particularly as it must be based entirely on the patient's description of unfamiliar symptoms. The aura of migraine is a form of transient ischaemic attack due to functional arterial narrowing, and can be distinguished only by its clinical context. The classical visual aura of migraine occurring for the first time in the fifth decade should be regarded as due to cerebrovascular disease, particularly if it is not followed by headache. The occurrence for the first time of focal migrainous symptoms in a woman on oral contraceptives should be interpreted as due to embolism and regarded as an imperative indication for the pill to be stopped.

'Little strokes' have long been recognized, and were formerly attributed to spasm of cerebral arteries. This explanation is untenable, since the rigid arteries of many of these patients are clearly incapable of any form of active contraction. There are two alternative explanations, vascular insufficiency and embolism. On the former theory the patient's cerebrovascular system is so precariously balanced that any temporary relative failure of flow such as might follow a fall in blood pressure causes ischaemia in areas with a supply that is normally just adequate. This can certainly happen, for focal symptoms may occur in Stokes–Adams attacks where the cardiac output temporarily ceases. Whether less drastic insufficiency is a frequent cause is more doubtful, but prolonged monitoring has shown that many patients with transient cerebral ischaemia have unsuspected brief episodes of cardiac dysrhythmia. One objection to the embolic theory is the stereotyped nature of the attacks. However, it is known from experiment that emboli repeatedly follow precisely the same pathway, however improbable this may seem. In the retina it has occasionally been possible to observe the passage of emboli through the arteries during an attack of unilateral blindness.

The emboli probably responsible for the majority of transient cerebral ischaemic attacks do not closely resemble the large coiled clots found at autopsy in those dying of pulmonary artery embolism, but are small fragments of platelets and fibrin that have formed on atheromatous plaques in proximal arteries. Such fragments are sufficiently plastic to cause temporary arterial obstruction, being eventually swept through the capillary bed.

Cerebral infarction

The causes of cerebral infarction appear to be identical to those of transient ischaemia. Atherosclerosis leads both to thrombosis and occlusion of cerebral or cervical arteries or to the formation of thrombosis that gives rise to emboli that occlude more distal vessels (Fig. 14, following p. 152). Large emboli can arise from the left atrium in patients with mitral valve disease and, much more rarely, in atrial fibrillation from other causes. It is presumably the duration of the ischaemia that determines whether the symptoms are transient or whether infarction occurs, but small infarcts are found so often at post mortem in patients never known to have suffered a stroke that the distinction which seems so important clinically may be more one of degree.

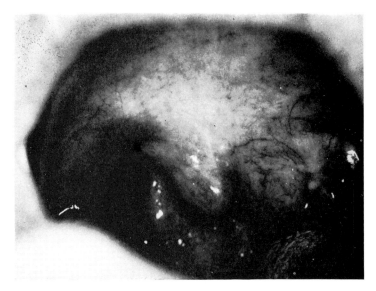

FIG. 7. Unmistakable paralysis of the left side of the palate. Minor deviations of the uvula are often misinterpreted and should be ignored.

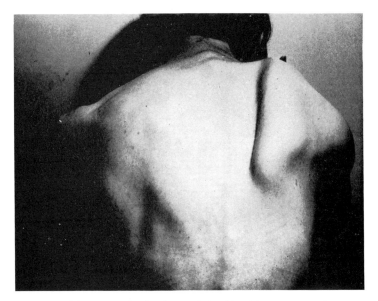

FIG. 8. Neuralgic amyotrophy showing paralysis of the right serratus anterior.

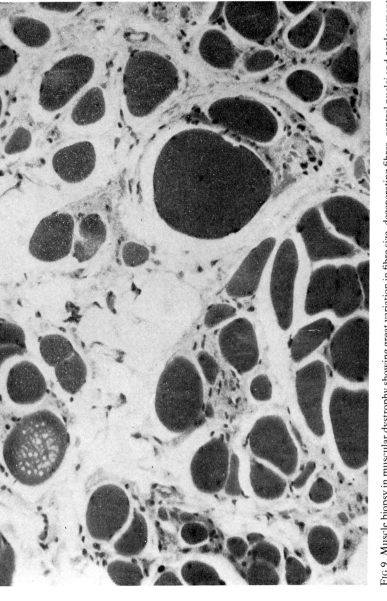

FIG 9. Muscle biopsy in muscular dystrophy showing great variation in fibre size, degenerating fibres, central nuclei and replacement with fat.

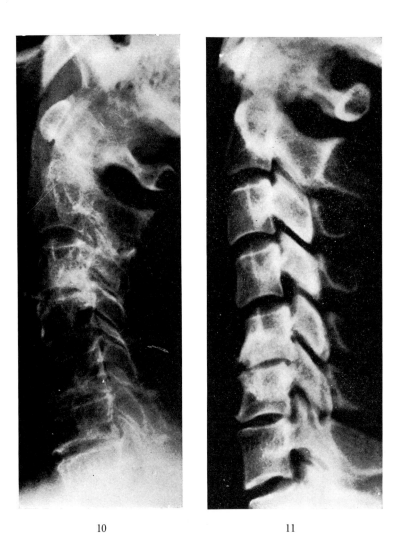

Fig. 10. Gross degenerative spondylosis without symptoms in a woman of 64.

Fig. 11. Spondylosis of lower cervical spine in a woman of 50, with narrowed disc spaces and marginal osteophytic lipping, causing progressive paraplegia.

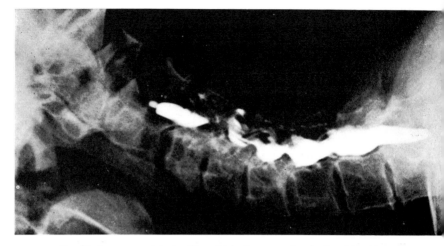

FIG. 12. Severe spondylosis with multiple disc protrusions in the mid and lower cervical regions, causing progressive spastic quadriparesis.

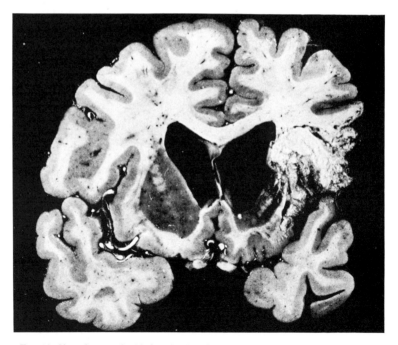

FIG. 13. Shrunken cerebral infarct in right frontal lobe: the white colour of the blood vessels is due to injection.

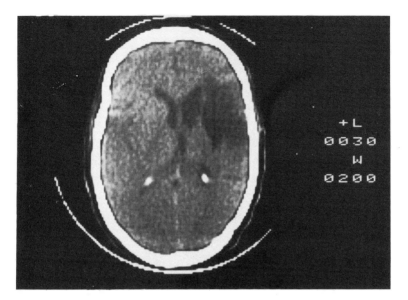

Fig. 14. CT scan showing an old infarct in the distribution of the right middle cerebral artery. The infarcted area is of low density and the lateral ventricle on that side is dilated because of the destruction of tissue.

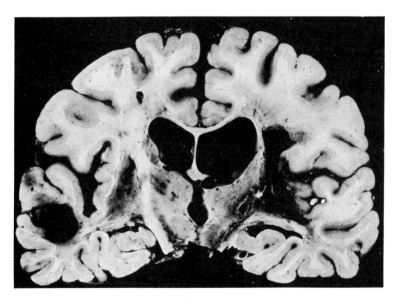

Fig. 15. Massive capsular haemorrhage in a severely hypertensive patient who also has a recent haemorrhage in the opposite temporal lobe and several other areas of softening.

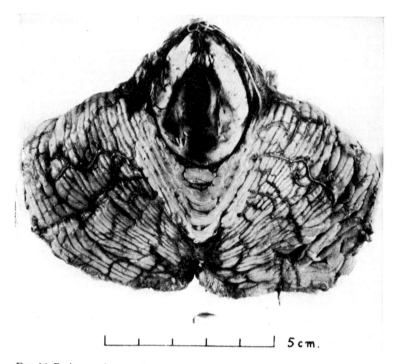

FIG. 16. Brain-stem haemorrhages secondary to massive capsular haemorrhage. Similar brain-stem changes may be seen in rapidly increased intracranial pressure from other causes such as neoplasm, and after severe head injury.

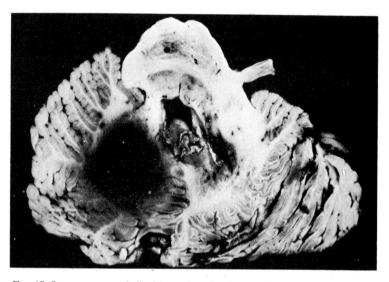

FIG. 17. Spontaneous cerebellar haemorrhage in a hypertensive subject, with ischaemic destruction of dentate nucleus on opposite side.

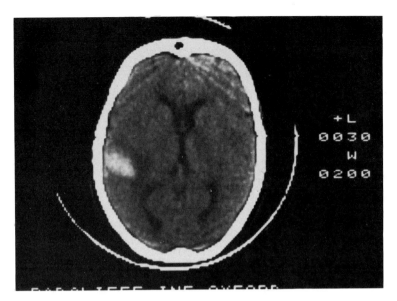

FIG. 18. CT scan showing primary intracerebral haemorrhage in left temporal lobe.

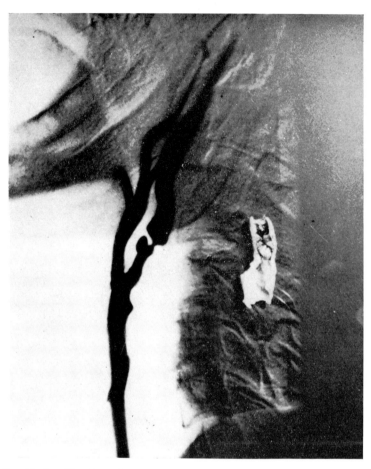

Fig. 19. Carotid angiography showing severe stenosis of the internal carotid artery in the neck with the atheromatous lesion removed at operation.

Fig. 20. Carotid angiogram after subarachnoid haemorrhage in a woman of 55, showing two saccular aneurysms on the circle of Willis, one arising from the origin of the posterior communicating artery and the other in the region of the anterior communicating artery. Aneurysms are multiple in about 15% of cases.

Fig. 21. Subarachnoid haemorrhage in a man of 59; vertebral angiography shows an angiomatous malformation in the posterior parietal region, supplied by branches of the left posterior cerebral artery and drained by grossly dilated veins into the superior longitudinal sinus.

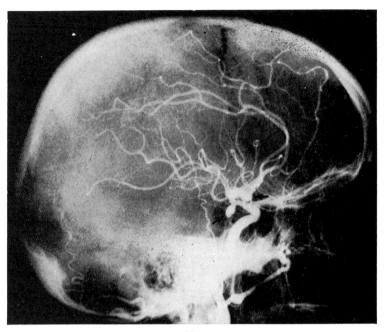

20

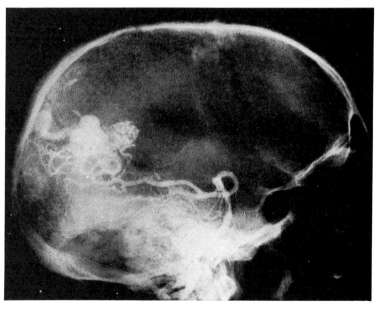

21

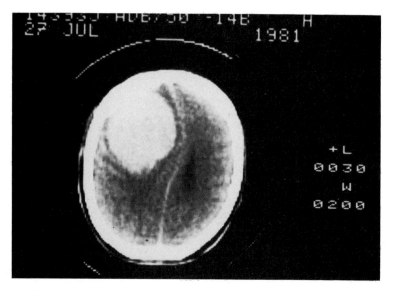

FIG. 22. A contrast enhanced CT scan showing a large left frontal meningioma. The falx cerebri can be seen to be displaced by the tumour.

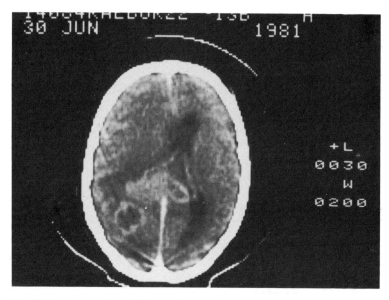

FIG. 23. A contrast enhanced CT scan showing a malignant glioma with many areas of different density involving both cerebral hemispheres posteriorly.

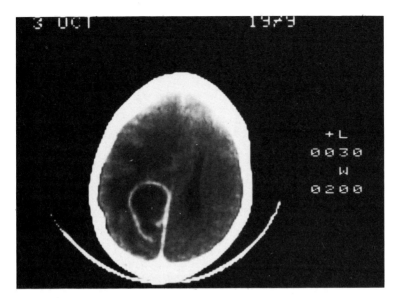

FIG. 24. A contrast enhanced CT scan showing an abscess posteriorly in the left hemisphere. In this case the infection was carried to the brain in the bloodstream.

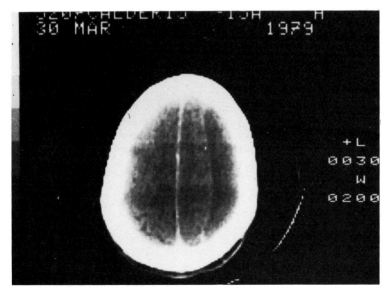

FIG. 25. CT scan showing a right-sided subdural haematoma. It can be seen that the difference in density between the contents of the haematoma and the brain is not marked.

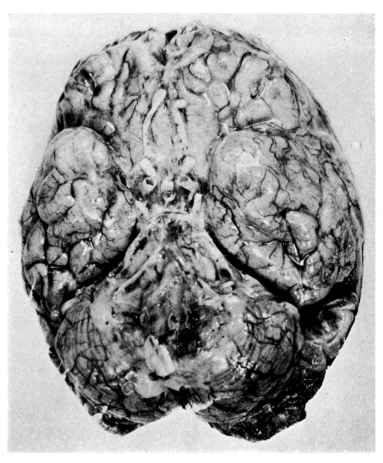

FIG. 26. Acute pneumococcal meningitis in a middle-aged woman: profuse basal exudate in an unrecognized case of 7 days' duration. Pneumococci were also isolated from the right middle ear and from a pelvic abscess associated with diverticulosis.

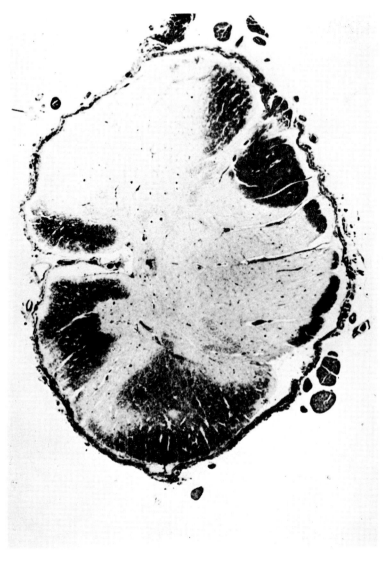

FIG. 27. Multiple sclerosis. A cross-section of the spinal cord stained black for myelin showing extensive confluent plaques.

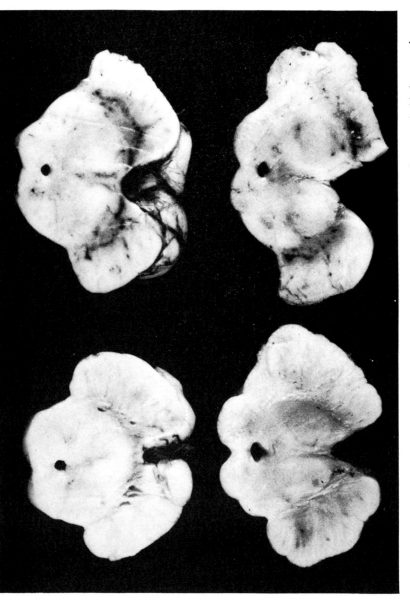

FIG. 28. The contrast between the depigmented substantia nigra in Parkinson's disease on the left compared with the normal.

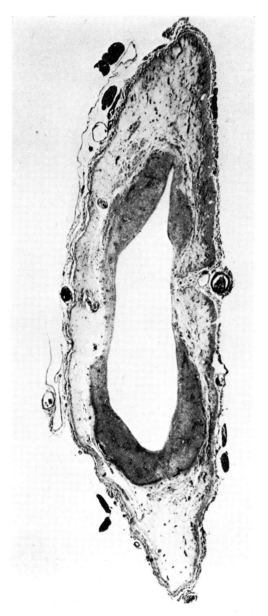

Fig. 29. Syringomyelia: transverse section of spinal cord in cervical region showing internal compression of cord substance by extensive central syrinx.

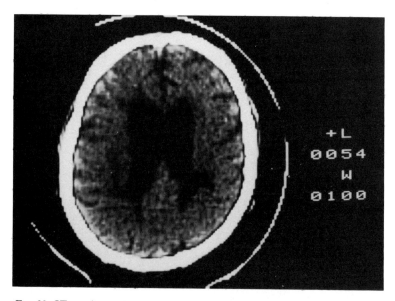

FIG. 30. CT scan in a patient presumed to be suffering from Alzheimer's disease. The lateral ventricles can be seen to be markedly dilated and the cerebral sulci are greatly widened.

The clinical effects of recognizable infarction differ from those of transient ischaemia only in their duration and in the persistence of signs of brain damage. The onset is rapid and sometimes abrupt, but the disability seldom reaches its peak immediately. A characteristic history is of weakness of one arm developing in the evening, followed by hemiplegia on waking the next morning. Infarction often occurs during sleep and the hour after waking is also a vulnerable time. Increasing severity of symptoms over several hours or days is sometimes called a 'stroke in progress' but this does not mean that some quite different process is operating. Fluctuation in the clinical course, with short-lived improvement followed by sudden deterioration, sometimes vividly suggests the ebb and flow of the collateral circulation in the ischaemic area around the infarct. The symptoms and signs naturally depend on the site and extent of the lesion, but the commonest presentation is the hemiplegic stroke.

Hemiplegia

Loss of function of the upper motor neurones, anywhere in their course from the precentral gyrus at the posterior end of the frontal lobe to the decussation of the corticospinal tracts in the medulla, causes a disorder of voluntary movement on the opposite side of the body. In the cortex the neurones extend over a considerable area and partial lesions are relatively common, but the fibres descending in the central white matter of the hemisphere converge on the internal capsule where they are closely packed and exposed to destruction from relatively small lesions. The fibres remain concentrated in the mid-brain and medulla but are more dispersed in the pons. Many types of cerebral lesion give rise to hemiplegia, but it is encountered in all its clinical variations in occlusive vascular disease.

Severe hemiplegia due to infarction usually implies an extensive lesion in the middle cerebral artery territory, since although the artery supplies an extensive area of cortex its deep branches also furnish the circulation of the internal capsule. Even with such severe lesions initial loss of consciousness is uncommon. The limbs may at first be flaccid, the eyes deviated away from the paralysed side and swallowing is difficult because of pharyngeal palsy. Tendon reflexes may be depressed but the plantar response is extensor. A severe stroke of this kind may prove fatal, and a declining level of consciousness strongly suggests dangerous cerebral oedema and brain stem compression. Previous cerebral infarction is also a poor prognostic sign, but in other circumstances improvement can nearly always be expected. Why this should be so is not immediately obvious but certain factors are clearly important. Ischaemic neurones around the infarct may survive through the establishment of collateral circulation. Cells paralysed by extensive oedema may recover. Some functions of the destroyed area may be taken over by undamaged neurones. Whatever the cause, voluntary movement and the spasticity characteristic of an upper motor neurone lesion develop concurrently. Dysphagia usually recovers within a few days. Proximal limb muscles recover first, followed by the distal muscles of the lower limb. Walking becomes possible with the leg in spastic extension, and movement at the shoulder and elbow returns, but useful movement of the fingers and hand is always delayed and is never restored after a severe hemiplegia. The arm is then held adducted and flexed at the elbow, with the fingers tightly curled into the palm. The speed of recovery varies greatly, but improvement may continue for weeks or months. Less severe degrees of weakness are common, and functional recovery may be excellent, but permanent damage is evident in increased reflexes on the affected side and often in impairment of fine finger movements. This loss of movements out of proportion to loss of strength is characteristic of the upper motor neurone lesion, and may be diagnostic in minor cerebral infarction affecting the arm alone. If infarction is limited to the cortical distribution of the anterior cerebral artery weakness is confined to the leg or even to the foot. The accompanying extensor plantar response distinguishes the syndrome from the commoner peripheral causes of foot drop.

Sensory loss is common in any severe hemiplegia, and this finding at the onset has little importance for the patient and no diagnostic significance. However, functional recovery from hemiplegia may be greatly impeded by persisting loss of postural sense. When the impact of a posteriorly situated lesion has been mainly on the sensory cortex or pathways power may recover fully and fine movements may be adequate, but only if the patient watches his hand. Unawareness of the position of the fingers in space is a severe disability. Following infarction of the non-dominant right hemisphere a characteristic and disabling feature is the tendency to neglect the affected limbs even if there has been good recovery of power and sensation. This arises from damage to cortical areas concerned with the appreciation of external space and of the patient's own body—the body image. Such patients appear not to use the left limbs to full advantage because they lack normal awareness of their existence.

Relatively severe but localized neurological deficits, such as isolated unilateral sensory loss, but with good recovery and with no disturbance of higher cerebral function can sometimes be related to small *lacunae* or cystic spaces in the brain stem or subcortical areas.

Apraxia

The slow and clumsy movements of the patient with an upper motor neurone lesion are sometimes wrongly referred to as apraxia. Although the movements are defective the patient obviously understands what he is trying to do and how to set about it. In apraxia there may be no general impairment of motor function but certain actions cannot be performed at all or even attempted. This may arise either because no concept of the necessary action can be formulated or because the idea cannot be translated into practice. An example commonly given is that of the patient who does not put out his tongue on request although he licks his lips spontaneously, though this is usually not due to apraxia but to failure to understand the order.

Many forms of purposive movement appear to be controlled by an area of the left parietal lobe around the supramarginal gyrus. A lesion here or interruption of the connections of this centre with the motor cortex causes apraxia. A left-sided lesion can therefore cause either bilateral apraxia or apraxia on the right side alone if only the connecting fibres on the left are involved. The fibres crossing to the right hemisphere in the anterior part of the corpus callosum can also be damaged in isolation, causing left-sided apraxia.

Apraxia involving the skilled movements of the upper limbs, such as holding a knife and fork, is comparatively rare and may be overlooked unless the patient is tested in the manipulation of common objects and the ability to imitate or copy gestures. Apraxia for walking and sometimes even for sitting is a severe disability. Apraxia for dressing without any difficulty for other actions is often seen in diffuse cerebral disease though it is probably due to parietal lobe damage.

Carotid artery occlusion

By far the commonest site of stenosis or occlusion of the internal carotid artery is just above the bifurcation of the common carotid. Stenosis is also common in the siphon, and indeed occlusion often involves the whole length of the artery between these sites. Occlusion may be symptomless, but without effective collateral circulation infarction will occur. This may be just like any other acute hemiplegic stroke, but there are sometimes distinctive features. The onset may be slowly progressive and the initial symptoms as sharply localized as difficulty in using the index finger. Disability may increase progressively by episodes each of which resembles a classical stroke. It would be convenient if carotid occlusion, and especially the distinction between obliteration and stenosis, could be defined with certainty on clinical grounds, but this has proved impossible. Only if the common carotid is blocked is there any detectable loss of pulsation in the neck. A systolic bruit heard over the artery high in the neck often indicates carotid artery disease, but it may be heard in both stenosis and occlusion. Horner's syndrome on the side of the lesion may accompany carotid occlusion but is an unreliable sign. The classical syndrome of the carotid artery, with unilateral blindness on the side of the lesion due to retinal ischaemia, accompanied by crossed hemiplegia, is very rare.

Vertebrobasilar syndromes

In the posterior cerebral artery territory infarction causes hemianopia. Initially there may be bilateral involvement with temporary total blindness which rapidly clears in one half-field. This is explained by the common origin of the two arteries as the terminal branches of the basilar. The onset is usually abrupt, and hemianopia is often not recognized by the patient, who complains merely of ill-defined difficulty with vision or who may be quite unaware of any visual disturbance. The hemianopia is often incomplete and may shrink to a quarter of the field or less, but improvement rarely continues for more than a few days.

The so-called *thalamic syndrome* is an uncommon but peculiarly distressing result of infarction of the sensory pathways, sometimes distal to the thalamus, in either the carotid or vertebral territories. Cutaneous sensory impairment on one side of the body is accompanied by very unpleasant pain, both spontaneous and induced by light touch or any contact with the skin. The syndrome often improves, as for example when it follows stereotaxic thalamic surgery, but it can persist, and responds hardly at all to any form of analgesic.

Infarction in the brain stem, with its crowded cranial nerve nuclei and descending and ascending tracts, and in the cerebellum, evokes a bewildering variety of clinical syndromes. Only rarely can these be attributed to infarction in the distribution of a single artery, and pathological examination confirms that lesions are often scattered and bilateral. Unilateral cerebellar ataxia may occur in isolation but is rare. Vertigo from infarction of the vestibular nuclei is a common feature, and unless it is accompanied by signs of damage to neighbouring structures it is clinically indistinguishable from vestibular neuronitis (Chapter 4). An occasional and interesting finding is internuclear ophthalmoplegia. On looking to one side the abducting eye moves but the eye that should adduct does not. However, the medial rectus is not paralysed, since it contracts when the eyes converge. This dissociation is due to interruption of the tract leading upward from the sixth nerve nucleus to that of the third, which normally subserves coordinated lateral gaze.

The classical syndrome attributed to thrombosis of the posterior inferior cerebellar artery is often quoted to illustrate the importance of memorizing diagrams of cross-sections of the medulla. The complete syndrome is rare, and comprises cranial nerve palsies and cerebellar ataxia on the side of the lesion with signs due to involvement of the spinothalamic and sometimes the pyramidal tracts on the opposite side, because the lesion is above the decussation of the tracts. The onset is with vertigo, vomiting and often numbness or pain in one side of the face. The infarct involves the descending root of the Vth nerve, causing loss of pain and thermal sense on the face. On the same side there is paralysis of the palate, pharynx and vocal cord from damage to the motor nucleus of the vagus, and a Horner's syndrome from interruption of the descending sympathetic pathway. Nystagmus is usually present. There is cerebellar ataxia of the limbs on the same side and a variable degree of loss of pain and thermal sensation on the opposite side of the body below the face. The prostrating vertigo is not prolonged, and the other symptoms and signs including the dysphagia improve gradually, except for the sensory loss which is often permanent and accompanied by unpleasant dysaesthesiae. There are numerous variants on this theme, the commonest being ipsilateral VIth and VIIth nerve palsies with crossed sensory loss.

The effects of occlusion of the basilar artery itself can rarely be compensated by collateral circulation. Fatal coma with flaccid tetraplegia may be preceded by rapidly advancing cranial nerve palsies, and particularly by dysphagia. Some patients survive for a few days or weeks in a distressing state known as the locked-in syndrome. No voluntary movements of the limbs or face are possible but the eyes can be moved in the vertical plane. The patient is conscious and able to respond to questions by moving the eyes.

Cerebrovascular dementia

Repeated infarction of large areas of brain is incompatible with life. Repeated small infarcts of a size that might cause no symptoms at all in isolation produce a cumulative effect. The common result is the syndrome of *pseudo-bulbar palsy*. This traditional and confusing term should give place to *supranuclear bulbar palsy* because the bulbar symptoms and signs result from bilateral lesions of the corticobulbar pathways. Speech is slurred and tongue movements are stiff and slow. Swallowing is difficult but never wholly impossible. The jaw jerk is usually increased.

Some degree of dementia is the rule, and is often accompanied by lability of emotional expression, so that crying is induced by reading of the misfortunes of strangers and foolish laughter provoked in embarrassing circumstances. Signs in the limbs may be limited to a diffuse increase in reflexes, and the plantar responses are usually flexor. The characteristic *marche à petits pas* with short tottering steps is seen with supranuclear bulbar palsy or in isolation.

Multiple cerebral infarcts may cause dementia, but seldom without a history of one or more minor or major strokes as well as clear evidence of damage to areas of the brain other than those mainly concerned with intellectual functions. Many patients diagnosed as suffering from arteriosclerotic mental deterioration are, in fact, instances of presenile dementia unrelated to arteriopathy.

The prognosis in diffuse cerebral infarction is uniformly bad.

CEREBRAL HAEMORRHAGE

Pathology

The common site of origin of massive spontaneous cerebral haemorrhage is deep in the hemisphere, extending into the internal capsule (Fig. 15, following p. 152). The extensive haematoma not only destroys the brain but causes acute swelling of the hemisphere, with resulting herniation of the under-surface of the temporal lobe through the tentorial opening. The brain stem is compressed and the resulting secondary haemorrhages are often fatal (Fig. 16, following p. 152). This is classical apoplexy, but smaller and less destructive haemorrhages are common. Fatal primary haemorrhage may also occur in the pons and cerebellum (Fig. 17, following p. 152). Hypertension in middle age is the usual cause, though apparently identical haemorrhage is very occasionally seen in young adults with normal blood pressure, possibly due to small vascular anomalies that escape detection at autopsy because they have been destroyed by the haemorrhage. Blood dyscrasias with defects in clotting mechanisms also account for occasional cases but the haematological condition is usually obvious. For practical purposes primary intracerebral haemorrhage is a complication of hypertension. The pathological basis is not, however, that of normal arteries giving way under increased pressure. An almost constant finding in known hypertensive subjects is the presence of minute aneurysms on small perforating arteries in the internal capsule and neighbouring structures. These aneurysms are apparently caused by hypertension and the risk of rupture is a constant threat to life.

Clinical features

A large haemorrhage into the cerebral hemisphere is rapidly followed by coma, with hemiplegia evident in extreme flaccidity of the limbs on one side. As brain stem compression increases the pupils dilate, and Cheyne–Stokes respiration heralds the end. Smaller haemorrhages are clinically indistinguishable from infarction except that initial coma is much more common. The coma of pontine haemorrhage is characterized by pinpoint pupils. In about 5% of patients in whom the site of haemorrhage is known the cerebellum is involved (Fig. 18, following p. 152). The clinical features are confusing. Headache and vomiting are common at the onset, followed by progressive decline in the level of consciousness, without hemiplegia or other focal signs.

The probability of death from a single cerebral haemorrhage is much greater than after a single infarct however large, but if consciousness is regained the prognosis for reasonable functional recovery is often unexpectedly good. Haemorrhage forces apart the fibres of the white matter, but infarction destroys them by anoxia. The distinction between the two forms of stroke is not very important unless active treatment is contemplated, and has proved unexpectedly difficult on clinical grounds.

Hypertensive encephalopathy is now uncommon, probably because effective hypotensive agents have made malignant hypertension a rarity. The term is used to describe a sudden catastrophic increase in the level of a previously high blood pressure, with convulsions, focal neurological signs and severe headache or disturbance of consciousness, apparently due to breakdown of the mechanisms that protect cerebral blood flow from changes in systemic blood pressure. The episode is brief and recovery unexpectedly complete, but such patients often have severe renal complications of hypertension. The syndrome can be caused by acute brain oedema and petechial haemorrhages, but an identical sequence of clinical events sometimes may be caused by localized cerebral haemorrhage, and hypertensive encephalopathy is often a rather speculative diagnosis.

INVESTIGATION AND TREATMENT

These two topics must be considered together. The object of investigation is to confirm the diagnosis where this is in doubt and to explore the possibility of treatment.

Investigation should obviously be adjusted to circumstances. The elderly atherosclerotic patient crippled by his third stroke requires no investigation at all. Initial investigation should always include routine blood tests for polycythaemia and syphilis and an ESR which will be raised in arteritis. Blood lipids should be estimated in young patients and diabetes excluded.

In the patient presenting with transient ischaemic attacks alternative diagnoses should be considered including migraine, focal epilepsy, the paroxysmal symptoms of multiple sclerosis and hypoglycaemia. All these conditions are very much less common than transient ischaemia and may be overlooked. The important decision is whether to carry out angiography and the answer must depend on the possibility of treatment being based on the results. Surgical treatment is available for internal carotid artery stenosis and for the much less commonly detected subclavian stenosis with or without steal from the vertebral distribution. Carotid artery disobliteration has been carried out on a very large scale with, unfortunately, little concerted attempt to assess the results. Before discussing the details it is important to consider what results are sought and what the aims of treatment are.

Transient ischaemic attacks are disturbing and frightening but unless they occur frequently are not disabling. Treatment might well be directed at abolishing the attacks but a far more important consideration is the prevention of cerebral infarction. A commonsense view would be that transient ischaemic attacks are a warning symptom of an impending stroke, but it is unexpectedly difficult to discover whether this is true. Prospective studies show that about 60% of patients with transient ischaemia will have a stroke within five years, so treatment directed to the prevention of infarction is a rational procedure.

There is general agreement that the ideal patient for carotid surgery is relatively young, with ischaemic attacks in the territory of one carotid artery and demonstrated stenosis of that artery (Fig. 19, following p. 152). Most surgeons would want to know that the other carotid was patent but would not require four-vessel angiography. At the other extreme is the elderly patient with diffuse atherosclerosis, ischaemic attacks in more than one arterial territory and perhaps clinical evidence of bilateral carotid disease from listening over the arteries. In general, patients approximating to the first description should be investigated by angiography with a view to surgery while those in the second category should not. Between these extremes clinical judgment must be exercised to avoid potentially harmful and useless investigation and to provide patients with their best chance of avoiding a hemiplegic stroke. Much will depend on the quality of the surgery available. Transient symptoms indistinguishable from those of vascular disease may also be caused by cerebral tumours, possibly by 'stealing' blood from the normal brain. A CT scan will resolve this difficulty.

The alternatives are to use anticoagulants with the idea of preventing the formation of clot that forms the source of emboli, or agents that prevent platelet aggregation. Anticoagulants, of which warfarin is now the most favoured, often appear to abolish transient ischaemic attacks when these have been very frequent, perhaps many times a day. Such patients are, however, a rarity and it is not known whether warfarin will prevent infarction, largely because of the difficulty in controlling clinical trials and the risk of cerebral haemorrhage. A common practice has been to use warfarin for a year and then to reduce slowly with a view to stopping. Some rebound return of symptoms may occur. Of the agents preventing platelet aggregation aspirin appears to be the most effective and there is now evidence that a daily dose of 600 mg will have an influence in preventing stroke in men with transient cerebral ischaemia as well as reducing or abolishing transient symptoms. Other 'antiplatelet' agents, sulphinpyrazone and dipyridamole, have not been shown to be effective.

In completed stroke investigation may be required to avoid diagnostic error. Most published series include a few patients with cerebral tumours but more important is the distinction from chronic subdural haematoma. CT scan will not always do this reliably but should be carried out if there are unusual clinical features such as fluctuating symptoms, especially drowsiness. The scan will also distinguish between cerebral haemorrhage, where the blood shows as a high density lesion, and ischaemic infarction which is low density. Haemorrhagic infarction may present difficulties. This distinction is not important unless treatment is contemplated which could be inappropriate or dangerous in the presence of haemorrhage.

The aim of treatment must be to prevent death in the acute stage and to reduce the eventual disability. Treatment must therefore be directed both to the prevention and reversal of cerebral oedema, the cause of death, and the reduction of the size of the infarct, the cause of the neurological deficit. These objectives clearly overlap to a large extent. Treatment directed at brain swelling has included dexamethazone and glycerol, both agents that reduce oedema related to cerebral tumour. They are, however, ineffective in oedema due to infarction and do not influence prognosis. There is also no evidence that diuretics are effective.

Numerous attempts have been made to improve the oxygen supply to the ischaemic area of the brain, but most presumed vasodilators do not have this action on cerebral vessels. The one agent known to have this effect is carbon dioxide, but, largely on theoretical grounds, it has been supposed that increasing the P_{CO_2} will dilate the normal vessels and not those in the ischaemic area which are paralysed, with the effects of 'stealing' blood and therefore of doing harm. No good trial of CO_2

inhalation has, however, been published. Anticoagulants are contraindicated in acute infarction except as a means of preventing further embolism in cases of mitral valve disease where the treatment should be started immediately. Theoretical objections to this are not borne out in practice. Operating on acutely blocked carotid arteries has a very high mortality and is positively harmful. Early surgical evacuation of an intracerebral haemorrhage is not helpful and later is unnecessary.

The attempt to find specific treatment has so far failed. The airway must be kept clear and food and fluid intake maintained. If swallowing is difficult a nasogastric tube should be passed. Physiotherapy or at least active and passive movements should begin as soon as possible. Blood pressure should be controlled as soon as the immediate fluctuations attendant on the stroke have subsided.

VENOUS THROMBOSIS

Cavernous sinus thrombosis is now a rare result of infective thrombophlebitis spreading along the communicating veins from the subcutaneous tissues of the face. Blocking of the venous drainage of the retina causes intense papilloedema, and the third, fourth and sixth nerves are paralysed as they traverse the sinus. The signs are usually bilateral since there is free communication between the two sides. This previously fatal and still dangerous condition responds to vigorous antibiotic treatment.

The lateral sinus is in close relation to the middle ear, but antibiotics have greatly reduced the incidence of thrombosis in otitis media and the resulting 'otitic hydrocephalus'. In this condition the volume of cerebrospinal fluid in the cranium is not increased, as the name suggests, but pressure is raised by impaired absorption of the fluid. Unless thrombosis extends into the superior longitudinal sinus the prognosis with adequate antibiotic therapy is good.

Thrombosis of the superior longitudinal sinus is a rare complication of the puerperium, not obviously related to infection. The high papilloedema and rapidly increasing coma are due to almost complete failure of absorption of cerebrospinal fluid, with extensive haemorrhagic venous infarction. Recovery from such a disaster is not to be expected and the condition is fatal.

Cortical thrombophlebitis also occurs in the puerperium and in the last weeks of pregnancy. Focal neurological signs, often including aphasia, develop acutely, usually without any disturbance of consciousness. The cerebrospinal fluid contains red cells but is not frankly blood-stained. The prognosis for full recovery is excellent, and this comparatively benign condition does not appear to be a precursor of superior longitudinal sinus thrombosis.

SUBARACHNOID HAEMORRHAGE

Blood may enter the subarachnoid space after primary intracerebral haemorrhage or haemorrhage into a cerebral tumour. But by far the commonest cause of spontaneous primary subarachnoid haemorrhage is rupture of an aneurysm of one of the arteries in the subarachnoid space, either those of the circle of Willis or its main contributing vessels and branches (Fig. 20, following p. 152). Most such aneurysms are congenital and occur at a point of arterial branching. Those that rupture are seldom as much as a centimetre in diameter and are otherwise quite symptomless. Other aneurysms are arteriosclerotic in origin, but cases resulting from syphilis and septic emboli (mycotic aneurysms) are not now encountered.

Vascular malformations are the only other common cause of subarachnoid haemorrhage. These angiomas consist of an arteriovenous shunt through a tangle of abnormal vessels and greatly dilated feeding arteries and draining veins (Fig. 21, following p. 152). Such congenital anomalies nearly always reach the surface of the brain or the ventricular wall at some point, and blood from a ruptured vessel therefore enters the subarachnoid space either directly or after passing through the ventricles. Haemorrhage from such lesions may be repeated, but its mortality is less than that of bleeding from aneurysm.

Subarachnoid haemorrhage occurs at any age, but the maximal incidence is in the fifth and sixth decades. It is one of the common causes of sudden death. Of those who survive, many rapidly or immediately become comatose. If consciousness is retained the cardinal symptom is sudden headache, generalized but rapidly spreading to the back of the neck and sometimes down the spine. Its severity varies but it is usually intense. Vomiting usually occurs at the onset.

Neck rigidity from meningeal irritation is an almost constant finding, but Kernig's sign is less common. The blood may not be confined to the subarachnoid space, and signs of focal damage to the brain may be present. The level of consciousness varies from deep coma through all degrees of confusion to complete lucidity. In severe cases subhyaloid haemorrhages are present in the retina, and papilloedema may develop. If an angioma is present a bruit may be audible over the carotid artery or orbit, and sometimes over a wide area of the skull. This differs from the bruit of occlusive vascular disease in being continuous, though with systolic accentuation.

Spinal subarachnoid haemorrhage is rare, and usually results from rupture of a spinal angioma, though occasionally from other tumours or in the course of polyarteritis nodosa. The initial symptom is a sudden agonizing pain in the back, but thereafter the syndrome is indistinguishable from that of cranial subarachnoid haemorrhage unless the cord is damaged at the time of the haemorrhage, when paraplegia may occur.

The diagnosis of subarachnoid haemorrhage is not often in doubt, but lumbar puncture is imperative to exclude meningitis unless subarachnoid blood has been shown on CT scanning. If subhyaloid haemorrhages are present lumbar puncture is unnecessary and as the pressure is then usually very high may be dangerous. If headache is mild, or in those unusual cases where the pain rapidly becomes localized to the distribution of the sciatic nerves due to irritation of the sacral roots, lumbar puncture will also confirm the diagnosis, but the indications for this are less obvious. For several days after the haemorrhage the cerebrospinal fluid is obviously blood-stained. Thereafter the number of red cells declines but the fluid becomes yellow from pigments formed from the liberated haemoglobin. Immediately following a subarachnoid haemorrhage from any cause the blood pressure is often raised to levels that would otherwise indicate important hypertension. This subsides in a few days and is no contraindication to investigation. The electrocardiogram may show transient changes similar to those of cardiac infarction.

A patient in coma from subarachnoid haemorrhage is in danger of dying. Without coma there is no danger from the presenting haemorrhage but a high risk of further haemorrhage which is often fatal or crippling. Of those who reach hospital alive and who are treated conservatively—which implies no active treatment at all—about 40% will die from the first or subsequent haemorrhage within eight weeks. Thereafter the risk of further haemorrhage is greatly reduced. This high mortality justifies and indeed demands urgent investigation and consideration of surgical treatment. If subarachnoid haemorrhage is to be investigated at all, this must be done as soon as the patient is judged fit for any operation that might be indicated. Waiting six weeks and then investigating the survivors is a waste of time and lives.

Patients in coma should not be investigated, since surgery has nothing to offer unless they regain consciousness. In all other patients under the age of sixty bilateral carotid angiography should be undertaken. If no aneurysm or angioma is found further haemorrhage is unlikely and the cause of the initial haemorrhage remains unknown. In such patients vertebral angiography should be carried out if the patient is young, or if there has been repeated haemorrhage, but few aneurysms will be found. If one or more aneurysms are shown in the carotid territory a surgical attack can be planned. Of the common sites aneurysm of the internal carotid, of the junction of the posterior communicating and carotid arteries, and of the middle cerebral artery fare relatively well. Aneurysm of the anterior communicating artery is the most dangerous, whether operated on or not. Even the most technically successful of operations may be followed by extensive fatal cerebral infarction. Occasionally an aneurysm in the vertebral artery territory is amenable to surgery. The risks of subarachnoid haemorrhage and of aneurysm surgery are greatly increased by spasm of the cerebral arteries which is responsible for focal neurological signs and even cerebral infarction. The spasm is apparently in response to some component of the subarachnoid blood. A further complication is hydrocephalus due to blocking of the arachnoid villi by blood. This can develop rapidly and must be suspected if there is increasing drowsiness. It can be successfully treated by a shunt.

The indications for attempting to remove a cerebral angioma are highly individual for each patient and surgeon. Small angiomas well away from the motor cortex and speech area can be completely removed, but large malformations are inoperable. The decision to operate is further complicated by the extraordinary natural history of cerebral angioma. Some such lesions remain asymptomatic throughout life, while others cause a single haemorrhage followed by a prolonged period of normal health. In other instances repeated, crippling and eventually fatal haemorrhage occurs. Epilepsy is a common symptom of unruptured angiomas which may occasionally be revealed as the cause by calcification of abnormal vessels seen in skull X-rays, or by a carotid or cranial bruit. Many patients bleeding from an angioma give a history of migraine, but this is of no diagnostic value since the migraine differs in no respect from that encountered in sufferers without such a lesion. The investigation of cases of atypical or complicated migraine in search of angiomas is in fact almost uniformly unsuccessful.

UNRUPTURED ANEURYSMS

Many intracranial aneurysms cause no symptoms. An unruptured aneurysm declares itself only when it is large enough to compress neighbouring structures. The only common site for this is the internal carotid artery behind the orbit, where aneurysm may produce the orbital fissure syndrome of progressive ophthalmoplegia with pain and sensory loss in the distribution of the first division of the trigeminal nerve. The sudden onset of a third nerve palsy usually results from haemorrhage rather than sudden expansion of the aneurysm, but large aneurysms behave as tumours and rarely rupture. Such lesions may be several centimetres in diameter and partly filled with blood clot, while calcification in the wall can sometimes be seen in X-rays of the skull. The only indications for operating on an aneurysm of this kind are intractable pain or compression of the optic chiasma.

GIANT-CELL ARTERITIS

This is a generalized arterial disease of unknown cause, originally known as cranial arteritis, affecting those above the age of fifty-five. It usually presents with headache, often in one temple but frequently spreading to the opposite side and to the occiput. The pain is due to an inflammatory reaction in the arteries of the scalp which are swollen, tender and sometimes occluded. There are many variants, since the impact of the disease may be mainly on the arteries of the neck or shoulders, with widespread pain, and larger arteries may also be involved. A common symptom of diagnostic value is claudication of the jaw muscles, the pain arising from ischaemia during chewing. The occlusion of the lumen is seldom important in superficial vessels (though gangrene of the scalp is occasionally seen) but occlusion of carotid, coronary or mesenteric arteries causes infarction. The local symptoms are accompanied by those of general ill-health—low fever, anorexia and loss of weight.

The disease is self-limiting and recovers spontaneously, but only after months or years of distress. Apart from the rare involvement of large vessels the most important complication is occlusion of the ophthalmic arteries. This may occur rapidly and may affect both eyes, causing total blindness. The appearance of the retina in the acute stage shows no distinctive features and the arteries may appear remarkably normal. The visual loss is nearly always permanent and is succeeded by primary optic atrophy resulting from ischaemia of the optic nerve.

The diagnosis must always be considered in an elderly patient with headache. The sedimentation rate is always raised, often to 80 mm, and if the clinical findings are unmistakable treatment should begin immediately. If doubt exists, biopsy of a scalp artery is nearly always confirmatory, showing the inflammatory exudate containing giant cells in the vessel wall. The inflammatory element responds rapidly to corticosteroids but the effects of arterial occlusion, including blindness, cannot be reversed. On 40 mg of prednisone a day, rapidly reducing to a tolerable maintenance dose, the pain subsides almost immediately. Treatment must be continued for many months but the dose can then be gradually reduced with a constant watch on the sedimentation rate. If this rises, or if symptoms return, the previous dose must be restored.

The diagnosis is often missed and is also sometimes made in error in elderly patients with headache and a raised sedimentation rate. The latter mistake can be corrected if the headache persists in spite of treatment, but failure to recognize or suspect the disease may end in the tragedy of irrecoverable blindness.

OTHER FORMS OF ARTERITIS

The central nervous system may be involved in systemic lupus erythematosus and polyarteritis nodosa. In both conditions symptoms arise from cerebral ischaemia and infarction due to arterial occlusion, the result of inflammatory and necrotic changes in the vessel wall. The majority of arteries affected are of relatively small calibre and occlusion of a major vessel such as the middle cerebral artery is less common. As these changes can occur anywhere within the brain the symptoms are naturally extremely varied. In addition to the usual focal signs of infarction of the cerebral hemisphere or brain stem, symptoms suggesting more widespread involvement occur and are liable to misinterpretation. Confusion and hallucinations may sometimes closely resemble primary psychiatric disease, particularly in disseminated lupus where another curious presentation is with chorea. Many of the symptoms are capable of complete remission with or without steroid treatment and are not easily attributable to cerebral infarction. The diagnosis of these forms of arteritis must usually rest on the presence of systemic evidence of disease.

Takayashu's disease is a form of arteritis that predominantly involves the aorta and its branches. It is mainly a disease of young women and causes symptoms due to narrowing or occlusion of the major blood vessels in the neck. In the early stages the ESR is raised and treatment with steroids will arrest the disease. The chronic stages are not amenable to treatment. Takayashu's disease is rare in Great Britain.

VASCULAR DISEASE OF THE SPINAL CORD

The incidence of spinal cord infarction is low but is likely to increase in an ageing population and with advances in methods of reviving the apparently dead. The techniques of thoracic and aortic surgery also expose the spinal cord to risk, because infarction is more often due to interruption of the blood supply from remote causes than to disease of the spinal arteries themselves. Severe aortic atheroma or dissecting aneurysm may obliterate the intercostal arteries from which much of the blood supply of the cord is derived, and there is a particular risk in operations in which intercostal arteries on the left side at the level of the diaphragm are at risk, since this is the site of origin of the arteria magna supplying a large area of the dorsal cord. Profound shock and cardiac arrest are also potential causes of cord ischaemia. As they enter the spinal canal the arteries may be compressed by articular disease that narrows the foramina, and the ascending and descending meningeal vessels may be involved in any disease process that narrows the spinal canal.

The classical clinical syndrome is attributed to thrombosis of the anterior spinal artery, but is more accurately described as due to infarction or ischaemia in the distribution of this artery. The onset is sudden, with pain in the back followed by weakness or paralysis of the legs. The degree and distribution of the weakness varies greatly and may be unilateral, but the essence of the syndrome is the loss of pain and thermal sensation with retention of sensation conveyed in the posterior columns, which are supplied by the posterior spinal arteries. If the cervical cord is affected lower motor neurone paralysis occurs in the upper limbs. The prognosis is unexpectedly good, and although permanent paraplegia can result, many patients make an excellent functional recovery. Transient ischaemic attacks of the spinal cord can also be recognized, producing paraplegia with complete recovery within a few hours. The extent to which chronic progressive ischaemia of the cord can result in symptoms is not fully known but this cause can be suspected in some patients with obvious aortic disease and weakness and wasting of the legs.

Further reading

Benson D.F. (1977) Neurological correlates of aphasia and apraxia. In *Recent Advances in Clinical Neurology II*, ed. W.B. Matthews and G.H. Glaser. Churchill Livingstone, Edinburgh and London.

Feinglass E.J., Arnett F.C., Dorsch C.A., Zizic T.M. & Stevens M.B. (1976) Neuropsychiatric manifestations of systemic lupus erythematosus. *Medicine (Baltimore)* **55**, 323.

Fisher C.M. (1965) Lacunes: small deep cerebral infarcts. *Neurology* **15**, 774.

Ford R.G. & Siekert R.G. (1965) Central nervous system manifestations of periarteritis nodosa. *Neurology* **15**, 114.

Hamilton C.R., Shelley W.M. & Tumulty P.A. (1971) Giant cell arteritis. *Medicine (Baltimore)* **50**, 1.

Hutchinson E.C. & Acheson E.J. (1975) *Strokes: Natural History, Pathology and Surgical Treatment*. Saunders, London.

Marshall J. (1976) *The Management of Cerebrovascular Disease*, 3rd ed. Blackwell Scientific Publications, Oxford.

Matthews W.B. (1978) The treatment of acute cerebral infarction. In *Recent Advances in Clinical Neurology II*, ed. W.B. Matthews and G.H. Glaser. Churchill Livingstone, Edinburgh and London.

CHAPTER 10
Space-occupying Lesions of the Central Nervous System

INTRACRANIAL PRESSURE

The adult skull is a rigid box and its contents, the cerebrospinal fluid, blood and semi-solid brain, are incompressible. No expansion within the skull is possible without destruction or displacement of the confining bones or of the normal contents. The consequences may be illustrated by the effects of an infiltrating cerebral tumour.

At first the tumour may destroy brain tissue without increasing the size of the hemisphere, and symptoms will be those of disordered function of the destroyed and threatened neurones which represent the localizing signs of the lesion. As the tumour proliferates the bulk of the hemisphere eventually increases, a process often accentuated by oedema. There is little extracellular space in the brain, and the sometimes massive swelling in the vicinity of a tumour is mainly due to accumulation of fluid in glial cells. The intracranial pressure rises.

The cerebrospinal fluid pressure is normally measured manometrically during lumbar puncture with the patient lying down. In these circumstances the pressure of from 80 to 180 mm of water recorded is probably a reasonable measure of the normal intracranial pressure. However, this is only because the head is level with the site of the puncture, and although such 'normal' pressures are clinically useful they have little direct relationship to the intracranial pressure during physical activity in the upright posture. This pressure, relative to the atmosphere, is a complex function compounded of the arterial pressure transmitted to the capillaries and the hydrostatic pressure of the cerebrospinal fluid. The pressure within the venous sinuses is of cardinal importance, since these contain a large and rapidly variable volume of fluid in communication with a reservoir outside the skull. If normal absorption is to continue the venous pressure must be maintained a little below that of the cerebrospinal fluid.

The expanding tumour displaces venous blood from the skull, increasing vascular resistance and capillary pressure. Secretion of cerebrospinal fluid continues against a considerable head of pressure which a needle inserted directly into a lateral ventricle may show to be 500 mm of water or more. Venous engorgement can be seen in the optic fundi. In part at least, this is due to local venous constriction in the arachnoid sheath of the optic nerve, and this is probably also the cause of the papilloedema or swelling of the nerve head that follows. The increased capillary pressure causes retinal haemorrhages radiating from the disc. Brief attacks of darkened vision (visual obscurations) may be precipitated by movement or stooping, and herald the threat of irreversible blindness. Stretching of the meninges causes the headache often associated with raised intracranial pressure described in Chapter 3.

Vomiting is not an early symptom of raised intracranial pressure, but may occur as an initial isolated symptom of tumours within the fourth ventricle. It may accompany the characteristic early morning headache of brain tumour, and is also encountered in an effortless projectile form when intracranial pressure is extremely high.

The skull vault is not distensible after the sutures have fused, but below the age of ten the sutures can be forced apart by intense or long-continued pressure. The circumference of the skull increases and a 'cracked pot' note on percussion can be detected with varying confidence by experts. In both adult and child the delicate bony structure of the anterior and posterior clinoid processes may be eroded by long-continued pulsatile pressure transmitted through the floor of the third ventricle.

The tumour may obstruct the flow of cerebrospinal fluid at the 'narrows' of the foramen of Monro leading from the lateral to the third ventricle, or at the aqueduct from the third to the fourth ventricle. Secretion continues and the obstructed ventricle dilates because of venous compression and eventually from destruction of brain tissue.

The cranial cavity is divided into communicating compartments by the relatively rigid vertical falx cerebri between the two hemispheres and the horizontal tentorium cerebelli overlying the posterior fossa. Expansion within one compartment displaces brain tissue into the narrow openings in these dural barriers. Thus a rim of the medial surface of the hemisphere may be forced under the lower edge of the falx. Much more important is the tentorial cone, in which pressure above the tentorium forces the lower surface of the temporal lobe on one or both sides into the tentorial opening. There the third cranial nerve may be compressed, and the resulting dilated pupil is a common sign of dangerously increasing pressure. The wedges of temporal lobe also compress the brain stem with its reflex centres that are essential to life. These may be destroyed by haemorrhage as a secondary effect of the compression and distortion.

The cerebellar cone, in which brain tissue is actually extruded from the skull through the foramen magnum is a less common result of increased intracranial pressure. The cerebellar tonsils are forced down and compress the medulla, often fatally. Palsies of the sixth cranial nerve are a common sign of less drastic distortion of the brain stem, often from remote causes—a false localizing sign. Lumbar puncture in the presence of high intracranial pressure carries a definite risk of precipitating fatal coning. If papilloedema is present lumbar puncture should be undertaken only with the specific purpose of excluding or confirming a reasonable suspicion of meningitis or subarachnoid haemorrhage.

If pressure continues to rise unchecked, consciousness is intermittently disturbed, either from compression of the alerting mechanisms in the brain stem or by a more general reduction of cerebral blood flow. As an agonal event the intracranial pressure may even exceed that in the capillaries.

CEREBRAL TUMOUR

Tumours within the cranial cavity are relatively common, and while the majority conform to their evil reputation in being both malignant and inoperable their recognition and management are important and often difficult. Even histopathologically benign tumours are potentially fatal by reason of their pressure effects.

The commonest primary tumour is derived from glial cells and varies greatly in malignancy and rate of growth. At one extreme is the astrocytoma Grade I that may infiltrate the whole of one hemisphere causing little increase in bulk and barely distinguishable under the microscope from a simple proliferative astrocytic reaction. Higher grades are more rapidly growing and more easily recognizable as tumours. Large cysts may be formed with smooth walls and often only a mural nodule of tumour. At the other extreme is the glioblastoma multiforme or astrocytoma Grade IV. The cut surface of the brain at post-mortem examination shows areas of amorphous tissue, old and fresh haemorrhages, and small cysts with ragged walls. Even in such rampant growth areas may be found in which the histological picture is that of a low-grade astrocytoma: a terminal increase in malignancy is a common event.

Whatever its grade, the adult astrocytoma is scarcely accessible to cure by excision, because the edges of the tumour cannot be defined and there are limits to the amount of brain that can be sacrificed. However, the juvenile cystic type of astrocytoma, almost confined to the cerebellar hemisphere in children, has a quite different natural history and can be wholly excised without recurrence.

The medulloblastoma is also a tumour of early life and again involves structures in the posterior fossa, especially the cerebellar mid-line. It is thought to be derived from glial cells and is truly malignant, often seeding metastases throughout the subarachnoid space. Such a deposit may, for example, cause a rapidly developing paraplegia.

The oligodendroglioma is an infiltrating but slowly growing glial tumour. The ependymoma, derived from the ventricular lining, is rare in the brain and seen more frequently in the spinal cord. The haemangioblastoma is probably not derived from nervous tissue. Although it arises within the cerebellar hemisphere it is benign and often associated with a large cyst.

Blood-borne metastases in the brain are the commonest form of cerebral tumour, and despite every precaution the neurosurgeon not infrequently finds a secondary deposit at operation instead of the expected primary growth. They may be derived from cancer at any site, especially bronchus and breast, and are found in every part of the brain. At autopsy single secondary deposits are exceptional, and six or more may be found when clinical evidence pointed to a single lesion. Metastatic tumours are much more clearly circumscribed than primary glial growths, but their number usually frustrates attempts at removal.

Tumours compressing the brain from without are usually benign, though for anatomical reasons they are often dangerous and difficult of access. The meningioma (Fig. 21, following p. 152) has an attachment to the dura, and is usually a rounded slowly growing mass, potentially removable. Occasionally it forms a diffuse thickening over a large area at the base of the skull—meningioma *en plaque*—technically impossible to excise.

Adenomas of the pituitary are relatively common tumours and most are derived from the chromophobe cells. Malignant pituitary tumours are rare. The craniopharyngioma is derived from embryonic remnants and forms a usually cystic tumour above the pituitary fossa.

Benign tumours, miscalled neuromas, arise from the sheath of the acoustic nerve (VIIIth cranial nerve) and much more rarely from the Vth nerve. They are best regarded as a form of neurofibroma.

Rarities gratifying to diagnose since they can be cured are the colloid cyst of the third ventricle and the papilloma of the choroid plexus, usually in one lateral ventricle.

An exception to the benign nature of these extrinsic tumours is the chordoma derived from the primitive notochord. In the skull this usually develops in front of the brain stem from the clivus.

Clinical features

The symptoms and signs of a cerebral tumour are largely dependent on its site. Certain forms of tumour have a predilection for certain sites, and the rate of progression may also afford some evidence of the nature of the growth. Confident anatomical and pathological diagnosis on clinical grounds alone is often correct, but there is a wide margin of error. It is clearly impossible to do more than describe a few of the more commonly encountered clinical presentations.

Any cerebral tumour may cause symptoms and signs of raised intracranial pressure, but this is not invariable. Exuberantly expanding tumours and those that block the flow of cerebrospinal fluid are most likely to do so, but unexpectedly some patients with massive or multiple tumours develop neither headache nor papilloedema. Any tumour growing in the vicinity of the cerebral cortex may cause epilepsy, most often major fits without warning, but most suggestively fits with a focal onset. In slow growing tumours epilepsy may be the only symptom for many years. The investigation of such patients is described in Chapter 17.

The meningioma is a slow-growing tumour of middle life and it might be expected that the clinical development would be similarly protracted. This is sometimes so, but although epilepsy may be of some years' duration, other symptoms have often been present for only a few months before the diagnosis is established and the tumour is often found to be large. Slow compression of the brain may be asymptomatic until a late stage, and then suddenly manifest only because of some acute disturbance of local circulation. A short history does not exclude a benign tumour. Conversely, although an astrocytoma is technically malignant, its progressive focal symptoms may develop over a prolonged period of time.

Frontal lobe. Tumours of the anterior part of the frontal lobes, particularly on the right side, may give rise to no recognizable localizing symptoms or signs until a late stage. A change in personality, with apathy and depression, dementia, or misplaced jocularity may be noticed but misinterpreted as a primary psychiatric disorder. Incontinence of urine or sometimes deliberate inappropriate micturition is common. In the left hemisphere encroachment on the third convolution causes dysphasia. Posterior extension involves the motor cortex with resulting hemiparesis.

Most such tumours are astrocytomas or secondary deposits, but a meningioma arising from the olfactory groove extends upwards into the frontal lobe producing as its local sign loss of sense of smell on the side of the tumour and in the case of large tumours unilateral optic atrophy from compression of the optic nerve. Olfactory groove meningioma is the classical cause of the Foster Kennedy syndrome of optic atrophy from pressure on the nerve in one eye and papilloedema caused by the general rise in intracranial pressure in the other.

Another favoured site for the growth of a meningioma is in the immediate neighbourhood of the superior sagittal sinus, usually anteriorly. The initial symptoms are those of involvement of the motor cortex on the medial side of one hemisphere, with focal fits beginning in the opposite great toe, but on occasion both sides may be compressed causing bilateral spastic weakness of the legs that may be misinterpreted as paraplegia of spinal origin.

Parietal lobe. Tumours of the parietal lobe encroaching on the sensory cortex cause loss of sensation on the opposite side of the body. The forms of sensation most often distributed are those involving some element of discrimination, sense of position, or the comparison of different stimuli, but more basic forms of sensation, including that of pain, may certainly be impaired.

Stereognosis, or the recognition by touch of objects placed in the hand, is a complex function obviously disturbed when common sensation is impaired. Astereognosis without impairment of other forms of sensation is a sign of damage to the sensory cortex. Loss of discrimination is conveniently demonstrated by the two-point test. On the palmar surface of the terminal phalanges it is normally possible to distinguish two points even when they are no more than 2 mm apart. If sensation is impaired by a lesion of the sensory pathways below the cortical level there may be inability to distinguish the two points even when they are 5 mm apart. Nevertheless a definite threshold can be established above which no mistakes are made. With a cortical lesion mistakes continue to be made and no threshold can be found.

The use of the affected limbs is impaired, partly due to lack of knowledge of their position in space, but often accentuated by disturbance of those functions of the parietal lobe concerned with appreciation of spatial relationships, both within the body and in relation to the external world. The 'body image', our awareness of the position, proportions and even existence of our own body appears to depend on an intact parietal lobe. Disorders of this essential awareness range from slight neglect of the limbs opposite to the side of the lesion to a total denial of their existence. In extreme cases it may even be claimed by the patient that they are part of some other person. Even minor degrees of neglect include lack of awareness or actual denial of disability. The lesser symptoms usually encountered include reluctance to use the arm, even though the strength is normal; falling away of the outstretched upper limb when the eyes are closed even when postural sense is but slightly impaired; and neglecting to attend to the affected limbs, like failing to tie the shoelace. The ability to name parts of the body may occasionally be lost, without any other evidence of aphasia. There is usually an accompanying lack of full awareness of external space, so that obstacles on the affected side are not avoided even when they are clearly seen.

An interesting disorder of sensory appreciation can often be detected —failure to recognize bilateral simultaneous stimuli. When symmetrical points are touched simultaneously only that on the normal side will be felt, even though sensation is normal when each side is touched separately. Like most forms of cortical dysfunction this sign, known as sensory extinction, is highly variable.

In addition to the awareness of space on one or other side, the parietal lobe of the hemisphere non-dominant for speech, normally the right, plays an important part in many complex functions concerned with orientation. In tumours or other lesions of this region a common symptom is that of being lost in familiar surroundings. Right and left are confused, and tasks such as laying the table or dressing become impossible. This disorder of spatial awareness can be shown by asking the patient to copy simple patterns, to arrange matchsticks, or to draw a house or a clock face. The nature of the task is understood, but absurd mistakes are made and characteristically covered by futile excuses such as a plea of lack of artistic skill in the patient called upon to draw a circle. The defect is known as constructional apraxia. The ability to manipulate numbers, which are arranged spatially in many peoples' minds, is also sometimes lost—acalculia, although this is more characteristic of lesions of the dominant hemisphere.

Neighbouring structures are often involved, notably the optic radiation. Even when no defect of the visual field can be detected by ordinary means there may be a failure to appreciate bilateral simultaneous stimuli, including gross movements.

Temporal lobe. The signs of a tumour in this region depend mainly on whether the side dominant for speech is involved. Progressive dysphasia occurs with any tumour of the left temporal lobe, but on the right side a tumour may be relatively or entirely 'silent' until symptoms of raised pressure develop. The lower fibres of the optic radiation sweep forward into the temporal cortex, so that hemianopic field defects are common. Temporal lobe tumours are often associated with epileptic manifestations and emotional disturbances, especially if the major hemisphere is involved. Precisely similar visual field defects are caused by tumours of the occipital lobe, but since the area of the visual cortex is small complete hemianopia usually develops. In a more anteriorly placed parieto-occipital lesion a failure to appreciate the significance of objects seen is more striking than hemianopia, though a half-field defect of some degree is usually present.

Tumours arising from the *pituitary gland* or its immediate neighbourhood may compress the optic chiasma from below. Although there are variations depending on the shape of the tumour and the position of the chiasma the usual result is that the decussating fibres are compressed. As these come from the nasal half of each retina the resulting hemianopia is bitemporal. This develops gradually, and the earlier stages are much less easily detected and interpreted, particularly when there is only slight loss of one upper temporal field. It is astonishing how often patients ignore progressive visual loss confined to one eye and how often their complaints are dismissed as trivial when they do seek advice. Progressive visual failure must have a cause and the cause must be found. Testing the visual fields by confrontation is an easy and essential test frequently and disastrously omitted. Visual failure proceeds beyond the temporal fields, even to total blindness. The optic discs show primary atrophy and even with large tumours papilloedema is not seen. A tumour at this site, and especially a suprasellar meningioma, may grow upwards and compress the frontal lobes.

Tumours of the pituitary itself cause prominent endocrine disorders, nearly all resulting from loss of function of the gland. Amenorrhoea may precede other symptoms by many years. In the male, impotence is an early symptom, followed by progressive loss of facial and body hair. The youthful almost unwrinkled face is characteristic. These secondary effects of failure to secrete gonadotrophins are common, but the more serious effects of failure to stimulate the adrenal cortex are rarely seen in chronic destructive lesions of the pituitary. The aim is naturally to diagnose these tumours as early as possible long before they have caused damage to neighbouring structures or severe irreversible endocrine disorders. Minute tumours are now being found that secrete prolactin, resulting in amenorrhoea and sometimes lactation. The only radiological change is slight asymmetry of the floor of the pituitary fossa.

The common adenoma of the chromophobe cells is usually simply destructive, though it is occasionally accompanied by excessive hormonal secretion causing acromegaly, which more frequently results from an adenoma of the eosinophil cells. Although other hormones are formed in excess, the main clinical effect is due to overproduction of the growth hormone. Before the epiphyses have fused gigantism results, but this is rare. In adult life abnormal bone growth is seen mainly in the lower jaw and in the hands and feet, which are broad and massive with tufting of the terminal phalanges seen on X-ray. The frontal sinuses are also greatly enlarged. The characteristically coarse facial appearance is mainly due to soft tissue overgrowth that is particularly well seen in the tongue. Internal organs such as the liver, spleen and heart may be enlarged. Acromegalics are often very powerfully built but eventually destruction of the gland leads to hypopituitarism. Signs of compression of the chiasma are not invariable. The adenoma may remain confined to the pituitary fossa, and mild and apparently static cases of acromegaly are not uncommon.

Basophil tumours of the pituitary are present in Cushing's disease but hardly ever declare themselves as space-occupying lesions, and treatment of the endocrine abnormality must be directed to the overacting adrenal glands.

The *craniopharyngioma* usually presents at an earlier age than the pituitary adenoma, most often in children. Growth may be retarded, puberty delayed, and the chiasma compressed. These lesions often contain radiologically visible flecks of calcium.

A tumour in one *cerebellar hemisphere*, usually an astrocytoma or a haemangioblastoma, causes progressive disability in the limbs on the same side. Loss of cerebellar function prevents the smooth coordination of movements. Such cerebellar ataxia results from a break in the link between the afferent flow to the cerebellum and the outflow to the motor centres, with an obvious failure to maintain and correct the posture of the limbs. The hand no longer moves steadily to its objective, but first overshoots and then is in turn overcorrected. If the outstretched arm is pushed aside it does not immediately return to its former position but swings past it and is once more overcorrected. These abnormalities are displayed when the patient touches his nose and the examiner's finger alternately, or runs his heel down his shin. Rapidly alternating movements may be affected before disturbance of larger movements is obvious. Various elements of this type of ataxia have been differently named, but all are signs of failure to coordinate sensory data with motor performance and of a resultant inability to maintain posture or to adjust to changes in posture.

A *mid-line cerebellar tumour*, usually a medulloblastoma, has a specific effect on walking and standing. The afferent flow from the vestibular nuclei is intimately concerned with the posture of the trunk, and is relayed to this area. At first the child's gait is ataxic and he lurches from side to side with the feet widely spread. Later, walking, standing, or even sitting unsupported become impossible.

Nystagmus is commonly though not invariably present in cerebellar lesions, but it is more typical of a lateral lobe than a mid-line lesion, and its character and direction are unreliable localizing signs.

The commonest tumour in the *cerebello-pontine angle* is an acoustic neurofibroma, and it produces a characteristic syndrome. Pressure on adjacent cranial nerves causes varying degrees of unilateral deafness and loss of vestibular nerve function; facial weakness and loss of sense of taste; and loss of the corneal reflex with sensory impairment on the face. In many cases the eighth, fifth and seventh nerves are involved in that order, the sixth at a later stage. Cerebellar involvement causes nystagmus and ipsilateral ataxia. Pressure on the pons may involve the long ascending and descending tracts, in particular the corticospinal tracts. By the time this syndrome has developed the opportunity for effective curative treatment has long passed. The aim is to discover these tumours while they are confined to the internal auditory meatus. This is not easy but suspicion must always be aroused by unilateral nerve deafness. As with visual failure a cause must be found and this is often neglected.

An infiltrating glioma of the *pons* causes an insidious but remorselessly progressive succession of cranial nerve palsies and long tract signs before there is any evidence of raised intracranial pressure (Fig. 23, following p. 152). This is especially surprising since most other expanding lesions in the posterior fossa readily obstruct the flow of cerebrospinal fluid by distorting the aqueduct or blocking the outflow from the fourth ventricle.

Diagnosis of cerebral tumours

Many intracranial tumours present with epilepsy, a diagnostic problem discussed in Chapter 17. Any patient with progressive signs suggesting a single lesion in the brain will naturally be suspected of having a cerebral tumour. Although patients in this group pose anxious problems the diagnosis is seldom difficult. The type of tumour may be suspected from its site and rate of development, and from the age of the patient. Thus the rapid onset of an ataxic gait and signs of raised intracranial pressure in a child strongly suggest a medulloblastoma. More gradual development and asymmetrical ataxia raise the hope of a juvenile astrocytoma of the cerebellar hemisphere. Chiasmal compression in a child suggests a craniopharyngioma and in an adult a pituitary adenoma, but other possibilities exist. The inexorable development of dysphasia and right-sided weakness in the middle-aged or elderly patient is strong presumptive evidence of a glioblastoma or a metastasis. All such conclusions are necessarily tentative.

To these patients who obviously demand investigation must be added an important group in whom the suspicion of cerebral tumour is much less obvious. This will include very few patients in whom the only ground for suspicion is a complaint of headache, since contrary to popular belief only a minute proportion of such patients have cerebral tumours. The patient with dementia, personality change, or depression may present formidable diagnostic difficulties. The unwitting treatment of a meningioma with electroconvulsive therapy sounds difficult to defend, but in practice such a mistake is sometimes unavoidable. In this type of patient the best chance of ultimately successful diagnosis lies in continued awareness that clinical features incompatible with an original diagnosis of primary psychiatric disease must have some other explanation.

Investigations should always include radiographs of the chest to exclude primary or secondary tumours. X-ray of the skull may show calcification in a tumour. Almost all forms of slowly growing tumour occasionally calcify, but there is a much higher incidence in the oligo-dendroglioma and craniopharyngioma. Erosive secondary deposits in the skull vault may indicate the nature of the cerebral lesion. The bone near the origin of a meningioma may be either thickened or eroded, and vascular channels in the bone may be unduly prominent. The calcified pineal gland may be pushed across the mid-line by lateral pressure.

The invention of computerized axial tomography (CT scanning) has revolutionized the investigation of patients suspected of having a brain tumour. The method produces a picture of the relative radiodensity of the structures in a transverse slice across the skull and brain. Increased density can often be enhanced by the intravenous injection of an iodine-containing substance that is selectively taken up by some forms of tumour and other abnormal structures. Not only is the technique harmless and only mildly unpleasant but it is much more informative than other methods. The anatomy of the lesion is usually displayed in some detail and the pathology can often be determined by the shape and other characteristics of the tumour.

With the exception of certain special techniques used in the discovery of small acoustic tumours and in a few other situations the CT scan has rendered all other techniques of investigating brain tumours obsolete. As the CT scan is not universally available some account of other methods is probably still necessary.

The electroencephalogram (EEG) is often abnormal, since slow activity is generated by damaged or oedematous brain in the vicinity of a tumour. The growth itself is electrically silent. A normal record does not exclude tumour and minor abnormalities can be misleading. A persistent focus of high voltage slow activity (delta) is fairly reliable evidence of a focal lesion, although not of its nature, but when this is present there are usually other obvious signs. In the anterior frontal lobes, however, a focus of this kind may be the only evidence of a tumour. A glioma or metastasis of recent origin is more likely to yield positive EEG findings than a longstanding meningioma or astrocytoma.

Echoencephalography, or the use of ultrasound in the exploration of the cranial contents, is sometimes helpful in the diagnosis of tumours. The mid-line structures of the forebrain can usually be reliably located, and these may be displaced by expanding lesions of the hemisphere. An equally harmless and far more rewarding investigation is the gamma-scan. A radioisotope, at present usually technetium, is given by mouth or by intravenous injection and is preferentially absorbed by some tumours and also by infarcts and certain other lesions because of local breakdown of the blood-brain barrier. The gamma radiation can be localized through the intact skull.

Carotid angiography was formerly an essential investigation in tumours above the tentorium. Distortion and displacement of arteries and veins often provide clear localizing evidence, and an abnormal circulation pattern may outline the tumour or even suggest its pathology. Tumours in the posterior fossa are not outlined by carotid angiography, but the investigation may still usefully reveal stretch of the anterior cerebral arteries due to dilatation of the lateral ventricles. Vertebral angiography is of less value in the investigation of posterior fossa tumours mainly because the pictures are difficult to interpret.

The techniques of outlining the ventricles and subarachnoid spaces with air, injected either by lumbar puncture or directly through a burr-hole into the lateral ventricle, are now obsolete.

It will be noted that lumbar puncture has not been included as an essential step in the investigation of a suspected cerebral tumour. Where intracranial pressure is raised the procedure is firmly contraindicated. If there is strong evidence of a progressive focal lesion lumbar puncture is unnecessary. If there is doubt as to the presence of an expanding lesion it may be useful in showing that the pressure is indeed raised, or it may reveal an increased cerebrospinal fluid protein content, confirming that there is at least some lesion requiring further elucidation. If CT scanning is available it is greatly to be preferred. A normal lumbar puncture and cerebrospinal fluid do not exclude any form of cerebral tumour, though the protein content is nearly always raised by an acoustic neurofibroma or an intraventricular tumour.

Precise pathological diagnosis of the tumour has a profound influence on possible treatment. Sometimes the pathology can be accepted as malignant from the history and physical and radiological signs. If a benign tumour is still thought to be a possibility it must be examined under a microscope. In some centres the practice of obtaining a fragment of the lesion through a burr-hole still obtains. The specimen is often valueless and the procedure has an appreciable mortality. It is better either to accept the radiological evidence or to conduct a more elaborate exploration.

Treatment

Any operation on the brain carries some risk of unexpected complications, and especially of infarction or haemorrhage. Many benign tumours can be excised with complete success, but there is a definite, although small mortality and morbidity even in the removal of meningiomas from the surface of the cerebral hemispheres. In general the more the brain has to be disturbed to reach the tumour the greater the risk of vascular damage, particularly of infarction in the distribution of the perforating branches of the anterior and middle cerebral arteries. Some meningiomas are so applied to the base of the skull that their removal would carry unacceptable risks. The acoustic neurofibroma is benign but the mortality is disappointingly high if operation is delayed until the onset of raised intracranial pressure. The craniopharyngioma is also benign and often cystic but complete removal is difficult because of its attachment to the hypothalamus in the floor of the third ventricle. Pituitary adenomas can be removed and blindness averted, but endocrine substitution therapy requires continued careful supervision. The neurosurgeon's problems are by no means solved by confirmation of the presence of a benign tumour.

Malignant tumours can seldom be excised but this does not mean that none are operable. It is pointless to attempt the partial excision of a rapidly growing glioblastoma, but removal of a cystic astrocytoma or partial excision (internal decompression) of a low-grade glioma may afford considerable relief of symptoms and a few years of life. Again multiple secondary deposits are best left alone, but an apparently single metastasis causing severe symptoms and markedly raised intracranial pressure can often be removed with great relief of suffering although seldom much prolongation of life. Rational palliative neurosurgery has much to offer.

Radiotherapy for cerebral tumours is disappointing and seldom achieves anything in tumours judged to be inoperable. There is a better theoretical case for radiotherapy after successful partial removal of a malignant tumour but its value is uncertain.

Symptomatic medical treatment of gliomas and metastatic malignant tumours with high intracranial pressure and much surrounding oedema of the brain is sometimes remarkably successful, although of course success is temporary. Dexamethasone, 5 mg six-hourly by mouth or by injection, reducing gradually to maintenance dose may result in an astonishing reversal of localizing signs and of evidence of raised intracranial pressure. This is, indeed, a great advance in the management of malignant tumours. If there is a response it can often be maintained for many months, and when deterioration occurs it is abrupt. This is greatly preferable to the lingering decline to a miserable end often seen before the introduction of steroid therapy.

Reduction of raised intracranial pressure by the use of intravenous hypertonic solutions is valuable in an emergency to improve a patient's condition sufficiently to permit investigation or operation. The effect is produced in a few minutes and lasts a few hours, but if a lasting reduction of pressure has not been achieved during this interval it is often followed by a recurrence or 'rebound' of increased pressure. An intravenous 30% solution of urea in doses of 30–90 g is the most potent agent for cerebral dehydration. It has the disadvantages of being extremely irritant to tissues at the point of infusion, and causing cardiovascular disturbances if administered too quickly. Mannitol 10–15% solution 3–500 ml intravenously, having a much larger molecule, has a less dramatic effect, but it is safer in use and is probably the most popular agent at present. Sucrose 50% up to 120 ml is a very swift and effective cerebral dehydrator in an emergency. Glycerol, 50 g in a 10% solution in glucose-saline has also been used. Both urea and glycerol may be given by mouth but with less benefit.

CEREBRAL ABSCESSES

Abscesses in the brain arise from direct spread of the infection from the middle ear or frontal sinuses, from penetrating wounds or from blood-borne infection. Lung abscess and bronchiectasis which were common sources of metastatic infection are now comparatively rare, but in congenital heart disease infection may reach the brain more easily since the blood may not pass through the filter of the lungs. Closed head injury may sometimes appear to cause brain abscess, perhaps because the damaged brain provides an area of lessened resistance to infection. When an organism can be identified it is usually either a staphylococcus or a streptococcus.

The common site of an otogenic abscess is in the temporal lobe, causing aphasia if the dominant hemisphere is affected and sometimes a hemianopia or an upper motor neurone palsy of the opposite side of the face due to involvement of the lowest part of the motor cortex. Pus from the ear may spread posteriorly into the cerebellar hemisphere, but clinical localizing evidence may be scanty. Frontal abscesses from sinusitis usually produce no focal signs unless they are very large, when hemiplegia occurs. In this situation the pus may spread extensively in the subdural space with an increased likelihood of epilepsy and even of status epilepticus. Metastatic abscesses may, of course, produce a great variety of focal symptoms depending on their site.

Intracranial pressure usually increases rapidly and the patient becomes drowsy or stuporose. There is seldom much fever or other systemic evidence of infection. Lumbar puncture *must* be avoided if an abscess is seriously suspected, because of the danger of coning, but if the cerebrospinal fluid is examined an increase in white cells to around 100 per mm^3 may be found and a few at least are polymorphonuclear leucocytes, although the fluid can be normal at first if the abscess is deeply situated. The left temporal lobe otogenic abscess is easy to diagnose, but frontal, metastatic, and subdural abscesses may be extremely difficult. The diagnosis must always be considered in a young patient with rapidly advancing evidence of a focal cerebral lesion or with raised intracranial pressure without local signs.

Cerebral abscesses are shown very well on the CT scan (Fig. 24, following p. 152) and other methods of diagnosis are not now required unless no scan is available. The EEG is often of real value in diagnosis since an abscess in the cerebral hemisphere is an acute lesion and almost invariably induces very high voltage slow discharges from the surrounding brain. The isotope brain scan will also reliably demonstrate an abscess in the cerebral hemisphere but cerebellar and subdural abscesses are less easily detected in this way. Carotid angiography may be used to localize cerebral abscesses but definite diagnosis depends on pus being found by the surgeon's exploring needle.

Treatment consists first in aspiration of the abscess, repeated if necessary. Failure to improve may be due to multilocular or multiple abscesses. Some surgeons excise abscesses immediately without aspiration. Massive systemic antibiotic treatment must be given, if possible adjusted to the sensitivity of the organism. Metronidazole may be required for anaerobic organisms, often present in brain abscesses. Antibiotics may also be injected into the abscess cavity, but the epileptogenic activity of concentrated penicillin must not be forgotten. The tendency to recurrence is the main indication for surgical excision after the lesion has been localized and sealed off by the above measures, but the condition is a serious one and the prognosis remains unexpectedly bad. Modern surgery and potent antibiotics often fail to prevent spreading or resistant infection and irreparable brain damage. The mortality cannot be much less than 50%. In those who recover the incidence of epilepsy is high.

BENIGN INTRACRANIAL HYPERTENSION

In this strange condition the intracranial pressure is greatly increased in the absence of any expanding lesion or any obstruction to the flow of cerebrospinal fluid. It predominantly affects women and is particularly apt to occur at times of physiological hormonal change—the menarche, pregnancy and the puerperium—and also in a separate subgroup of fat young women. It can occur in the male and also in children of both sexes. The effect of hormonal changes is shown by the intracranial hypertension that develops in some children on long-term corticosteroid treatment, particularly after a change of dose.

The symptoms and signs are those of raised intracranial pressure; headaches, visual obscurations, papilloedema and sixth nerve palsies. In general the symptomatic disturbance is less severe than from a similar rise of pressure due to tumour. Consciousness is not disturbed nor life threatened, but vision is at risk and may occasionally demand urgent unilateral or bilateral subtemporal decompression. Unrelieved, the severe papilloedema may cause rapidly progressive and irreversible blindness.

The diagnosis may be suspected on clinical grounds, but there are obvious serious risks of overlooking other causes of high pressure. Many a 'pseudo-tumour', as the condition was once described, has proved all too genuine. The CT scan shows small, apparently squeezed ventricles, without distortion. This is not therefore 'hydrocephalus', since there is no increase in the quantity of cerebrospinal fluid. The raised pressure is probably due to diffuse swelling of the brain itself, speculatively related to increased capillary permeability. In a few instances a similar syndrome arises from obstruction to the venous outflow from the cranial cavity due to venous or venous sinus thrombosis—a rare complication of infective processes in the middle ear, face, or sinuses.

Once the radiological findings of benign intracranial hypertension have been established treatment can be directed to lowering the pressure without fear of unpleasant consequences. In this disorder coning does not occur on lumbar puncture, and repeated puncture lowering the pressure to normal on each occasion has been used successfully in treatment. Less traumatic is the use of the diuretic chlorthalidone with potassium supplements. Progress can be monitored by plotting the size of the blind spots which are enlarged by the papilloedema. Treatment must often be prolonged and recurrence is possible.

TUMOURS OF THE SPINAL CORD

Most tumours involving the spinal cord occur by compression from outside, and in contrast to the brain intrinsic tumours are rare. The intrinsic astrocytoma encountered is slow-growing and extensively invasive rather than destructive. The ependymoma may form a cyst extending through many segments of the cord, and contains fluid of high protein content. The filum terminale, the vestigial remnant of the spinal cord in the lumbar and sacral canal, may be the site of a solid ependymoma.

Extrinsic tumours are often benign, the commonest being the neurofibroma growing from a nerve root, and the meningioma. Either may form a smooth usually rounded tumour, sometimes with an extension through the intervertebral foramen to form a 'dumb-bell' mass. The common malignant tumour is metastatic carcinoma from virtually any site. Such a growth often forms a constrictive collar outside the dura, sometimes obviously growing from a deposit in a vertebral body. Myeloma is also a relatively common cause of cord compression. The rare chordoma occurs in the cervical and sacral regions. It is malignant and often rapidly growing.

Clinical features

The symptoms and signs of spinal cord compression are those of progressive dysfunction of the ascending and descending tracts and of the motor and sensory roots at the level of the lesion. Their understanding comprises a straightforward exercise in applied anatomy and physiology, but misinterpretation is common. The effects of traumatic spinal cord lesions were described in Chapter 5. Those of compressive lesions naturally vary according to the site and nature of the compression. The two common diagnostic problems are those of the chronic and of the acute lesion.

CHRONIC COMPRESSION

Chronic spinal cord compression is likely to be due to benign and entirely curable causes, and removal of a spinal neurofibroma or meningioma may be followed by complete recovery even of severe paraplegia. Failure to make the diagnosis exacts a comparable penalty.

Root pain may be an early symptom, particularly of neurofibroma. In the arm this is indistinguishable from that caused by cervical spondylosis but it is at any rate usually recognizable as root pain. Pain from compression of a dorsal root is felt in one side of the chest or abdomen and there are obvious opportunities for misdiagnosis, especially since the neural origin of the pain is seldom betrayed by accompanying paraesthesiae or sensory loss. The patient may be saved from laparotomy only by recognition that the pain is related to change of spinal posture or to coughing, which raises pressure in the spinal canal by venous compression. When the pain follows the sloping distribution of the dermatome from back to front or is in a bilateral girdle distribution it is more easily recognized.

Compression of the corticospinal tract causes spastic weakness, nearly always asymmetrical and progressive over months or years. If the lesion is cervical the arm on the side of the lesion may be first affected and then the ipsilateral leg, but there is much variation. Paraesthesiae of the type due to disease of the posterior columns (Chapter 3) are common, but a complaint of loss of sensation is rare in the early stages. Failure of normal bladder control is increasingly common as the disease progresses. At any stage a fall or similar slight trauma may cause severe aggravation of the paraparesis.

Once the initial and often sadly hesitant step in diagnosis has been taken in that the progressive difficulty in walking is recognized as the result of spinal cord disease, the cause must be determined. Although there are numerous causes of progressive spastic paraparesis the problem is mainly that of distinguishing spinal cord compression due to tumour from multiple sclerosis, cervical myelopathy due to spondylosis, or subacute combined degeneration. An absolute distinction may not be possible on clinical grounds but a very careful search must be made for loss or blunting of cutaneous sensation and in particular for any suggestion of an upper level of sensory loss. A tumour compressing the spinal cord from one side may produce a partial Brown–Séquard syndrome, though nearly always with bilateral extensor plantar responses.

An intramedullary tumour, growing within the cord, may encroach on the spinothalamic tracts from their internal aspect, thus damaging recently entered fibres and sparing those from lower segments with preservation of sensation in the sacral segments (so-called sacral 'sparing' or 'escape'). Investigation rarely reveals a spinal tumour in the absence of definite cutaneous sensory changes, and conversely a persistent sensory level of this kind is very uncommon in multiple sclerosis. Café-au-lait patches or other evidence of cutaneous neurofibromatosis may suggest a spinal neurofibroma. X-rays of the spine sometimes provide useful information. The canal may be widened due to erosion of the inner surfaces of the pedicles of the vertebrae by a slow-growing tumour. An intervertebral foramen may be enlarged by a neurofibroma. Often enough, however, spinal tumour presents as spastic weakness and loss of vibration sense with neither clinical nor radiological pointers to a specific cause.

In these circumstances it was traditional practice to use Queckenstedt's test for spinal block, demonstrated by the failure of jugular compression to induce a pressure rise in a manometer attached to a lumbar puncture needle. This is not a very reliable test and has been largely replaced by myelography which must be regarded as an obligatory investigation where there is any possibility that a spinal cord lesion might be due to compression.

The method now used in Britain is to inject a water-soluble iodine-containing substance metrizamide by lumbar puncture and to screen its passage through the subarachnoid space. The interpretation of this investigation is difficult, but a complete obstruction in the spinal canal is easily demonstrated. It is often possible to advance a reasonably accurate opinion on the cause of the block and as to whether it arises from a lesion within the cord or from compression by tumour within or outside the dura. Although it is an essential investigation in spinal cord disease, myelography must not be regarded as merely a simple screening test. It is uncomfortable, and although any but trivial side-effects are very rare it is sometimes followed either by a sterile meningeal reaction or by a complaint of discomfort in the lower limbs: it is no investigation for the amateur.

The treatment of spinal neurofibroma or meningioma is in no doubt; they must be excised as soon as possible. The treatment of intramedullary tumours is naturally more difficult. Excision is often impracticable and may result in paraplegia. Prolonged remission may follow simple surgical decompression of the spinal cord.

Myelography may reveal lesions other than tumour. The arteriovenous malformation or angioma can present with progressive paraparesis, perhaps punctuated by one or more subarachnoid haemorrhages. At least some of the damage to the spinal cord is due to compression from the large pulsating vessels bound to the cord by the arachnoid membrane: their removal is sometimes beneficial.

A prolapsed dorsal intervertebral disc may narrow the spinal canal and compress the cord. The clinical presentation is indistinguishable from that of other forms of chronic compression, and the diagnosis may be made only by myelography or at operation. The results of operation are often disappointing, no doubt because of the precarious blood supply of the dorsal cord. There is grave risk of post-operative paraplegia unless the operative approach is deliberately planned to allow access to the disc without disturbing the spinal cord.

ACUTE COMPRESSION

The diagnostic problems and management of acute spinal cord compression present quite different problems. Paralysis advances rapidly over the course of a few days, accompanied by subjective numbness up to a definite level, and by retention of urine. The differential diagnosis is between acute compression of the cord by tumour or abscess, acute relapse of multiple sclerosis, transverse myelitis, or infarction of the cord. Apart from evidence of more widespread disease of the nervous system in multiple sclerosis, or of carcinoma elsewhere, there is no certain clinical guide to diagnosis. An X-ray may show vertebral collapse due to a secondary deposit. There is no time for deliberation over the possible meaning of any change in the cerebrospinal fluid, and a myelogram should be done immediately. The results of operative decompression of the commonest cause of this syndrome—extradural compression of the dorsal cord from carcinoma—are poor, but if anything is to be attempted it must be done before the spinal cord lesion is complete.

Acute epidural staphylococcal abscess is rare. It is sometimes associated with superficial sepsis, but may arise for no discernible reason, when a severe constitutional disturbance and possibly some local tenderness may be the only suggestive evidence of the cause of spinal cord compression. Diagnosis is scarcely possible without operation. Unfortunately the cord may be permanently damaged even if it is treated with the utmost despatch.

Acute Pott's paraplegia due to a tuberculous cold abscess is now rare, but chronic progressive paraparesis is still sometimes encountered, associated with severe angulation of the spine from old tuberculosis, and usually responds well to appropriate surgical measures.

THE CAUDA EQUINA

Tumours in the spinal canal below the first lumbar vertebra compress the cauda equina, the leash of nerve roots extending below the termination of the cord. The symptoms and signs are therefore entirely those of lower motor neurone and posterior root involvement. Root pain is of sciatic distribution and often bilateral. Weakness and wasting of the glutei and sensory loss in sacral dermatomes escape detection in routine examination with the patient on his back. The reflex arcs controlling the sphincters are interrupted, and retention of urine with overflow is common. At the level of the first lumbar vertebra the terminal portion of the cord, the conus medullaris, is compressed. Clinically this is scarcely to be distinguished from a lesion of the cauda equina, except that sphincter dysfunction is often the earliest symptom.

Further reading

Northfield D.W.C. (1973) *The Surgery of the Central Nervous System*. Blackwell Scientific Publications, Oxford.
Weisberg L.A. (1975) Benign intracranial hypertension. *Medicine (Baltimore)* **54,** 197.

CHAPTER 11
Infections

The impact of acute and chronic bacterial infection on the nervous system and its coverings has been greatly modified by chemotherapeutic agents and antibiotics, and notable advances have also been made in the prevention of viral infection. Nevertheless, morbidity and mortality are still higher than might have been hoped and such infections can present formidable diagnostic and therapeutic problems.

MENINGITIS

Pathology

Although the dura mater is occasionally involved in localized purulent infection, for practical purposes meningitis implies infection of the leptomeninges, the pia and arachnoid membranes, the subarachnoid space and the cerebral ventricles. Acute and subacute bacterial infection produces a severe inflammatory reaction with a purulent exudate in the cerebrospinal fluid. The infection can seldom be confined to the meninges and certainly in fatal cases it is found to have spread into the substance of the brain and spinal cord, notably around the blood vessels. In purulent meningitis the exudate consists of polymorphonuclear leucocytes, while in tuberculous meningitis chronic inflammatory cells are more prominent. Dense organized exudate may be formed over the base of the brain and over the convexity and in the spinal canal, particularly in tuberculous infection. Cranial nerves may be involved in this exudate, which may persist after infection has cleared and obstruct the flow or absorption of cerebrospinal fluid and cause hydrocephalus. Damage to the central nervous system results from direct invasion of bacteria and from thrombosis of cerebral veins and arterioles.

The inflammation in viral meningitis is much less severe. It is not purulent and no organized exudate is formed, but the meningitis is usually secondary to viral infection of the brain. Perivascular cuffing with inflammatory cells is common to all forms of fatal meningoencephalitis.

Clinical features

Certain clinical features are common to all forms of meningitis in the adult but are greatly modified by the severity and speed of evolution of the disease. Headache is almost invariable and usually severe, but in mild cases it differs little from that of any febrile illness. In bacterial infections, if untreated, and rarely in virus infections, the level of consciousness is increasingly disturbed, progressing from slight drowsiness and restless confusion to deep coma. Focal damage to the brain may occur in any form of meningitis, and cranial nerve palsies, particularly of the VIth nerve, are common.

Signs of *meningeal irritation* are present in the adult and usually in children. Of these neck rigidity is the most reliable. Normally it is possible to flex the neck so that the chin almost reaches the chest, although in the elderly movement is more restricted. In meningitis passive neck flexion is limited to a greater or lesser degree. In extreme examples, now seldom seen, the head is retracted in opisthotonos, and in severe infections the neck can be flexed only a few degrees. Less severe degrees of neck rigidity are not easy to recognize with certainty, and since to overlook bacterial meningitis may be to miss the opportunity of effective treatment the decision can be an anxious one. Kernig's sign is not very helpful. If the thigh is flexed to 90° in a young person it is normally possible to extend the knee almost to a straight line with the thigh. In severe and obvious meningitis the extension is limited by muscle spasm and the sign is positive. However, when neck rigidity is in doubt Kernig's sign is seldom positive.

In infants, meningitis develops with none of the signs familiar in the adult, though below the age of 12 months distension of the fontanelle may give a clue. In a baby a severe illness for which there is no obvious immediate cause is an indication for a lumbar puncture.

Errors in the diagnosis and management of meningitis, attended by grievous consequences for the patient, are still lamentably common. Before describing specific infections in detail some attention should be paid to this general problem. Not only must the different kinds of meningitis be recognized but meningitis must be distinguished from other infections and from other causes of meningeal irritation. Decisions must be reached rapidly and with as much certainty as the evidence allows for there is little time for vacillation and urgent definitive measures must be taken.

In the management of acute infections the general practitioner is subjected to almost intolerable pressure to use antibiotics in the absence of precise diagnosis. In banal infections this policy is naturally successful, although unnecessary, and no doubt many potentially serious infections are also cured in this way. If the infection so treated with inadequate uncontrolled administration of antibiotics is, in fact, bacterial meningitis, the results are deplorable. Symptoms may be partially masked so that the diagnosis of meningitis is further delayed and the gravity of the illness may not be recognized until irretrievable brain damage is sustained. Even small doses of antibiotics that scarcely affect the severity of the infection may prevent the isolation of the responsible organism from the cerebrospinal fluid. The reaction in the subarachnoid space may be so modified that the nature of the meningitis may remain in doubt. In any infection, or indeed in any unexplained ill-health, examination for neck rigidity is obligatory and, if found or suspected the cerebrospinal fluid must be examined without delay. To give antibiotics in ignorance or to await events that are likely to be disastrous are both inexcusable. It is difficult to think of a more justifiable use of a hospital bed than to investigate suspected meningitis.

The clinical features of bacterial and viral meningitis differ in significant respects. In virus infections fever is seldom high, constitutional disturbance may be relatively slight and there may be signs of some specific infectious fever. Such features are, however, inadequate for differential diagnosis, as purulent infections may sometimes cause remarkably little disturbance while mumps meningo-encephalitis, for example, can be prostrating.

An occasional source of confusion is *meningism* in acute infections not involving the meninges. Signs of meningeal irritation may occur in pneumonia and other serious infections, apparently due to an increase in cerebrospinal fluid pressure. Lumbar puncture shows that there is no cellular reaction and the chemical composition of the fluid may be unusually dilute.

Subarachnoid haemorrhage is readily mistaken for meningitis and such patients are often admitted to fever hospitals. The history is, of course, usually distinctive but the onset of symptoms from haemorrhage is not always immediate and in any case, no very precise account will be obtained from a stuporose patient. The initial clinical confusion is relatively unimportant provided the need for verification is recognized and acted on at once.

Raised intracranial pressure of such degree as to cause coning of the cerebellar tonsils results in neck rigidity and even sometimes a positive Kernig's sign. This is uncommon but must be considered as a possibility in patients with signs of meningeal irritation, with or without papilloedema, but with no fever. Far more harm is done by failing to diagnose meningitis early than by the rare fatality following lumbar puncture in undiagnosed posterior fossa tumours. If the puncture is performed only after a rational assessment of the relative risks and benefits little harm will result.

The treatment of specific forms of meningitis is described below but a general principle can be drawn from an examination of the failures in the treatment of bacterial meningitis. The chief enemy of success is lack of resolution—infirmity of purpose. To pile one antibiotic on another and yet to withdraw each agent before it could have proved effective is a prescription for disaster. Decisions reached after reasoned consideration of the evidence should be steadfastly adhered to unless superseded by fresh information.

Purulent meningitis

Neisseria meningitidis, the meningococcus, is the commonest cause of purulent meningitis in the adult. It is spread by droplet infection and in the past often occurred in devastating epidemics in confined populations, but is now sporadic. The clinical course varies from a hyperacute illness producing stupor and delirium within a few hours to an insidious onset with increasing fever and headache for ten days or longer, particularly in the elderly. The organism is present in the blood stream, and meningococcal septicaemia sometimes occurs without meningitis but with fever and polyarthralgia. Apart from the usual signs of meningitis the only striking feature of meningitic cases is a petechial or purpuric rash.

Pneumococcal meningitis (Fig. 26, following p. 152) is usually secondary to infection elsewhere, the bacteria being carried from the lungs to the meninges in the blood stream or spreading directly from an infected frontal sinus or middle ear. It is a constant threat in patients who develop a leak of cerebrospinal fluid into the nasopharynx following a fracture of the base of the skull or a lesion of the cribriform plate. The illness is severe, convulsions are common, and the patient is often in coma by the time the diagnosis is made.

Streptococcal meningitis is also commonly the result of spread of local infection, usually from the middle ear. Staphylococcal meningitis is rare and there may be no obvious source of entry. Following neurosurgical operations accidental infection with *Pseudomonas pyocyaneus* sometimes produces a low-grade but persistent meningitis, which may prove extremely troublesome. *Listeria monocytogenes* may cause meningitis in adults on immunosuppressant therapy, particularly following renal transplantation and also affects newborn babies.

In children *Haemophilus influenzae* meningitis is an important form of infection, less often seen in the adult, and in the newborn *E. coli* meningitis may occur.

In purulent meningitis, unmodified by treatment, the cerebrospinal fluid appears milky or even more opaque, but when antibiotics have been given it may be no more than faintly cloudy. The fluid must be sent for bacteriological examination and blood can also be taken for culture at the same time. A precipitin reaction is also available for the detection of meningococcal and pneumococcal antigen in blood and cerebrospinal fluid. The white cell count in the fluid ranges from approximately 500 to 10 000 per mm^3, the protein is greatly raised and sugar reduced or absent. Bacteria may be identifiable on the direct smear. In treated cases the changes are often much less marked and not easily distinguishable from those of tuberculous or viral meningitis. In obscure cases where the diagnosis or the cause of meningitis is in doubt the level of glucose in the cerebrospinal fluid may be important. Glucose is reduced or absent in bacterial infection but is nearly always normal in viral meningitis. It is also reduced if the blood glucose is low and thus should be estimated at the same time. A cerebrospinal fluid level of less than half the serum level is suspect.

Treatment must not be delayed until these results are known. If the fluid obviously contains pus and the patient is gravely ill 10 000 units of the intrathecal preparation of benzylpenicillin in 10 ml of sterile physiological saline should be injected through the lumbar puncture needle. This dose must never be exceeded: penicillin in high concentration causes status epilepticus and necrosis of the brain and spinal cord. In children the maximum intrathecal dose is 5000 units.

The great majority of adults with purulent meningitis will have either meningococcal or pneumococcal infection and both organisms are sensitive to penicillin, chloramphenicol and ampicillin. Intravenous benzylpenicillin 2 megaunits every 4 hours should be given initially, plus either chloramphenicol 1.0 g every 6 hours intravenously or ampicillin 2.0 g every 6 hours by the same route. Both these latter agents are effective against haemophilus influenzae.

If the laboratory finds an organism sensitive to penicillin, chloramphenicol should be stopped. Intravenous therapy should be continued until obvious improvement results when intramuscular penicillin can be given and continued until five days after clinical recovery. If the patient is known to be allergic to penicillin, sulphadiazine 200 mg/kg/day up to a total of 8 g/day should be given, at first intravenously. The cerebrospinal fluid may be examined again after a few days but minor abnormalities may persist for some time and are not a cause for concern. The results of treatment in meningococcal infections are generally excellent and the duration of the disease is often less than that of the common cold. Irreversible damage may, however, have been sustained before the infection has been eliminated and the occasional sequelae include epilepsy, mental retardation, deafness and optic atrophy.

If pneumococcal meningitis is confirmed penicillin by intravenous drip should be continued to a dose of 12 megaunits a day or even higher and with this regime intrathecal penicillin is probably not necessary. With these very high doses there is certainly some risk of penicillin intoxication but the results of treatment of pneumococcal meningitis are relatively so poor that this must be accepted. Provided that the patient was not in deep coma at the time of diagnosis recovery is usual but residual damage is unfortunately common and this remains a dangerous disease.

Haemophilus influenzae meningitis should be treated either with ampicillin 150–250 mg/kg/day injected in divided four-hourly doses into an intravenous infusion or with chloramphenicol 100 mg/kg/day intravenously or intramuscularly initially followed by oral administration.

If the patient plainly has purulent meningitis and no organism can be found ampicillin is again probably the best form of treatment. Streptococcal meningitis should be treated as pneumococcal infection but treatment must often be modified according to bacterial sensitivity. Staphylococcal meningitis must be treated with a penicillinase resistant form of penicillin or with cephaloridine. The prognosis in these last two infections is rather better than in pneumococcal meningitis. Patients who should be treated with penicillin but who are known to be sensitive to this agent should be given chloramphenicol 4–6 g/day.

Pseudomonas pyocyaneus meningitis is seen only as a dreaded complication of cranial surgery and is peculiarly resistant to treatment. Streptomycin and sulphonamides are sometimes successful. Although the organism is sensitive to the toxic antibiotic polymyxin this is seldom an effective therapeutic agent.

Meningitis in the newborn is often due to *Listeria monocytogenes* or to *E. coli*. The former responds well to penicillin but the latter requires chloramphenicol or ampicillin.

Meningococcal meningitis is infectious and the patient should be isolated. Family contacts should be given a course of a sulphonamide drug.

Tuberculous meningitis

This scourge is now comparatively rare in Great Britain but is still rife, particularly in children, in countries where tuberculosis has been inadequately controlled. It results from rupture of a small tuberculoma into the subarachnoid space, either during generalized miliary tuberculosis or as the result of a blood-borne focal cerebral lesion. In the adult active tuberculosis is commonly present elsewhere.

The history is more prolonged than in purulent meningitis but is otherwise similar. The familiar features of headache and fever are combined with those of chronic infection: anorexia, constipation, loss of weight, and night sweats. The insidious onset may conceal the gravity of the illness until more insistent signs appear: cranial nerve involvement, drowsiness increasing to coma, or evidence of focal cerebral damage such as hemiparesis. A subacute form occurs that cannot be distinguished on clinical grounds from purulent meningitis. The physical signs are those of any meningitis but evidence of tuberculosis may be found in the history or on X-ray. In miliary tuberculosis tubercles may very occasionally be seen in the choroid of the eye. These are round white patches, about half the size of the optic disc. They should be sought only after the pupils have been dilated and are easily missed. Active tuberculosis may be present in lung or bone, or miliary tuberculosis may be seen in the chest X-ray, but often no source is evident.

The cerebrospinal fluid may appear faintly opalescent or may be clear. A fine clot sometimes forms on standing. The white cell count is raised to 100 or 200 per mm^3, both polymorphs and lymphocytes being present. The protein is usually around 1.5 g l^{-1} (150 mg/100 ml) but sometimes much higher. In an established case the sugar is nearly always below 40 mg per 100 ml (2.2 mmol/l) but it is important to appreciate that in the early stages a normal figure must never be regarded as excluding this diagnosis. The tubercle bacillus must be sought assiduously since positive diagnosis is of the utmost importance. If no bacilli can be found after exhaustive examination of a direct smear further samples of fluid must be obtained on the succeeding days, but there are unfortunately many cases where the infective agent is found only later on culture or after guinea-pig inoculation.

Diagnosis cannot wait for this useful but delayed confirmation for treatment is urgent. The distinction from viral meningitis can often be made on clinical grounds since tuberculous meningitis is a progressive disease while viral meningitis almost invariably improves rapidly: the protein content of the spinal fluid is the most important single aid to differentiation, a figure above 80 mg per 100 ml casting grave doubt on viral aetiology. However, there is often some uncertainty at the height of the illness. The cerebrospinal fluid sugar is only very occasionally reduced in aseptic meningitis, notably in lymphocytic choriomeningitis. If the sugar is low and the clinical state is deteriorating anti-tuberculous treatment must be given. This will involve treating a small number of patients with carcinomatous meningitis due to direct invasion of the meninges by a malignant growth, for here also there is a chronic deteriorating clinical course together with a mixed pleocytosis and reduction or disappearance of the spinal fluid sugar: expert cytological examination may reveal malignant cells.

Provided the patient is not in coma or has not developed focal cranial nerve or cerebral signs when treatment begins, mortality should be very low, but permanent brain damage may already have occurred. All therapeutic agents of any value in the treatment of tuberculous meningitis can have serious toxic effects. These risks have to be accepted but with care can be kept to a minimum. Streptomycin 1 g daily by intramuscular injection in the adult is still regarded by many as an essential element in treatment. Intrathecal streptomycin should not be given routinely but in comatose patients or when deterioration continues after 10 days on routine treatment 50–100 mg should be given by lumbar puncture for six days a week for two weeks. In children the intramuscular dose of streptomycin is 40 mg/kg in a single daily dose. Isoniazid should always be given up to 400 mg a day in divided doses or in children 20 mg/kg. In addition either rifampicin 450–600 mg a day or ethambutol 15 mg/kg should be given.

Streptomycin damages the VIIIth nerve, particularly the vestibular nerve, although when prolonged intrathecal treatment was the rule permanent deafness was the usual result. If there is a favourable response streptomycin can be stopped after three months and provided other effective agents are being given should also be stopped if vertigo or imbalance develop. Isoiazid causes peripheral neuropathy and more rarely encephalopathy in subjects who metabolize the drug slowly. The symptoms are usually sensory with paraesthesiae in the extremities. If the clinical condition allows, the dose of isoniazid should be reduced and treatment with pyridoxine begun. Rifampicin may cause liver damage and ethambutol can affect visual acuity and colour vision and the possible development of these toxic effects must be regularly and specifically monitored. Para-aminosalicylic acid (PAS) should not be used as it often causes vomiting and it is doubtful whether steroids have the effect originally claimed of preventing organization of arachnoid adhesions.

If all goes well some improvement will be evident after a week. Fever begins to subside, headache is less and the patient more alert. Signs of focal brain damage will persist but clinical evidence of infection will resolve after a few weeks. Appetite returns and weight is regained and signs of meningeal irritation are no longer present. The decision on when to stop treatment is difficult. It is best to err on the side of caution and a course of less than six months of oral treatment will often prove inadequate. Repeated examination of the cerebrospinal fluid is not an entirely reliable way of assessing activity of the disease, but a persistent increase in the cell count should be taken to mean that treatment must continue.

The duration of treatment must be judged by the clinical response. After streptomycin has been stopped other drugs must be continued for at least a year. The composition of the spinal fluid is a very unreliable guide since its protein content usually continues to rise even after treatment is instituted, and it seldom returns to normal until several months after the infection has been overcome.

In a few cases where organized exudate causes foraminal or subarachnoid obstruction to the flow of spinal fluid a steady rise of intracranial pressure may demand surgical intervention. Burr-holes are made and this permits the administration of streptomycin through an intraventricular catheter as well as the relief of pressure.

It is important to remember that especially in a patient who has been vaccinated with BCG the onset of tuberculous meningitis may be so mild as to be quite indistinguishable from a viral infection, with a lymphocytic pleocytosis and normal sugar content in the spinal fluid. These cases present a difficult diagnostic problem and when rapid recovery does not occur in a doubtful case it should be treated as tuberculous.

Aseptic meningitis

Many infective agents other than bacteria can cause meningitis. It is convenient to group these as 'aseptic' in the sense that no organism can be cultured, and also because the clinical syndrome caused by different agents shows only minor variations. The onset is usually as acute as in purulent meningitis, but the symptoms are less severe and evidence of focal brain damage or disturbed consciousness is uncommon.

Meningitis is now rarely seen in secondary syphilis, but every case deserves a Wassermann or VDRL flocculation test. Weil's disease, due to infection with *Leptospira icterohaemorrhagica*, is caught from rats or their excreta, and meningitis sometimes forms the major component of the illness. The more familiar features are jaundice and renal damage. Canicola fever, contracted from pet dogs and due to infection with *L. canicola*, causes a comparatively mild illness, though headache may be severe for several days. Conjunctival injection is common in both forms of leptospiral infection, which responds to intramuscular penicillin.

Viral meningitis accompanies invasion of the central nervous system by neurotropic viruses that cause encephalitis or myelitis, but in many infections meningeal irritation is the basis of most of the symptoms and signs. In lymphocytic choriomeningitis the infection is caught from mice—in a recent example the patient had domesticated the mice in her flat to the point where she could feed them by hand. The meningeal stage is often preceded by a respiratory illness lasting a week. The meningitis is unpleasant but anxiety is soon relieved by rapid recovery. The cellular exudate in the spinal fluid is entirely lymphocytic, reaching several hundred per mm^3. The diagnosis can be confirmed in retrospect by transmission to laboratory mice or by a rise in serum antibodies.

An almost identical syndrome can result from infection with the viruses of mumps, poliomyelitis and infectious mononucleosis, and with Coxsackie and Echo viruses of various types. In the absence of distinctive symptoms diagnosis must rest entirely on virology. Specimens of stool and spinal fluid should be sent to the laboratory and two specimens of serum taken ten days apart should be tested for a rising titre of antibody. There is no effective treatment for viral meningitis, but the meningeal element of neurotropic virus infections is benign and without sequelae.

ENCEPHALOMYELITIS

Many of the agents that cause aseptic meningitis may also evoke an acute disease of the central nervous system with meningitis as an unimportant component. The clinical picture of viral encephalitis is that of rapidly increasing drowsiness and headache with a wide variety of signs of localized disease of the brain and spinal cord. Differentiation from the demyelinating form of acute disseminated perivenous encephalomyelitis associated with the exanthemata (Chapter 12) is difficult, and it is not known how often an identical clinical syndrome is due to direct viral invasion of the brain. Of the common diseases infectious mononucleosis and mumps appear most likely to produce symptoms in this way. In particular mumps meningitis may be accompanied by cranial nerve palsies, especially deafness, and infectious mononucleosis can present with one or more major fits and only vague ill-health to suggest an infective cause.

There are more specific forms of virus encephalitis. The severe forms of arthropod-borne encephalitis familiar in Japan, the United States and Central Europe, are not encountered in Britain. Encephalitis lethargica that swept the world in the decade following the First World War is now rare and perhaps does not occur at all. The characteristic features were disorders of sleep rhythm and of conjugate eye movements, both bespeaking brain stem involvement, but the clinical variation was remarkable. No virus was isolated by the techniques then available. Prolonged coma was often fatal and many survivors were mentally impaired or subsequently developed Parkinsonism (Chapter 13). In some patients the long interval between the acute illness and the sequelae suggests the possibility of chronic infection.

Rabies is contracted from the bite of an infected dog or other animal. The incubation period is up to three months. The initial symptom is usually pain at the site of injury followed by mental distress and by the characteristic pharyngeal spasm on attempting to drink, and by terminal paralysis. The disease is almost always fatal but can be prevented by a course of vaccine begun as soon as possible after the bite. No case of rabies has been contracted in Britain for many years.

POLIOMYELITIS

Poliomyelitis is in decline all over the world and at present it can be hoped that general vaccination will lead to its eradication. The virus is widespread and is transmitted by personal contact and by contamination of food and water. The incidence of infection as detected by antibody studies established that most of those affected had no symptoms and of those who did most developed no more than a mild aseptic meningitis. Nevertheless, where the endemic infection rate was high or where epidemics involved adult populations unprotected by previous infection the total number of cases of paralytic poliomyelitis was formidable.

The virus has a predilection for the anterior horn cells and the equivalent cells of the cranial nerve nuclei. The onset is with mild headache, slight fever and often a sore throat. After a day or two symptoms subside, to return more severely after a brief interval. Pain now involves the neck, back and limbs. There are signs of meningeal irritation and it is at this point that paralysis may occur. It does not follow any distinctive pattern and varies in severity from mild weakness of a single muscle group to catastrophic paralysis. Weakness increases and spreads for two days or a little longer and then all signs of active infection subside. At the height of the illness there may be 50 to 100 white cells per mm^3 of spinal fluid, mostly polymorphs at first, with a later substantial rise in the protein level.

In the absence of an effective antiviral agent the aims of treatment are limited. Physical exertion must be kept to a minimum since it undoubtedly increases the risk of severe paralysis. Pain must be relieved and weak muscles must not be stretched. Spontaneous improvement is often striking and continues for at least six months after the acute illness. The affected limbs naturally show the characteristic features of a lower motor neurone lesion with wasting, hypotonia and loss of deep reflexes.

Apart from the tragedy of a paretic limb the main danger in poliomyelitis is respiratory or bulbar paralysis, or a combination of both. Increasing weakness of respiratory muscles is shown by apprehension and shallow breathing, and assisted respiration is immediately necessary. If the patient cannot swallow, secretions in the mouth enter the trachea and if he cannot cough they block the bronchi. Infection and pulmonary collapse inevitably follow. Simple preventive measures allowing secretions to flow out of the mouth can be life-saving in any patient who cannot swallow. He should lie prone, with the head turned to one side and, if possible, the foot of the bed or stretcher raised. As soon as possible the more sophisticated aid of a respiratory care unit should be sought. Bulbar paralysis demands postural drainage, careful hypopharyngeal suction, and nutrition via a nasogastric tube: inability to maintain an adequate airway, pulmonary collapse or infection, or abductor paralysis of the vocal cords demand urgent tracheostomy—especially the last. Respiratory paralysis, on the other hand, requires assisted respiration either with an iron-lung type of body respirator or where, as often, the trachea has been intubated or tracheostomy performed, by means of a positive-pressure respirator.

The infectious nature of the disease should not be forgotten and barrier nursing should be enforced in the acute stage.

HERPES SIMPLEX ENCEPHALITIS

In recent years the importance of the virus of *Herpes simplex* as the cause of an extremely dangerous form of encephalitis has been recognized. In its familiar role as the cause of trivial 'cold sores' on the lips and elsewhere, herpes simplex is chiefly remarkable for its propensity to produce recurrent lesions in precisely the same site. It was next incriminated as the cause of a rapidly fatal form of haemorrhagic encephalitis in infancy. Herpes simplex encephalitis in the adult is an acute illness presenting with the headache, fever and impaired level of consciousness that are common to many infections of the nervous system. Sometimes the onset is explosive, with focal or generalized fits. Meningism is slight or absent. Papilloedema may be present and there are often signs of focal brain damage, especially to one or both temporal lobes, or hemiplegia. The spinal fluid pressure is often increased, and the fluid contains a moderate excess of white cells and usually also of red cells, though rarely enough to cause blood-staining obvious to the naked eye. Although its onset and evolution are usually less acute, clinical differentiation from cerebral abscess is sometimes impossible, and the resemblance is intensified if carotid angiography shows gross evidence of swelling in one temporal lobe. No pus is found at operation but biopsy shows necrosis accompanied by the perivascular inflammatory cells common to all forms of encephalitis. The temporal lobes are nearly always most affected and may be almost totally destroyed. Mortality is at least 40% and, although good recovery has been recorded, survivors may be intellectually impaired or otherwise incapacitated. It is not known how often less severe and unrecognized infection occurs, nor is it clear what determines this devastating change in the behaviour of the virus. Skin lesions do not accompany the encephalitis, which in most cases is probably due to reactivation of a previously latent infection.

The use of antiviral agents, first idoxuridine and later cytosine arabinoside and then adenosine arabinoside has been disappointing and there is no clear evidence that mortality or morbidity is reduced even when diagnosis is established and treatment begun without delay. The new agent acyclovir appears more promising. Rapid diagnosis can be achieved by brain biopsy which confirms the encephalitis and permits isolation of the virus. Antibody titres are of value only in retrospective diagnosis. High doses of dexamethasone to counter brain oedema have been claimed to be as effective as attempts at more specific forms of treatment.

HERPES ZOSTER

The virus of *herpes zoster* appears to be identical with that of varicella, except for its neurotropic habit. The infection may be widespread throughout the central and peripheral nervous systems but the clinical signs are usually those of involvement of one or more posterior root ganglia or equivalent ganglia of cranial nerves, and the skin of the affected dermatome. Pain is the first symptom and may be present severely for up to four days before the appearance of the characteristic vesicular rash, thus providing ample opportunities for misdiagnosis. Osler said that the man who could unfailingly recognize pre-herpetic neuralgia had nothing more to learn in medicine, and the condition is often mistaken for cardiac infarction, gallstone colic or appendicitis. The rash, nearly always strictly localized to one or two adjacent dermatomes, is easily overlooked on the pharyngeal wall, on the palate or in the auricle.

In most cases after several weeks of pain and discomfort the rash heals, and there are no sequelae apart from fine residual scars and some superficial sensory loss in the affected area. Occasionally there is clinical evidence of spread of the infection. Particularly in the upper limb motor neurones may be involved causing a poliomyelitis-like syndrome with persistent weakness and wasting. Cranial nerve palsies are rare with the exception of the facial nerve. It used to be thought that facial palsy in shingles resulted from zoster of the geniculate ganglion on the minute sensory component of the nerve. Certainly a herpetic eruption can sometimes be seen in the meatus, on the drum or behind the auricle, but equally it may be present in areas quite remote from the facial nerve. Prognosis for full recovery of this form of facial palsy is less good than in idiopathic Bell's palsy.

Shingles of the ophthalmic division of the trigeminal nerve is particularly distressing as the pain is often severe and there is danger of corneal ulceration.

Specific antiviral treatment consists of the local application of 5% idoxuridine several times a day, but this cannot unfortunately be used in the eye. Otherwise treatment can be no more than symptomatic for the relief of pain and the prevention of secondary infection of the vesicles. There is some evidence that high doses of corticosteroids given within a few days of onset may help to prevent the dreaded sequel of post-herpetic neuralgia. This is common in the elderly who are in any case particularly prone to shingles. Long after the rash has healed constant severe demoralizing pain persists. The skin is hypersensitive and is therefore protected by the patient to the point of sitting immobile. Depression is a common accompaniment and suicide not unknown. Early and effective analgesia is imperative. Some benefit may ensue from repeated freezing of the painful area with a cooling spray or from the periodic application of a rubber vibrator. Surgical interruption of the pathways involved in pain sensation is entirely ineffective though it is still attempted by a few optimists. Effective analgesia with drugs reduces the effort required to combat the deadly inactivity that assails these unfortunate patients: they can be reassured that the condition almost invariably clears up over the course of months.

Herpes zoster may be 'symptomatic'; that is to say it may affect a posterior root that is involved in some other disease, such as compression, or infection or injury from many causes, including radiotherapy.

OTHER VIRUS INFECTIONS

Virus infection of the central nervous system may therefore present as an acute illness producing a well-defined clinical syndrome, or it may remain latent to be activated by partly recognized agents. Infection may even involve the fetus, and it is now known that both intrauterine rubella and congenital cytomegalovirus infection are important causes of microcephaly and mental deficiency.

Progressive multifocal encephalopathy occurs as a terminal event in reticuloses and is thought to be due to invasion of the nervous system by a polyoma virus to which immunity has been lost. There are symptoms of severe and progressive damage to the cerebral hemispheres and cerebellum.

Benign myalgic encephalomyelitis is the name applied to an epidemic disease, usually occurring in institutions, particularly among nurses and other medical workers. There is no direct evidence that this is a virus infection, and indeed it has been claimed that it is a form of epidemic hysteria induced by fear of poliomyelitis. There is mild fever, pain in the limbs, tremulous voluntary movement and sometimes paresis without definite reflex changes. The spinal fluid is entirely normal. The acute attack is certainly attended by depression and anxiety, and the characteristic relapses during succeeding months or years become increasingly difficult to distinguish from psychogenic disorders.

Recent evidence indicates that the rare condition known as subacute inclusion body encephalitis or *subacute sclerosing panencephalitis* is caused by measles virus. The disease occurs between the ages of 5 and 20. The early symptoms are quite non-specific and usually consist of a deterioration of school performance and lack of interest and energy, often attributed to neurosis or sloth. Increasing clumsiness and evident dementia are sometimes interpreted as catatonic schizophrenia. Often the disease is in an advanced stage by the time it is recognized. The child is severely disabled by rigidity and by frequent involuntary movements. These are quite characteristic and take the form of brief lapses of posture or myoclonic contractions of stereotyped muscle groups every few seconds. Diagnosis is assisted by the EEG which shows frequent periodic high voltage triphasic slow wave complexes. The spinal fluid is normal except for a rise in its gamma-globulin content, estimation of which has largely replaced the Lange gold test: this yielded a paretic curve (e.g. 5544332100). These children have all had measles in the past except for a few who have received measles vaccine, and there is now strong evidence that the virus persists in the brain. The disease is progressive and fatal and there is no known treatment.

Certain obscure 'degenerative' diseases of the nervous system may be due to transmissible agents known as slow viruses. These are little understood but differ from the ordinary concept of a virus in many properties, notably their resistance to chemical and physical agents. Kuru, a disease found only in the hill people of New Guinea, is apparently transmitted by the curious and obsolescent ritual custom of eating deceased relatives. It has been transmitted to the chimpanzee by injection of a suspension of brain tissue. More significantly, similar transmission of Creutzfeldt-Jakob disease has also been achieved, though there has in the past been no suggestion that this rare disease of middle age might be due to an infective cause in man. It presents as subacute dementia with myoclonus, rigidity and paralysis. The concept of 'degenerative' disease has long ceased to be reputable in all specialities but neurology, and ignorance is usually more artfully concealed. This unexpected finding seems to present another breach in the formidable array of systematized degenerations of the nervous system.

NEUROSYPHILIS

Syphilitic infection of the nervous system is no longer common, no doubt because of more effective treatment of the early disease, but also because nearly everybody is treated with penicillin from time to time for incidental infections. The classical syndromes have been obscured and often present in modified or fragmentary forms.

Treponema pallidum invades the nervous system in the primary stage of the disease, but there are no early symptoms unless a tissue reaction is evoked in the secondary stage, when aseptic meningitis may occur and occasionally local signs such as a sixth cranial nerve palsy. Infection then becomes latent and may never again cause symptoms. Sometimes it is latent from the beginning. Serological tests are positive and are a potent cause of diagnostic confusion in the patient who later develops unrelated neurological disease.

Meningo-vascular syphilis is a form of tertiary disease usually occurring within five years of infection. The essential lesions are endarteritis and perivascular inflammation in the meninges. Very rarely indeed the chronic inflammatory reaction may form a space-occupying mass or gumma. The most characteristic lesion is that in the leptomeninges, which may produce a bewildering variety of symptoms. Headache is common and often associated with cranial nerve palsies, particularly of the third and sixth. The optic nerves or chiasma may be involved in basal meningitis. Involvement of the cerebral vessels causes mental deterioration and focal signs including hemiplegia and aphasia. The spinal cord may be involved in gummatous infiltration of the dura or in spinal leptomeningitis, resulting in progressive paraplegia or occasionally in an acute lesion (transverse myelitis) due to occlusion of the anterior spinal artery.

In this and in all forms of late neurosyphilis, overt or latent, pupillary abnormalities are common. The fully developed condition is the Argyll Robertson pupil which is small and irregular, and does not react to light but reacts on convergence. Both pupils are usually affected, but unequally. The iris is often atrophic and fades to a pale blue. Less well-defined abnormalities such as minor irregularities in outline and a diminished response to light are more difficult to interpret. The responsible lesion is probably in the upper mid-brain but a more peripheral site has been suggested. The Argyll Robertson pupil is a valuable physical sign but it is not pathognomonic of neurosyphilis: it has been described as a curiosity in many conditions, notably diabetes, hypertropic polyneuritis, sarcoidosis and injury to the orbit.

General paresis, or general paralysis of the insane (GPI), develops about 7 to 15 years after primary infection. The inflammatory reaction is less intense than in meningo-vascular disease and endarteritis is not a typical feature. The frontal and parietal lobes are generally shrunken and there is considerable loss of cortical neurones. Spirochaetes were found in sections of the brain in untreated cases but these are no longer seen. The clinical syndrome now encountered is often one of simple mental deterioration not immediately distinguishable from the commoner and less specific forms of presenile dementia. The grandiose delusions and euphoria previously so common are rare today. Epileptic fits and transient attacks of hemiplegia or aphasia are frequent. Tremor of the hands and tongue and slow slurred speech are characteristic. As the disease advances spastic weakness of the legs develops and the final stage is one of helpless paralysis and dementia.

Tabes dorsalis may develop even longer after the primary infection, sometimes as long as 20 years, and very often no history of venereal disease can be obtained. The essential lesion is atrophy of the dorsal spinal roots and therefore of the dorsal columns of the spinal cord which are extensions of fibres from the posterior root ganglia. There is little inflammatory reaction and the mechanism of this remarkably selective degeneration is not understood.

The symptoms are diverse. The onset is usually with lightning pains, so called from their sudden lancinating character. A brief jab of pain strikes into a localized point of one leg with such severity that the patient can be seen to wince. This is repeated in the same spot at frequent intervals for several minutes, when it may cease or move to a new site. More prolonged sickening pains occur and also constricting girdle pains around the trunk. Tabetic crises are due to spasm of smooth muscle and are usually intensely painful. The commonest is the gastric crisis comprising abdominal pain and ceaseless vomiting, lasting for several days and sorely tempting to the surgeon.

Other symptoms are more easily explicable in terms of loss of sensory function. The gait is ataxic because of loss of sense of position, and the patient is helpless with the eyes closed as in washing the face, or in the dark. Even in daylight he staggers and lifts his feet high off the ground. Romberg's sign consists of inability to retain balance with the eyes closed and the feet together. Patients with advanced tabes may fall very heavily unless supported.

Sensation from the bladder and bowel is interrupted so that both voluntary and reflex control is lost. The bladder becomes large and atonic and there is dribbling incontinence from retention with overflow. Painless ulcers on the feet are common. Particularly in the lower limbs the joints are often painlessly destroyed. In the typical Charcot joint, bone destruction is accompanied by osteophyte formation, with gross deformity and sickening crepitus but quite without pain. The lumbar spine may collapse to the point where root compression adds to the disability.

Cranial nerves may be involved. Optic atrophy is common and moderate bilateral ptosis with compensatory wrinkling of the brow is characteristic.

Examination confirms the presence of extensive sensory loss. Postural sense is lost in the legs and there are areas of loss of superficial pain sense most commonly on the feet, the inner borders of the arms, the sternum, and often the nose and forehead. Deep pain as tested by squeezing the Achilles tendon is absent. There is no paralysis, but the muscles are hypotonic so that passive hip flexion is possible to an extreme degree and the knees may hyperextend. Tendon jerks are absent but the plantar reflexes are normal.

Elements of tabes and general paresis occasionally coexist, so that mild dementia, absent tendon jerks and extensor plantar reflexes are found together with other signs in differing combinations.

The diagnosis of the full syndrome of tabes dorsalis should present no difficulty, but when its impact has been modified by incidental antibiotics it may present as a single symptom. Painless retention of urine, painless swelling of an ankle joint, a perforating ulcer of the foot or unexpectedly severe changes in X-rays of the lumbar spine may all be due to unsuspected tabes of which significant but unobtrusive confirmatory signs may be found on careful examination.

Optic atrophy in isolation is a third form of late neurosyphilis. It is bilateral and of primary type with small pale discs, and progresses to blindness.

In meningo-vascular syphilis the Wassermann reaction and VDRL are usually positive in blood and spinal fluid, and in general paresis the spinal fluid is always positive. In tabes dorsalis serological tests including treponema immobilization may be negative in apparently untreated cases. In active neurosyphilis the spinal fluid contains an excess of white cells up to 100 per mm³ and the protein is moderately raised, especially its gamma-globulin component. Hence the Lange curve is of the paretic (5544332100) or 'luetic' type (3455432100). In tabes an entirely normal fluid is sometimes found even when the clinical course suggests progressive disease: this may be seen some years after apparently successful and effective antisyphilitic treatment, and is possibly caused by secondary ischaemic changes due to atherosclerosis in healed lesions.

The standard treatment for all forms of neurosyphilis is procaine penicillin 600 mg by intramuscular injection daily for 21 days. This should be preceded by 3 days of prednisolone 40 mg a day to prevent the rare but dangerous Herxheimer hypersensitivity reaction. The response depends on how far the patient's symptoms are due to inflammatory changes and how far to irreversible loss of neurones. In meningo-vascular syphilis uncomplicated by severe mental change or by spinal cord infarction complete recovery can be expected, though pupillary changes will be permanent. General paresis also responds to early treatment but complete recovery is rare, some degree of mental dullness persisting. If treatment is delayed little improvement can be expected. The signs of tabes cannot be reversed by treatment and even arrest of the disease cannot be ensured. Optic atrophy also continues to progress in spite of treatment. The need for repeated courses of treatment is problematical. The spinal fluid is the best guide to active syphilitic infection of the nervous system and its cell and protein content return to normal very rapidly. On the other hand the Wassermann reactions may remain positive indefinitely in both blood and spinal fluid. In general continued deterioration, fresh symptoms or evidence of active inflammation in the spinal fluid are accepted indications for a further course of treatment.

Congenital neurosyphilis

The brain may be extensively damaged *in utero* by infection from the mother, in whom the disease may be latent. Surviving infants may be mentally or physically retarded and suffer from a variety of spastic cerebral palsies. The later development of juvenile general paresis or tabes is now a great rarity. The symptoms and signs are similar to those of the acquired disease in the adult, but in a child of 13 they can very easily be misinterpreted. The pupils are often distinctive: they are fixed to light but widely dilated, in contrast to the constricted Argyll Robertson pupil of the adult. Congenital tabo-paresis is a rare cause of a rather characteristic syndrome of fits, dementia, and catatonia.

Congenital infection with *toxoplasma* is a relatively uncommon cause of mental deficiency and hydrocephalus, often with epilepsy and cerebral calcification. Choroido-retinitis is usually present. The acquired disease in the adult is rare and presents as a subacute encephalomyelitis, often with papilloedema. Lymph glands are enlarged and the spleen may be palpable. The clinical diagnosis is obviously difficult but should be suspected if there is a rash or eosinophilia. Specialized serological tests are fairly reliable and the organism can be cultured from the spinal fluid. Pyrimethamine (Daraprim) is thought to be an effective treatment if given in a prolonged course, but it carries a risk of haemolytic anaemia.

Cryptococcae meningitis

Meningitis due to *Cryptococcus neoformans (Torula hystolytica)* is mostly seen in patients with chronic reticuloses, though primary cases are increasingly recognized even in Britain. The onset is gradual over several weeks or months with the usual symptoms and signs of meningitis, and often with papilloedema. There may be no pleocytosis in the spinal fluid, but the encapsulated yeasts can often be identified in fresh spinal fluid stained with black ink. Diagnosis can be confirmed by serological tests, mouse passage, and growth on suitable media. In other patients there is a sharp cellular reaction in the fluid. Treatment with amphotericin B by intravenous infusion is occasionally successful but the drug is toxic.

TETANUS

Tetanus is due to infection with the anaerobic spore-bearing organism, *clostridium tetani* which proliferates in wounds but which does not enter the nervous system. Since active immunization with tetanus toxoid gives highly effective protection the disease is now entirely preventable. It exerts its effects through the powerful exotoxin which enters the central nervous system mainly if not wholly by ascending the peripheral nerves. This occurs directly from the infected wound and indirectly following spread of the toxin in the blood stream. Its effect is to greatly increase reflex excitability, causing persistent muscular contraction augmented by an afferent stimulus.

The incubation period is from two days to several weeks but commonly around seven days. In the generalized form the initial symptoms are inability to open the mouth (trismus) and powerful spasm of the neck muscles. In severe cases this rapidly spreads to involve the face, limbs and trunk. The lips are drawn back into the fixed *risus sardonicus*, the abdominal muscles are board-like, and rigidity is periodically increased by painful spasms which impede respiration. Inability to swallow, asphyxia, heart failure, severe hypertension and hyperpyrexia are potentially fatal complications. Milder forms of generalized tetanus are more common and less dangerous.

In localized tetanus the spasm is confined to muscles in the neighbourhood of the wound. Continuous or intermittent contraction of the muscles of one limb, without other neurological signs, and often without an obvious wound, is usually misdiagnosed. The spasm may persist for weeks and its origin is infrequently revealed by trismus and other more characteristic features.

Tetanus is highly lethal and even with expert modern treatment it is still dangerous. Antitoxin is generally regarded as valuable and is given in a single massive dose of 200 000 units intravenously. There is a risk of immediate anaphylactic shock and it is to be hoped that human tetanus immune globulin will become generally available. The abolition of muscle spasm with curare and artificial respiration through a tracheostomy are life-saving measures, ideally undertaken in a special unit. Chlorpromazine may control spasm in less severe cases and especially when assisted respiration is not available it can be given by intravenous drip. Treatment must be continued until the paroxysms have stopped, but some degree of rigidity may persist for weeks. Overaction of the sympathetic system appears to be responsible for some of the more alarming complications such as hypertension, and can be treated with alpha and beta blocking agents.

Where the wound of entry can be detected all foreign matter and dead tissue must be removed since it may furnish a source of toxin. In 20% of cases no wound or other mode of entry can be identified.

Further reading

British Medical Journal (leading article) (1977) Partly treated pyogenic meningitis. **1**, 340.
Caterall R.O. (1977) Neurosyphilis. *Brit. J. Hosp. Med.* **17**, 585.
Illis L.S. & Gosling J.V.T. (1972) *Herpes Simplex Encephalitis*. Scientifica, Bristol.
Hughes R.A.C. (1980) Infections of the nervous system. *Medicine*, 1654.
Jefferson A.A. & Keogh A.J. (1977) Intracranial abscesses. *Quart. J. Med.* **46**, 389.
Lancet (leading article) (1976) Treatment of tuberculous meningitis. **1**, 787.

CHAPTER 12
The Demyelinating Diseases

The myelin sheath of both central and peripheral axons is naturally involved in any generally destructive process. The concept of primary demyelinating disease implies that myelin is destroyed leaving the axons intact. A group of diseases can be identified in which this occurs although this is a much simplified description of the pathology. Of this group, by far the most important is multiple sclerosis.

MULTIPLE SCLEROSIS

The name of the disease is derived from the appearances of the chronic process at autopsy, when scattered areas of glial scarring or sclerosis can be seen within the central nervous system. The peripheral nervous system is spared, apparently because of differences in the chemical composition of myelin, but the optic nerves are developmentally part of the central nervous system and are frequently involved. The sclerosis is the end product of a pathological process that begins, as far as can be determined, with small collections of lymphocytes around veins within the substance of the brain and spinal cord, accompanied by destruction of the myelin sheath, forming sharply defined areas known as plaques (Fig. 27, following p. 152). In the acute lesion there is considerable oedema and the active spreading edge of the plaque contains the lymphocytic reaction. Within the plaque the oligodendrocytes that form and maintain the myelin sheath are either absent or abnormal in form. The axons remain intact at this stage but in chronic lesions they too are destroyed. Gliosis occurs early in the development of the plaque.

The plaques are not distributed in any strictly systematic way but show a marked predilection for certain sites, including the optic nerve, the cervical spinal cord and the white matter surrounding the lateral ventricles. Their number and extent vary within wide limits but plaques can probably always be identified in both brain and spinal cord. Even in disease of very long duration, plaques with the characteristics of fresh lesions can usually be seen.

Clinical features

Multiple sclerosis is predominantly a disease of young adults. Apparently typical cases are occasionally seen in children under the age of ten, but the peak age of onset is around 30. Undoubted multiple sclerosis can present, apparently without preceding symptoms, as late as the sixth or seventh decade and may even be an incidental finding at autopsy in patients who have died of old age without known symptoms of the disease. Females are more commonly affected in a ratio of 3:2. The presenting symptoms are naturally varied as plaques can occur anywhere within the central nervous system but in the great majority of patients the onset takes one of the following forms: optic neuritis, weakness of the legs, sensory loss or diplopia.

The onset of optic neuritis is with pain in one eye, particularly on movement, accompanied by blurred vision which deteriorates for several days. The degree of visual loss varies from slight impairment of appreciation of colour to complete blindness but usually central acuity is reduced to 6/60 or less with retention of the peripheral field. This central scotoma is the characteristic visual field defect and results from demyelination of the axons from the area of the retina around the macula. These fibres comprise more than half the optic nerve and are placed centrally so that they are almost inevitably involved in a plaque within the nerve. The optic disc usually appears normal, when the condition is known as retrobulbar neuritis, or may be swollen. Retinal haemorrhages occur but are rare. Pain in the eye subsides within a week or two and vision then begins to improve. The usual outcome is virtually complete restoration of vision, although in severe attacks considerable loss may be permanent. Following an attack of optic neuritis, and in many patients with multiple sclerosis in whom a history of visual loss cannot be obtained, the optic nerve head becomes pale, particularly on the temporal side containing the fibres from the macula. Optic neuritis seldom affects both eyes simultaneously but recurrent episodes are common.

Weakness of one or both legs is another common mode of onset. It may be gradually progressive, particularly in older patients, or may increase rapidly, often being temporarily much worse during mild exertion. The weakness is of upper motor neurone type, with increased tendon reflexes and extensor plantar reflexes. Occasionally multiple sclerosis can present with acute paraplegia with complete loss of motor and sensory functions below the mid-dorsal level.

Sensory symptoms at the onset of multiple sclerosis usually involve the legs. A sensation of tingling or numbness begins in the feet and in the course of a few days spreads up to the waist, including the perineal region. There is no disability, except that the sensation of passing water and vaginal sensation may be lost. Physical signs are difficult to elicit, the patient saying that it feels as if there is something between the examiner's pin and her skin, but there is no definite sensory loss. This can easily be misdiagnosed as hysteria. A quite different form of sensory involvement results in a complaint of a 'useless hand', not from weakness but from loss of postural sense.

The other common presenting symptom is diplopia, usually identifiable as due to a partial VIth nerve palsy. Other less common initial symptoms include retention of urine, vertigo, trigeminal neuralgia, dementia and even occasionally epilepsy or stupor.

From this description it might be supposed that the onset is always with symptoms that could arise from a single lesion within the central nervous system. While this is often so, the disease is sometimes clearly 'multiple' from the onset, with combinations of symptoms such as optic neuritis and paraesthesiae in one hand, or diplopia and weakness of the legs.

Course

The recovery of vision after an attack of optic neuritis described above is an example of a characteristic feature of multiple sclerosis, that of remission. Following the initial symptoms, particularly in relatively young patients, full recovery within a few weeks is to be expected. The subsequent course is unpredictable. In some fortunate patients, particularly those in whom symptoms are confined to the visual and sensory systems, repeated relapses of the disease occur, followed by complete remission, so that even after five or more years there is no disability and no physical evidence of the disease apart from pallor of the optic discs. In others, especially where the onset has been with weakness of the legs, full recovery does not take place after the first attack and subsequent relapses leave increasingly severe disability. Between the benign type and those patients who never experience complete remission lies the majority of patients with moderately severe disease. Here the course is with repeated relapse and remission, at first with full recovery, but after perhaps the third or fourth relapse some disability persists, usually slight weakness of the legs or an ataxic gait. Disability increases after subsequent relapses and eventually, after five years or more, remission no longer occurs. There may now be a prolonged stage of apparent quiescence during which the patient has persistent symptoms but can function almost normally. The typical physical signs at this stage would include nystagmus on lateral gaze, slight ataxia of the upper limbs and spastic weakness of the legs with loss of vibration sense but no loss of cutaneous sensation. Control of the bladder will be imperfect, with urgency and occasional incontinence. Sexual impotence in the male is usual by this stage.

Eventually slow deterioration will become obvious. Walking becomes increasingly difficult and recourse must be had to aids and eventually to a wheelchair. The hands become increasingly ataxic and tremulous, particularly on attempted voluntary movement—intention tremor. Incontinence becomes persistent. Visual acuity is seldom much reduced by nystagmus and internuclear ophthalmoplegia make reading difficult. Both these abnormalities of ocular movement as seen in multiple sclerosis are due to lesions in the posterior longitudinal bundle and are described in Chapter 4. Eventually mild dementia occurs in virtually all severe cases of multiple sclerosis and it is these patients who are sometimes euphoric, in that they have a positive sense of well-being in distressing contrast with their helpless state. Not unnaturally depression may also occur.

In many patients who develop multiple sclerosis in the fourth or fifth decade or later the disease is progressive from the onset and usually takes the form of paraplegia with little or no evidence of cerebral disease.

The final outcome is difficult to predict. A small proportion of patients have a severe form of multiple sclerosis, usually with a transverse spinal cord lesion, and die within five years. A rather larger number will die within 15 years of the onset from the usual hazards of the severely disabled—bedsores, urinary and pulmonary infection. Many patients will, however, live for 25 years or longer after their first symptoms and those with the benign form may remain without serious disability.

Certain symptoms that may occur at the onset or during the course of the disease should be described in more detail. A feeling like an electric shock passing down the back and legs on flexing the neck (Lhermitte's sign) is highly characteristic although it can occur in other forms of spinal cord disease. Severe vertigo unaccompanied by tinnitus or deafness may be incapacitating for as long as three weeks. Deafness is said to be rare in multiple sclerosis and is certainly never persistent but quite often occurs in acute relapses. Aphasia and hemianopia, once thought to rule out a diagnosis of multiple sclerosis, are both seen occasionally.

A group of symptoms different in character from those already described are the curious paroxysms that seem to be the result of excessive neuronal activity rather than of loss of function. Of these the best known but not the most common is trigeminal neuralgia which is described in Chapter 4. Other paroxysms include dysarthria, often combined with ataxia and paraesthesiae of the face and upper limbs, and tonic painful spasms in which the limbs on one side adopt a posture resembling that of tetany. All these symptoms occur frequently, many times a day, but are brief, lasting no more than two minutes. They may be triggered by overbreathing or by sensory stimulation of the limbs or possibly by movement.

Diagnosis

The diagnosis may often be suspected during the first attack of the disease, particularly when this takes one of the typical forms. For example it is known that 85% of patients with optic neuritis eventually develop multiple sclerosis. The clinical diagnosis should, however, whenever possible, be based on the multiple nature of the lesions and their remitting course. This means evidence of damage in more than one site in the central nervous system, involving two or more separate episodes. Very often, by the time these criteria are met the diagnosis is not in any serious doubt, but when relapses are spread over many years or are but partially remembered by the patient difficulty can still arise. The progressive case presents a more difficult problem and there may be no method of distinguishing on clinical grounds between paraplegia due to multiple sclerosis and that due to spinal cord compression. Persistent cutaneous sensory loss is rare in multiple sclerosis but its absence is insufficient evidence on which to dismiss a spinal cord tumour. Investigation to exclude other diagnoses is therefore frequently necessary even if clinical suspicion is strong. A myelogram should be done in all cases of progressive paraplegia without obvious cause.

Confirmatory tests of the diagnosis of multiple sclerosis are now available, although not always applicable. The cerebrospinal fluid is abnormal in about 50% of cases with an increase of total protein to a maximum of 1.0 g l^{-1} (100 mg/100 ml) or an increase in lymphocytes, usually to around 20 mm^3 but occasionally rising to 50 mm^3. These changes are non-specific. The proportion of the total protein made up by gamma-globulin is above 20% in about two-thirds of multiple sclerosis cases. This again is non-specific but if neurosyphilis is excluded there are few other causes of such a change that could be confused with multiple sclerosis. More refined methods of separating the protein fractions promise much superior diagnostic results. Over 90% of patients show an oligoclonal globulin pattern but the test is not yet generally available.

An entirely different diagnostic approach has been based on recording average cerebral and spinal electrical potentials evoked by sensory stimulation. The method studied most fully is that of stimulating each eye in turn with an alternating chequerboard pattern while recording the evoked potential over the back of the head. Normally a positive wave with a latency of around 100 ms can be recorded. In many patients with multiple sclerosis this wave is delayed or absent. The diagnostic significance of this finding is that delay may be found in patients with no clinical evidence of a lesion of the visual pathways. The delay is presumed to be due to demyelination and thus provides evidence of *multiple* lesions in, for example, a patient with progressive paraplegia.

The value of the test based on the effect of unsaturated fatty acids on the motility of the patient's red cells in a magnetic field is still controversial. It has been claimed that this method is highly reliable in the diagnosis of established disease and will also detect children who will develop multiple sclerosis in adult life. This has not been shown to be true.

Pathogenesis

The cause of multiple sclerosis is not known. Any satisfactory theory must take into account certain facts about prevalence of the disease. In Britain and Northern Europe and Northern USA the prevalence is around 50/100000, whereas in many tropical countries it is doubtful whether it occurs at all. Multiple sclerosis does not follow any clear genetic pattern but there is a considerably increased incidence among first-degree relatives. There is also an association with certain HLA tissue types but these differ in different parts of the world.

Recent theories of causation have centred on persistent virus infection, autoimmunity and lipid metabolism. A slight increase in measles antibodies has been found but no convincing isolation of a virus. A disturbance of immune reactions is suggested by the possible animal model of experimental allergic encephalomyelitis, a perivenous demyelinating disease induced by injections of brain antigen. This model is more convincing now that a relapsing and remitting form of the experimental disease has been confirmed. The possibility of a disorder of lipid metabolism arises primarily from the altered composition of the brain lipids reported in multiple sclerosis, but has been much elaborated. These theories are not mutually exclusive but no convincing pattern has yet emerged.

Even the immediate cause of the symptoms is not entirely clear. It is often presumed that they result from the effect of demyelination in slowing or blocking axonal conduction. If this is so it is not clear how remission could take place as remyelination is not known to occur. No doubt the swelling in the acute plaque also plays a part but this could not be the whole explanation. Following recovery from optic neuritis apparently perfect vision can be accompanied by a pale optic disc and marked abnormality of visual evoked potentials, presumably indicating persistent demyelination but with no loss of function. The paroxysmal symptoms probably arise from abnormal spread of excitation between axons deprived of their myelin.

Treatment

The treatment of multiple sclerosis is an emotive topic. Many regimes have been earnestly promoted on insufficient evidence and eventually abandoned. The aims of treatment would be to prevent relapse and to induce remission or improvement of the chronic state. Owing to the natural history of the disease the results of treatment can only be assessed by elaborately controlled clinical trials. There is certainly no known curative treatment. It has been claimed that the regular consumption of sunflower seed oil has a slight effect in reducing the duration and severity of relapses but this is only demonstrable on a statistical basis in a large group and is most unconvincing in individual patients. The gluten-free diet was advocated on the basis of a single very striking case but has proved unhelpful. Other forms of long-term treatment under active investigation are based on extensive immunosuppression but the essential control trials have not yet been published. Dorsal column stimulation from epidural electrodes is under trial as a method of improving chronic disability.

For the acute severe relapse, treatment with ACTH 40 units twice a day, followed by a smaller dose for another one or two weeks can be given and there is some evidence that this will speed remission. Side-effects are common and oral potassium should be given. Equivalent doses of corticosteroids may also be used. This treatment does not influence long-term prognosis and continuous steroid treatment should be avoided.

Symptomatic treatment for spasticity and bladder dysfunction should be given when necessary. There is no good agent for the relief of spasticity in the ambulant patient and indeed to reduce tone may be to reduce the effectiveness of the legs as props in walking. In the severely disabled baclofen will often reduce or abolish extensor or flexor spasm. The management of the neurogenic bladder is described in Chapter 5. Physiotherapy is helpful to the patient recovering from relapse but has little place in long-term management.

Treatment must also include the advice given to the patient and relatives. Most neurologists would not pronounce the diagnosis after a single attack because of the possibilities of error or of prolonged remission. By the time there are permanent symptoms the patient should be told the diagnosis. Unfortunately, effective advice on how to avoid relapse is not possible, but it is usual to warn against fatigue and intercurrent infection. There is some increased risk of relapse in the puerperium and clearly a large family is undesirable but multiple sclerosis is not an absolute bar to pregnancy. Multiple sclerosis in parent and child is quite rare and it is correct to state that the risks of direct inheritance are small.

Patients with multiple sclerosis should be seen and examined at regular intervals, partly to ensure that no diagnostic error has been committed and partly to assess their need for symptomatic treatment and support.

ACUTE DISSEMINATED ENCEPHALOMYELITIS

This is a very rare neurological complication of various infections and inoculations, seen in a characteristic form a few days after vaccination against smallpox, during fading of the rash in measles and chickenpox, and even more often after apparently non-specific respiratory infections. The rarity of the syndrome must be stressed: it occurs, for example, only once in every 30 000 vaccinations. A similar pathological picture, characterized by perivenous exudation and infiltration, can be produced by the injection of sterile extracts of nervous tissue in experimental animals, where it is known as experimental allergic encephalomyelitis. The identical nature of the clinical and pathological syndrome as it occurs in these various clinical contexts, the frequent absence of spinal fluid changes other than a rise in gamma-globulin content, and the similarities between the human and animal lesion strongly support the hypothesis that even when it follows a virus infection this condition is not due directly to viral invasion but is the result of an autoimmune reaction to some element of central myelin.

Acute encephalomyelitis of this type may affect the brain or spinal cord, or both; on occasion there may even be some nerve root involvement. Where the cord is affected the usual picture is that of an acute transverse myelitis. This often occurs at the mid-dorsal level, leading to flaccid paralysis of the lower limbs with loss of sensation and urinary retention, and because of the level of the lesion the abdominal muscles are usually also paralysed. Perception of vibration and positional sense are sometimes retained in the presence of otherwise global sensorimotor paraplegia, and this has led to the suggestion that the condition arises primarily from segmental occlusion of the anterior spinal artery, possibly dependent on an acute allergic arteritis. This is probably the commonest form of acute transverse myelitis. This clinical picture of acute or subacute paraplegia may also result from quite different causes and a myelogram is an essential investigation to exclude spinal cord compression from extradural abscess or spinal tumour. Neurosyphilis should also be remembered as a possible cause, although now extremely rare. Despite its catastrophic onset, transverse myelitis may show remarkable recovery over a period of weeks or months, and even in some severe instances residual disablement may be minimal. This is probably the case where the lesion is truly segmental and where much of the disturbance is due to initial inflammatory oedema. There is, however, a much more unfavourable group of cases where the cord is damaged in its length below the lesion. In these instances the expected return of reflex activity below the lesion does not occur within days or a few weeks, and the spinal fluid changes tend to be more pronounced, often with a considerable increase in cell and protein content. Especially where the onset has been less acute the condition approximates to the uncommon and irrecoverable lesion described by French writers as subacute necrotic myelitis.

Occasionally, patients with acute transverse myelitis manifest some signs of encephalitis, and in occasional encephalitic cases there is concurrent evidence of some cord involvement. Pathologically, the changes are in most cases patchily diffused throughout the central nervous system, but clinically most present as predominantly myelitic or encephalitic syndromes.

The cardinal sign of this as of all other forms of encephalitis is impairment of consciousness, which may vary from slight drowsiness or confusion to rousable stupor or even to deep coma. On the whole the latter has an unfavourable prognosis. It is an everyday observation that, unlike the stupor of cerebral tumour, that of encephalitis or meningitis often tends to be restless and noisy, sometimes with repetitive screaming. Any combination of focal neurological signs may be found. They may be evanescent, and show a marked tendency to recover. On the other hand, in a small number of cases focal deficits such as hemiplegia may persist. Hemiparesis may be unilateral or bilateral, and cranial nerve palsies, optic neuritis, and cerebellar syndromes may all be encountered, the last especially after chickenpox.

Acute disseminated encephalomyelitis is a disease of childhood, adolescence and early adult life. Although it is often diagnosed in the middle-aged and elderly, the diagnosis in these circumstances is usually incorrect. There is an appreciable mortality, though since many cases remain undiagnosed, being dismissed for example as 'toxic measles', it is difficult to state a figure. However, when it occurs death usually ensues within a matter of days. There are occasional patients in whom the illness lasts for several weeks, but these are exceptional and often recovery is only slightly less rapid than onset. There is suggestive evidence that the condition responds to treatment with corticotrophin or steroid hormones given early and in massive dosage.

A small subgroup, some cases of which probably belong amongst these conditions, is acute haemorrhagic leucoencephalitis. Again this has every appearance of arising as a non-specific complication of a considerable variety of acute infections and possible antigenic insults. It was seen in its most characteristic form as a rare complication of the treatment of syphilis with organic arsenical drugs, and has been reported after treatment with sulphonamides. However, it has also complicated infections where no drug therapy has been given. It differs from the forms described above in that its onset is usually at the height of infection, and that it is a fulminating and usually fatal illness. It now seems likely that some cases of this syndrome are instances of herpes simplex encephalitis (see Chapter 11).

It has already been said that acute disseminated encephalomyelitis furnishes an example of the demyelinating lesion at its simplest. We know from autopsy observation that patchy perivenous demyelination in the white matter characterizes cases that survive for a few weeks. We also know that this is reversible, since careful histological examination of the nervous system of a few such patients some years later has failed to reveal any evidence of neurological damage. In approximately 10% of those diagnosed initially as having acute disseminated encephalomyelitis, subsequent relapses declare the case as incontestable multiple sclerosis. Whether this means that the initial diagnosis was wrong or that the two diseases are facets of the same process is at present undecided. Neither an encephalitic nor a transverse myelitic onset is common in multiple sclerosis, but both occur in a minority of cases, and episodes of either kind may punctuate the established chronic disease.

NEUROMYELITIS OPTICA

Alternatively named Devic's syndrome, this condition in its classical form comprises a biphasic demyelinating disease manifest in bilateral optic neuritis followed after a longer or shorter interval, typically of a few months, by an acute transverse myelitis. The sequence may be foreshortened or reversed.

The symmetrical pattern of the disease is noteworthy, and probably results from the intensity and widespread dissemination of the lesions. This pattern of demyelinating diseases is uncommon in temperate climates but frequent in such hot countries as those of East Asia. On the other hand, Devic's syndrome may complicate acute specific fevers, where it must be regarded as a manifestation of acute disseminated encephalomyelitis, and it may also occur during the course of classical multiple sclerosis.

The situation is further complicated by the fact that some neurologists, especially in Japan, use the term neuromyelitis optica to describe practically any combination of optic neuritis with spinal cord disease, including many cases that would undoubtedly be regarded elsewhere as straightforward instances of multiple sclerosis.

SCHILDER'S DISEASE

This extremely rare condition of children is now known to occur in two quite distinct forms, previously confused under the vague heading of *diffuse sclerosis*. One form is genetically determined and is associated with adrenocortical atrophy. The other is sporadic and is characterized by massive, well-defined, progressive and usually symmetrical demyelination in the white matter of the cerebral hemispheres. The process may begin anywhere in either hemisphere and this is reflected in the variable march of symptoms. Fits, headaches, cortical blindness, hemianopia, optic neuritis or atrophy, and mental deterioration are common features and in most cases a fatal outcome is heralded within two to three years by a state of quadriplegic decerebrate rigidity and dementia. Treatment is valueless. The sharply defined margin of advancing demyelination recalls the plaque of multiple sclerosis, and indeed some have regarded it as a juvenile analogue of the commoner disease.

Further reading

British Medical Bulletin (1977) **33**.
McAlpine D., Lumsden C.E. & Acheson E.D. (1972) *Multiple Sclerosis: A Reappraisal*, 2nd edn. Churchill Livingstone, Edinburgh and London.
Matthews W.B. (1980) Multiple sclerosis. *Medicine*, 1664.

CHAPTER 13
Diseases of the Basal Ganglia

The idea of control of voluntary movement by the cerebral cortex by way of the pyramidal tract is easy to grasp, at least in crude outline, and the negative and positive symptoms of paralysis and spasticity arising from injury to this system are also comprehensible. From experiments in animals, however, it is known that apparent 'voluntary', or at least coordinated movement is possible after section of the pyramidal tracts: alternative motor systems clearly exist. The definition of these as 'extrapyramidal' is obviously imprecise, and although the clinical features that result when they are implicated in disease are often highly characteristic, they are not well understood. The structures most clearly identifiable as the extrapyramidal motor system are the masses of grey matter known collectively as the basal ganglia.

The relevant anatomy is described in Chapter 1, but the interconnections of the extrapyramidal system must be briefly recapitulated. These are intricate, incompletely understood, and often in dispute. The main pathways appear to be as follows: from the motor cortex to the caudate nucleus and putamen; from the putamen and substantia nigra to the globus pallidus; from the globus pallidus to the ventrolateral nucleus of the thalamus and the descending reticular formation, and eventually to the motor neurones of the spinal cord. The subthalamic nucleus is connected both to the globus pallidus and to the reticular formation. The entire system has important links with the cerebellum and thence indirectly back to the motor cortex.

Explanation of symptoms caused by disorders of these interlocking structures is hampered not only by their complexity, but also by difficulties in interpreting the pathological material. Severe clinical disease may be accompanied by no more than slight and diffuse evidence of neuronal degeneration, while sharply localized lesions may sometimes produce no symptoms at all. Before attempting to understand the underlying disorders of physiology the clinical syndromes must be recognized.

PARKINSON'S DISEASE

Parkinson's disease or paralysis agitans is a relatively common disease of unknown cause, affecting more men than women and usually beginning between the ages of 40 and 70. Genetic factors do not seem to be important.

One of the cardinal symptoms and often the earliest, is tremor. Characteristically this begins in one hand, at first only under conditions of mild stress in public, but it increases until it is almost incessant. Spread to the leg on the same side is usual and also to the opposite limbs, but asymmetry often persists. The movement is rhythmic with a frequency of about six per second and it can be seen to be due to alternating contraction of opposing groups of muscles, as in any form of tremor. At first it is less marked or absent during voluntary movement of the limb, though it may be augmented by vigorous movement of the other limbs and often by walking. A 'pill-rolling' movement of the thumb and index finger is common, but much more ample movements of the proximal segments of the limbs also occur. Tremor of the head and jaw is also common. Although the involuntary movement has surprisingly little effect on function, its persistence is often almost intolerable.

The major disability is a complex disorder of voluntary movement, akinesia. Movements become slower and less facile. This is noticed first in fine manipulations such as writing and fastening buttons or shoelaces. Writing becomes small and cramped, and the time needed to dress is much increased. Other early symptoms include difficulty in rising from a chair, slowness in walking, generalized fatigue, and muscular aching. As the disease advances movement is increasingly restricted so that using a knife and fork, washing, dressing, getting in and out of bed and even turning over in bed become difficult and eventually impossible. The ability to walk may be relatively preserved but there is often difficulty in making the first step, or in turning round. Falling is common and may be preceded by *festination* in which the patient is impelled to break into a tottering run.

The speech may become low-pitched and almost inaudible and in a few patients swallowing is difficult. Increased salivation may lead to dribbling.

The great majority of patients with Parkinson's disease are depressed to a degree far in excess of that found in other forms of comparable disability. This is easily overlooked in the concentration on the more obvious physical symptoms.

Examination reveals many features unnoticed by the patient. The face is curiously immobile, without the normal frequent slight changes in expression and with infrequent spontaneous blinking. The face is often shiny with excessive sebaceous secretion. Even in its mildest form this melancholy 'Parkinsonian mask' can be recognized across the room.

Persistent involuntary blinking when the glabella is repeatedly tapped by the examiner's finger has been claimed as diagnostic but false results are frequent.

The stance and gait are also characteristic, the posture being one of flexion with the head and back bowed and the arms held partially flexed at the elbows, wrists and metacarpo-phalangeal joints. The arms do not swing on walking, and in early cases this failure to swing one arm may be diagnostic. Short gliding steps are taken, and when the patient attempts to turn, the feet may become 'stuck to the ground' for several seconds.

There is no paralysis or weakness, but initiation of movement is difficult, and repeated movements such as opening or closing the hands rapidly fatigue. It is well-authenticated that in grave emergency life-saving movements can be performed with normal speed and vigour.

Except in very early cases *rigidity* can be detected. In its minimal form it can be felt on passive flexion and extension of the wrist or elbow as a slight recurring catch followed by relaxation—the 'cog-wheel' effect. In more advanced disease plastic or 'lead pipe' rigidity is present, consisting of marked resistance throughout the full range of passive movement of the joint. Rigidity is often accompanied by pain. The tendon jerks are normal and the plantar reflexes flexor. Constipation is often troublesome but bladder dysfunction is exceptional.

The progress of the disease is highly variable. At one extreme an annoying tremor of one hand may persist almost unchanged for a decade or more, and at the other the patient may become helpless within a few years. The severe form terminates in virtual immobility. Another variable factor is the effect on mental function. In most patients this is unimpaired, but in a few there is progressive dementia which must be carefully distinguished from the depression that is almost an integral feature of Parkinson's disease.

Post-encephalitic Parkinsonism as now encountered is a late sequel of encephalitis lethargica and presents some distinctive features. The symptoms often remain unilateral and rigidity is disproportionately severe. Ocular symptoms and signs are common. Blepharospasm, in which the eyes are involuntarily closed, may be so severe as almost to prevent useful vision. In oculogyric crises the eyes are involuntarily fixed in conjugate deviation, usually upwards, often for many hours. Pupillary abnormalities, ocular palsies, increased tendon jerks and extensor plantar reflexes may be evidence of more widespread damage from the original infection, and mental changes are common.

Arteriosclerotic Parkinsonism is often diagnosed in elderly patients with paralysis agitans, but in fact arteriosclerosis plays no part in the aetiology of the disease. If the term is to be used at all it should be confined to those cases where repeated small 'lacunae' or cystic sequelae of small haemorrhages occurring in the course of hypertensive arterial disease have resulted in a clinical state which includes some degree of plastic rigidity and a tottering gait. There are also obvious signs of corticospinal tract involvement, and classical Parkinsonian tremor does not occur.

Drug-induced Parkinsonism is entirely similar to the idiopathic form but is seldom severe and tremor is less prominent. The expressionless or grimacing faces and stooping posture of the inhabitants of chronic mental hospital wards are often due to prolonged medication with phenothiazines or reserpine. The condition is nearly always reversible when the drug is withdrawn.

The diagnosis of an established case of Parkinson's disease should present no difficulty but in the early stages there are many sources of error. Difficulty in writing may cause confusion with writer's cramp, and pain in the limbs may lead to orthopaedic referral. Difficulty in rising from a chair may suggest weakness of proximal leg muscles. Distinction from other forms of tremor may be difficult, but that most commonly mistaken for Parkinsonism—essential tremor—is absent at rest.

The pathological changes are curiously slight (Fig. 28, following p. 152). The most consistent appear to be loss of nerve cells from the substantia nigra and of myelinated fibres from the globus pallidus. In the idiopathic form inclusion bodies are found within the cells of the substantia nigra and elsewhere.

The symptomatic treatment of Parkinson's disease was based for many years on drugs with an atropine-like or anticholinergic action. The use of these drugs had no physiological basis at that time, and indeed there was no agreement even as to whether their site of action was central or peripheral. The synthetic agents, of which benzhexol, ethopropazide, orphenadrine and benztropine are probably the best, undoubtedly have a beneficial effect on rigidity, and movement is thereby somewhat facilitated, but they do not help the tremor. In severe cases on treatment for many years the benefit may seem to be minimal unless the drug is stopped, when complete immobility demonstrates the true extent of the disease. The dose of benzhexol is from 6 to 30 mg a day in divided doses, increasing to the maximum tolerated. Orphenadrine is given as 50 to 100 mg thrice daily, and ethopropazide in the same dose. Benztropine is a cumulative drug and must be given as a single evening dose of 1–2 mg. All these agents act like atropine in drying the mouth, causing blurred vision and hallucinations and confusion as well as retention of urine from prostatism. The antiviral agent amantadine was accidentally found to help the symptoms of Parkinson's disease, probably through an anticholinergic action. The dose is 100 mg a day, increasing to twice this dose. Initial improvement is often not maintained.

Treatment has now been placed on a more rational basis. The basic observation was that in Parkinson's disease the concentration of dopamine is grossly reduced in the putamen and caudate nucleus. It was known that drugs that induce Parkinsonism either deplete the basal ganglia of dopamine and other catecholamines or block their receptors. Evidence accumulated that the symptoms of Parkinson's disease are due, wholly or in part, to destruction or loss of function of a tract passing from the substantia nigra to the striatum and liberating dopamine as a predominantly inhibitory transmitting agent. It was therefore a logical step to attempt to restore normal concentrations of dopamine in the basal ganglia.

Dopamine itself cannot be used as it does not pass the blood-brain barrier, but its natural precursor levodopa can enter the brain and is also absorbed when given by mouth. It has proved the most effective medical treatment yet developed but requires careful management. It is still uncertain whether treatment should be given for early mild symptoms or reserved until incapacity has increased. The relief obtained in early cases often shows clearly that the symptoms were less 'mild' than had been supposed, chronic fatigue having been accepted as natural. The initial nausea and vomiting and the gradual introduction necessary when levodopa is given alone are avoided by the addition of an inhibitor of decarboxylase, the enzyme that breaks down dopa in peripheral tissue. This permits a lower total dose but a higher concentration in the brain. These combined preparations (Sinemet, Madopar) should now be universally employed. Treatment should begin with 100 or 125 mg with enzyme inhibitor three times a day, with food, increasing if all is well to 250 mg thrice daily, the average dose, after a week. Patients already established on levodopa can be switched to a combined preparation overnight, 1 g being approximately equivalent to 250 mg with enzyme inhibitor. It is impossible to predict the response. Early cases often do well but even severely disabled patients may show astonishing improvement. In favourable cases it may be virtually impossible to detect any sign of the disease, a result never achieved with earlier methods of treatment. Some fluctuation in the course of the day is usual and in some patients this is severe and inexplicably sudden—the 'on/off effect'. Previous treatment with anticholinergic drugs should be continued, but not in uncomfortably high dosage, and amantadine is also a compatible drug.

The main limiting factor in the use of levodopa is the development of involuntary movements quite different from those of Parkinson's disease. This *dyskinesia* may be due to the action of dopamine on denervated cells in the basal ganglia—a form of denervation hypersensitivity—as it does not occur in normal subjects. The movements take many forms: grimacing, restlessness, chorea and fluctuating rigidity being among the commonest. Probably all patients with Parkinson's disease develop dyskinesia if the dose of levodopa is high enough and many will tolerate some abnormal movements for the sake of the relief from Parkinsonism.

Not all patients respond and there is an unfortunate group who become exceedingly sensitive to the drug so that a minute increase in dose causes distressing dyskinesia while the slightest reduction leads to the return of incapacitating Parkinsonism. The change from the underdosed to the overdosed state and the reverse may take place with startling suddenness, the so-called on/off effect. In serious cases the changes appear to bear no relation to the timing of doses of levodopa and no effective means of control has been developed. The use of the dopamine agonist bromocryptine in combination with Sinemet has sometimes seemed to be of limited benefit. Among the other numerous side-effects the most important are those on the cardiovascular system. Postural hypotension can be troublesome and cardiac failure and ischaemic heart disease may be aggravated. Even more serious are the mental side-effects: nightmares, confusion, hallucinations, agitation and even occasionally mania. Reduction of dosage is essential.

The idea of simple replacement therapy with dopamine is almost certainly over-simplified. The interaction between different therapeutic agents is not fully understood but there are obvious indications that acetylcholine and dopamine have opposing actions in the basal ganglia. A curious effect of practical importance is that pyridoxine completely abolishes the activity of levodopa.

All forms of medical treatment, including levodopa, have far more effect on rigidity and akinesia than on tremor which may persist when other symptoms are relieved. In carefully selected patients stereotaxic surgery can be remarkably effective. The surgeon's aim is to place a small lesion in the ventrolateral nucleus of the thalamus or in the pallido-thalamic fibres, but success is not always closely linked with the presumed site of the lesion. The theoretical basis, which will be discussed below, is insecure but interruption of the efferent flow from the extrapyramidal system seems to be the essential factor. Contraindications to operation are dementia, hypertension, arteriosclerosis, or severe impairment of gait, speech or swallowing. Tremor can be entirely cured and rigidity relieved, but akinesia may even be aggravated. Serious complications such as hemiplegia and mental confusion are now very rare.

※

Our knowledge of the pathogenesis of other diseases affecting the basal ganglia is less substantial, and the site and nature of the responsible lesions are often conjectural.

CHOREA AND ATHETOSIS

Chorea is characterized by fleeting involuntary coordinated but purposeless movements. These occur without repetitive sequence and may involve any group of muscles. Grimacing, rolling of the eyes, twitching of the limbs and movements of the head occur unpredictably. Voluntary and automatic movements are interrupted so that breathing is jerky and dysarthria may be severe. Postures cannot be maintained and it is characteristic that the tongue cannot be held protruded. The limbs are hypotonic and although the tendon jerks are preserved a tap on the patella tendon may set up a pendular movement if the leg is allowed to hang free, or relaxation may be interrupted by a choreic twitch.

Almost identical involuntary movements may occur from very different causes. Huntington's chorea is described in Chapter 16, and here there is severe degeneration of the caudate nucleus, but many other structures are involved. Sydenham's or *rheumatic chorea* (St. Vitus' dance) is a disease predominantly of children. It usually presents with involuntary movements, often unrecognized or for many weeks attributed to wilful misbehaviour. Writing and school work are early affected. In addition to the choreic movements the limbs may be weak and severely hypotonic. Where weakness is more conspicuous than involuntary movement serious diagnostic difficulty may arise, especially if the condition is mainly or entirely unilateral. Additional signs are often present, notably hyperpronation of the outstretched hands.

There is seldom any simultaneous evidence of acute rheumatism involving the joints, there is no fever and the ESR is not raised. The rheumatic origin of the disease is betrayed by the typical cardiac lesions that may ensue, but active carditis can seldom be detected during an attack of chorea. It is traditional to treat these children at rest in bed for many weeks but it is impossible to adduce evidence of resulting benefit. Drug treatments in vogue in the past have usually proved harmful, and mild sedation during severe episodes is all that can be attempted. Recovery is almost invariable but may be delayed for many months, and relapse is common. Prolonged prophylaxis against streptococcal infection is advised in rheumatic fever and should logically be imposed following an attack of chorea.

Chorea gravidarum is rheumatic chorea in pregnancy and is now a mild disease probably not associated with fresh cardiac lesions. Certainly maniacal chorea with intractable and exhausting movements and extreme mental excitability is no longer seen.

In the occasional fatal case of chorea examined at post-mortem no lesion of the brain has been found, showing that this is potentially a completely reversible disorder of function. This is confirmed by the rare and similarly recoverable development of chorea in polycythaemia vera and following the use of oral contraceptives.

However, the inclusion of chorea among the symptoms of disease of the basal ganglia receives some support from the association of apparently related involuntary movements with established focal lesions. *Athetosis* in its fully developed form consists of comparatively slow writhing movements, predominantly of the arms, face and tongue. These are exacerbated by attempted voluntary movement which is therefore clumsy and inaccurate. A characteristic feature is the posture of the outstretched arm, adducted at the shoulder and partially flexed at elbow and wrist with strong extension of the fingers, but interrupted by slow contractions. In many patients more rapid movements are also present and it is usual to speak of choreoathetosis.

Athetosis is uncommon, and is seen as a form of congenital cerebral palsy, as a rare progressive disease of unknown cause developing in adolescence, and in a less conspicuous form accompanying residual hemiplegia due to cerebral infarction. The responsible lesion is often difficult to localize, but damage to the putamen is thought to be the essential factor. Medical treatment of athetosis is unsuccessful since anticholinergic drugs are ineffective and diazepam only marginally helpful in soporific doses. Nor is stereotactic surgery consistently helpful in this form of involuntary movement.

OTHER FORMS OF INVOLUNTARY MOVEMENT

Hemiballismus is a rare but dramatic form of involuntary movement, nearly always of sudden onset and due to infarction of the subthalamic nucleus—a precise localization unique in the study of the basal ganglia. Incessant ample and violent irregular movements of the limbs on one side soon exhaust the patient and cause local injuries. The movements can almost always be stopped immediately by 25 to 50 mg of chlorpromazine thrice daily by mouth, and in most cases the disorder remits spontaneously after several weeks. Persistent cases can be relieved by thalamotomy.

Spasmodic torticollis is less of a rarity. It may certainly occur as part of some widespread disease, particularly as a sequel of encephalitis lethargica, but it is generally encountered as an isolated symptom. It usually begins between the ages of 20 and 50 and affects both sexes without evidence of inheritance. Early symptoms are often ignored and when the patient seeks advice the head is involuntarily and frequently turned forcibly to one side, or occasionally backwards. This can easily be prevented by the observer, or indeed the patient, opposing the movement by light pressure on the chin, although relief is short-lived. Those unfamiliar with the condition confidently diagnose hysteria or malingering but this is hardly ever correct. In severe cases the head becomes almost permanently turned to one side, held in this position by intense and painful muscular contraction and not by fixed deformity of the neck. The condition causes great distress, often made worse by injudicious psychiatric or orthopaedic treatment.

As with many important but non-fatal diseases the pathology of the common form of spasmodic torticollis unassociated with other obvious disease is almost unexplored. In the only thoroughly investigated patient with spasmodic torticollis as an isolated symptom in whom full neuropathological study was possible no lesion was found. This must not be taken as supporting an hysterical cause as disordered function is not necessarily detectable with the microscope. A disorder of neurotransmitter mechanisms is highly probable but none has been detected.

Attempted treatment has ranged through psychotherapy, hypnosis, negative feedback and rigid collars to a great variety of drugs, but none have proved reliable. Some patients obtain partial relief from diazepam or anticholinergic drugs and physiotherapy may help the pain from the muscle spasm. Surgery should be reserved for severe disability. Simply cutting the sternomastoid muscle is not enough, since all the muscles of the neck are involved in this complex disorder of posture. Section of the upper three cervical roots on one side and the upper four on the other is a formidable procedure: it does not result in a normal neck but is received with gratitude by the patient. Stereotaxic surgery on the basal ganglia is also helpful but the lesions inflicted must be bilateral. In most patients this is a tendency towards natural improvement over many years, but complete remission is uncommon.

Torsion dystonia is a rare condition usually seen as a progressive and totally disabling disease of adolescents, occasionally familial, rarely subject to spontaneous arrest. It may also occur in patients with Wilson's disease (Chapter 14) but in most examples no cause is found and, remarkably enough in a crippling and eventually fatal disease, no significant abnormality can be found on microscopic examination of the brain. The condition often begins with the child walking on the ball of the foot, at first intermittently. Ultimately the muscles of the trunk and of the proximal and distal segments of the limbs are involved in continuous writhing spasms, producing scoliosis and grotesque distortions. In adults it may be preceded by spasmodic torticollis. Apart from occasional success with levodopa, drugs are useless but early stereotaxic surgery is sometimes dramatically beneficial.

Drug-induced involuntary movements are now a common emergency in casualty departments. Phenothiazine and related compounds in excess, or in ordinary therapeutic doses in susceptible subjects, may induce the sudden onset of the most bizarre and alarming contortions. Trismus, forced gaping of the mouth, spasmodic protrusion of the tongue, oculogyric crises and neck retraction are the commonest patterns but the trunk and limb muscles may also be involved. The patients are often young and may have been experimenting with drugs, but as it is not generally known that even a single dose of such compounds as prochlorperazine and perphenazine can sometimes produce these calamitous effects, hysteria is often diagnosed and regrettably treated by injection of a phenothiazine. The correct treatment is the intravenous injection of 5 to 10 mg of diazepam, repeated if necessary.

Involuntary movements of a different type may develop insidiously during protracted treatment. Parkinsonism has already been mentioned. Highly characteristic is the strange condition known as *akathisia* in which there is extreme restlessness and a constant need to move. This subsides, although not always rapidly, when the responsible drug is withdrawn, but another relatively common complication, writhing movements of the lips and tongue, may persist indefinitely. Similar movements sometimes develop in elderly people who have never received phenothiazines, and minor degrees are common, often annoying the relatives more than the patient. No relevant lesions have been identified in the brain. So-called tardive dyskinesia is a major problem in the treatment of schizophrenia. Some relief can be obtained by using even larger doses of phenothiazines but this is obviously undesirable. Tetrabenazine is also partially effective but is a depressant drug.

There is no evidence that the common condition *essential or hereditary tremor* is due to disease of the basal ganglia, but it must often be considered in the differential diagnosis of involuntary movement. Tremor begins at any age from the second decade onwards but is rare in children. The hands are primarily affected in such actions as writing or holding a cup. Like other involuntary movements it is worse in company and is all too readily attributed to emotional tension. Its severity usually increases slowly, and it may occasionally become a serious disability especially to those who have to appear in public. A fine tremor of the head may develop. If the patient can be persuaded to relax completely there is no tremor, but it appears immediately the hands are held up, particularly if the elbows are flexed. It is faster than the tremor of Parkinson's disease, beating at eight to ten per second. There is undoubtedly often an element of intention tremor but none of the other signs usually attributed to cerebellar disease. There is no rigidity and no alteration in reflexes but it is not surprising that the condition often gives rise to fears of multiple sclerosis or Parkinson's disease.

Dominant inheritance is often strongly evident and marked tremor in old age is probably an expression of the disease, but otherwise nothing is known of its cause. Anticholinergic drugs are ineffective and treatment with sedatives inappropriate in a life-long minor disability. A characteristic feature is that the tremor is rapidly but temporarily abolished by moderate doses of ethyl alcohol. The α-sympathetic blocking agent propranolol affords symptomatic relief in many patients. Thalamotomy is known to abolish the tremor but can only be contemplated when disability is unusually severe.

Writers' cramp is not, as far as is known, due to any disorder in the extrapyramidal system but is a form of involuntary muscular contraction that may cause diagnostic confusion. It affects exclusively those whose work involves writing, although the literary effort involved may be no more than noting an occasional sale. Writing is at first tremulous but later the pen is gripped with increasing force and the 'cramp' can be seen to involve contraction of all the muscles of the limb. Writing becomes impossible and the pen may fly from the hand. The function of the hand for all other activities, even the finest manipulations, is entirely normal, a point of diagnostic importance.

Like many other unfamiliar and peculiar symptoms writers' cramp is usually diagnosed as hysteria, but it does not respond to suggestion, hypnosis or psychotherapy. Far more important is to exclude Parkinson's disease, spastic weakness, or essential tremor all of which may present with difficulty in writing. Other occupational cramps are now rare and an isolated inability to use the left hand when playing the violin is the only other form likely to be encountered. These disabilities appear to be 'functional' disorders in the true sense of the word, in which the most recently acquired and most difficult forms of dexterity involving rapid movement are lost. Success has been claimed for a form of aversion therapy in which the patient receives an electric shock if his hand strays from its original path, but in general the occupational cramps are incurable.

The four conditions, spasmodic torticollis, torsion dystonia, essential tremor and writer's cramp have several features in common. They are without established morbid anatomical basis and show some tendency to occur together in different combinations. It should be remembered that even Parkinson's disease was for long classified as a 'neurosis'.

A strange form of involuntary movement with an established pathology lying rather beyond the accepted confines of the basal ganglia must be mentioned here. *Palatal myoclonus* consists of almost rhythmic rapid contractions of one side of the soft palate. The movement usually spreads to the other side or may involve the face, larynx and diaphragm, and sometimes other muscles. It follows infarction of the brain stem or head injury, and isolated cases have been described in many diseases. It is said to be the only involuntary movement to persist during sleep. The responsible lesion involves the dentate and olivary nuclei.

Myoclonus is merely a descriptive term, loosely applied to sudden shock-like muscular contractions due to many different causes. The common form of myoclonic epilepsy is described in Chapter 17. Much more widespread and often continuous myoclonus without any constant localization occurs in a number of rare diseases such as the lipidoses and familial myoclonic epilepsy, in which there is diffuse neuronal loss, particularly from the cerebellum. As a transient episode myoclonus can occur in acute infections, in uraemia and other metabolic disorders including overdosage with intravenous penicillin. A form of action myoclonus interfering with voluntary movement is now encountered with increasing frequency in patients surviving cerebral anoxia due to cardiac disease.

THE NATURE OF BASAL GANGLIA SYNDROMES

There is general agreement that interpretation of the disorders of motor activity due to disease of the basal ganglia in terms of disordered physiology is formidably difficult. Agreement does not proceed beyond this point. The rarity of strict correlation between the site of identifiable lesions and resulting symptoms has already been noted. This is less disconcerting if the concept of the reversible biochemical lesion undetectable by conventional microscopy is invoked, as indeed it must be to explain the drastic but temporary effects of drugs. It is also helpful to remember that however complex the anatomical network and multiplicity of presumed transmitter substances, neurones can act only by excitation or inhibition.

By analogy with the effects of dysfunction of the corticospinal or pyramidal pathways, those of extrapyramidal disorders must be divided into negative and positive symptoms. The former, directly due to loss of excitatory neurones, must include the loss of normal motor activity, notably the akinesia of Parkinson's disease. Not only is 'voluntary' activity impaired but also many actions normally performed without conscious effort, such as swinging the arms or standing upright. An unproven but attractive theory is that what is lost is the control of the extrapyramidal system over the activity of the fusimotor neurones. Perhaps the corticospinal system initiates movement by excitation of alpha motor neurones, while the extrapyramidal system acts primarily by altering the rate of fusimotor firing and only secondarily and as the result of reflex action activates the prime movers, the alpha motor neurones and their motor units. The loss of normal righting reflexes in Parkinson's disease and in hemiballismus, and similarly the hypotonia of chorea and the uncoordinated movements resulting from lesions in the subthalamic region can also be interpreted as negative symptoms.

The great majority of symptoms in extrapyramidal disease are, however, clearly positive, representing excessive neuronal activity and apparently indicating release from normal inhibition. In Parkinsonian rigidity stretch reflexes are enhanced, although in a manner different from that seen in spasticity in that tendon jerks are not increased and the response to slow stretch is distinctive. The flexed posture of Parkinson's disease and the more severely disabling postural defects in other forms of dystonia may be explained in principle, if not in detail, by excessive and disordered activity of less easily observed reflexes entering at different levels of the extrapyramidal system. The afferent impulses for the righting reflexes largely responsible for the maintenance of normal posture arise at many sites: the labyrinth, the eyes, the joint and muscle receptors, particularly of the neck, and surface contacts of the body. Obviously either exaggeration due to failure of inhibition, or loss of these reflexes due to failure of facilitation or interruption of reflex arcs could result in a diversity of motor disabilities.

It is the involuntary movements that are particularly hard to understand. One school of thought maintains that there are centres of neuronal activity normally discharging at a frequency of about five per second and prevented from causing rhythmic muscular contraction by the activity of the extrapyramidal system. Evidence is conflicting, and an alternative view is that involuntary movements are a sign of reflex disorders similar to those causing rigidity but less severe. It is comparatively easy to envisage a reflex origin for the continuous muscular contraction of Parkinsonian rigidity that might be interrupted by the interplay of stretch reflexes and mutual inhibition at spinal level from opposing muscle groups, with the production of rhythmic tremor. The reflex origin of the violent movements of hemiballismus can be understood as due to total loss of reflex control of posture of the limbs, and a comparable disorder of the complex reflexes controlling posture of the head could reasonably be invoked in spasmodic torticollis. A similar origin for the writhing movements of athetosis, the sudden grimaces of chorea or the extraordinary contortions of phenothiazine intoxication is far less credible.

The effect of stereotaxic surgery in alleviating tremor and rigidity and certain other forms of involuntary movement and dystonia can therefore be seen as due to interruption of the major outflow from the extrapyramidal system, apparently carrying mainly excitatory impulses, thus reducing or abolishing the exaggerated reflex activity. The most effective lesions are precisely placed to achieve this purpose, in the globus pallidus, the ventrolateral nucleus of the thalamus or their connecting fibres. Symptoms that can reasonably be attributed to loss of excitatory functions such as akinesia, disorders of gait, balance, speech and swallowing could scarcely be alleviated by further destruction of neurones and, apart from some relief from abolition of rigidity, improvement in these functions does not occur following operation. It is to be hoped that levodopa and other agents yet to be discovered may act by restoring normal function with relief of both positive and negative symptoms.

Further reading

Marsden C.D. & Parkes J.D. (1973) Abnormal movement disorders. *Brit. J. Hosp. Med.* **10,** 428.

Marsden C.D. & Parkes J.D. (1977) Success and problems of long-term therapy in Parkinson's disease. *Lancet* **1,** 345.

Pallis C.A. (1971) Parkinsonism: natural history and clinical features. *Brit. Med. J.* **3,** 683.

CHAPTER 14
Metabolic Disease

The concept of the biochemical lesion of the nervous system has always been exciting and is of increasing importance. A change in the biochemical environment can produce a disorder of function that is at first fully reversible if normal conditions are restored but proceeds to irreversible structural damage if it continues. The search for such potentially curable metabolic causes of disease has been eagerly pursued, and although those identified in man have seldom proved as sharply defined as in the experimental animal, a measure of success has been achieved.

DEFICIENCY DISEASES

Pure dietary deficiencies are a rarity in developed countries, and where starvation is rife lack of protein and carbohydrate rather than vitamin deficiencies dominates its clinical expression.

Dietary thiamine (aneurine, Vitamin B_1) deficiency produces beriberi in the presence of an adequate carbohydrate intake. The syndrome is one of severe polyneuritis often associated with cardiac failure and oedema. If not too advanced it is fully reversible. Thiamine is concerned in the oxidative decarboxylation of pyruvate, an essential metabolic activity in many tissues, particularly the brain. It was naturally hoped that many forms of polyneuritis and other nervous disease might prove to be due to secondary disorders of pyruvate metabolism. This led to the rational but unrewarding administration of thiamine to patients with all forms of polyneuritis and, by insensible degrees, to the unthinking use of costly polyvitamin preparations in subjects of paraesthesiae from any cause, and eventually in functional nervous disorders. Except for alcoholic neuropathy and Wernicke's encephalopathy (Chapter 6) there is no evidence that vitamin B_1 is helpful in any disease other than beriberi. Because of the action of thiamine in the chain converting glucose into energy, the levels of pyruvate in the blood after a loading dose of glucose have been extensively studied in polyneuritis. Apparent defects in pyruvate tolerance have been reported, but consistent results cannot be obtained and the examination is of no practical value.

Pyridoxine (vitamin B_6) is concerned in amino-acid metabolism. It is essential for the biosynthesis of adrenaline and noradrenaline as well as for γ-aminobutyric acid, which inhibits neuronal activity. Accidental dietary deficiency has caused epilepsy in infants, and rare instances are known of frequent convulsions in the newborn that are controllable only by the administration of quantities of pyridoxine greatly in excess of normal requirements. The possibility of pyridoxine-dependent epilepsy has been investigated in infantile spasms (Chapter 17). Although disturbances of tryptophan metabolism have been found that might be attributed to failure of effective action of pyridoxine, such fits cannot be controlled by massive doses of the vitamin.

Peripheral neuropathy induced by isoniazid may be partially preventable with pyridoxine, but it is not invariably effective.

The role of vitamin B_{12} in the metabolism of the nervous system is largely unknown. There is increasing evidence that the detoxication of ingested or inhaled cyanide is an important function, but this is unlikely to be its only mode of action. By far the commonest form of deficiency is failure of absorption due to lack of intrinsic factor in the gastric juice. Neurological complications are common in pernicious anaemia, though they are often mistakenly attributed to the anaemia itself, while they sometimes precede any abnormality in the peripheral blood. There is a very low serum B_{12}, and almost invariably bone marrow changes even when the blood count is normal in every respect. A mild degree of dementia, in most patients amounting to no more than slight forgetfulness and lack of concentration, is very common. Severe degrees occur, usually with little or no anaemia, and are clinically indistinguishable from other forms of dementia. Since the condition is reversible with B_{12} replacement the possibility should always be considered in the diagnosis of mental disorders of organic type.

Subacute combined degeneration of the spinal cord is relatively uncommon. It was named before its cause was recognized, because of the characteristic loss of myelin in both the posterior and lateral columns of white matter. The patients usually belong to the middle-aged or elderly age group of pernicious anaemia, and the symptoms may be erroneously attributed to senility. In younger patients without anaemia the condition may be disastrously mistaken for multiple sclerosis.

The presenting symptoms are usually sensory and begin in the feet. Mild 'pins and needles' sometimes increase to persistent and exceedingly unpleasant burning paraesthesiae, spreading up the legs and even to the trunk. Paraesthesiae in the fingers are less obtrusive and are rarely the initial symptom. Motor symptoms develop later, although in some patients they predominate throughout. There is increasing difficulty in walking, damage to the corticospinal fibres being aggravated by sensory ataxia. Without treatment weakness increases until walking is impossible. Sphincter disturbance is uncommon.

The physical signs are those of ataxic and spastic weakness of the legs, with profound distal loss of postural and vibration sense and some loss of cutaneous sensation in severe cases. There is concurrent peripheral nerve damage, evident in tenderness of the calf muscles and in loss of the ankle jerks in spite of obvious evidence of damage to the upper motor neurone.

Treated in time the condition is reversible, although annoying paraesthesiae may persist. A patient still able to walk can be cured, but once he is bedridden the prognosis is uncertain. Severe damage cannot be repaired since the biochemical lesion has caused permanent structural changes. The importance of early diagnosis is evident. In every patient with unexplained paraparesis the possibility of B_{12} deficiency must be considered. If the vitamin has already been given as a placebo, as often happens in neurological disease regarded as incurable, the serum level will be useless and the bone marrow probably normal. If pernicious anaemia is to be excluded or confirmed, a Schilling test of absorption of B_{12} labelled with radio-cobalt must be done, before and after oral administration of intrinsic factor.

Visual failure and optic atrophy also occur in pernicious anaemia, presenting as impaired vision with a central scotoma or one extending from the fixation point to the blind spot. This has been closely linked to the function of B_{12} in detoxicating cyanide, as it is virtually confined to smokers.

Treatment of B_{12} deficiency in any form comprises simple replacement by injecting large doses. One thousand micrograms of hydroxocobalamine daily for a week is clearly far more than is needed but there is no point in being niggardly. Thereafter injection can be weekly for a time and then monthly, reducing to 100 micrograms but persisting indefinitely.

Comparable spinal cord disease is exceedingly uncommon in other forms of B_{12} deficiency.

Deficiency of folic acid has been suspected as a cause of both peripheral neuropathy and spinal cord disease, but this has not been confirmed. From the neurological point of view it is of interest that several anticonvulsants can induce deficiency.

Deficiency of nicotinamide is one of the main factors in the production of *pellagra*, of which the chief neurological feature is dementia, sometimes associated with polyneuritis. In malnutrition of such degree multiple deficiencies are the rule, and pellagra is not now believed to be a simple nicotinamide deficiency. Hartnup disease, a familial aminoaciduria, resembles pellagra in a number of respects.

INBORN ERRORS OF METABOLISM

The nervous system and skeletal muscle are involved in many inborn errors of metabolism, of which new forms are continually being discovered. These errors are genetically determined, and many have been detected in only a few families where a rare recessive gene has been contributed by each parent. The combination in the homozygous children produces overt disease, often rapidly lethal. In general the transmitted defect is one of enzyme activity, and this in turn is the consequence of a gene defect. Absence of an enzyme can cause deficiency of the metabolite next in the chain, or an accumulation of metabolites before the block. Either situation, or both, can cause spreading disruption of other enzyme systems, and where the final clinical effect is understood at all it may be difficult to explain in terms of the biochemical anomaly. Some metabolic errors are known in detail, but in others only an abnormal end-product can be recognized. Determined attempts have naturally been made to unearth inborn errors of metabolism in such genetically determined diseases as the hereditary ataxias and Huntington's chorea, but, until recently, without success (Chapter 16).

Wilson's disease (hepatolenticular degeneration) is a rare recessively inherited condition in which a metabolic error of fascinating complexity has been partially unravelled. Symptoms usually begin in the second or third decades. In many children there is a history of hepatic disease, transient jaundice or progressive liver failure. An episode of haemolytic anaemia may also occur as an early sign. Neurological symptoms sometimes develop without clinical evidence of liver disease, but there is much variation. In children these are often increasing rigidity, tremor on action or at rest, and disorders of gait and posture. A characteristic sign in advanced cases is a constant and inappropriate grin. Swallowing becomes difficult and death may result within a few years from inanition, hepatic failure, haemorrhage from oesophageal varices, or coma of uncertain cause. In the young adult the disease may be more benign, showing itself for many years only by a tremor of the hands that is both static and intentional.

A pathognomonic sign of the disease is the Kayser–Fleischer ring of green to golden pigment on the posterior aspect of the cornea just internal to the limbus. The ring may be partial and difficult to see, demanding slit-lamp examination.

In the brain there is widespread destruction of neurones, concentrated in the lenticular nuclei in the more acute forms. There is multilobular cirrhosis in the liver.

The underlying metabolic defect involves the trace element copper. This is normally transported from the gut to the liver where it is incorporated into a specific plasma globulin of unknown function, caeruloplasmin. Copper is eventually excreted in the bile. In Wilson's disease the formation of caeruloplasmin is defective. Copper thus accumulates in the liver and is carried in the blood in loosely bound form to be deposited in the brain, kidneys, cornea and other organs. Excretion in the bile is reduced while urinary excretion is increased but not sufficiently to prevent a life-long state of positive copper balance. The hepatic and cerebral damage are due to copper poisoning and the almost invariably occurring aminoaciduria is probably the result of the deposition of copper in the renal tubules. The diagnosis can be confirmed by low serum copper and caeruloplasmin levels with increased urinary copper, although as this is a trace element the daily excretion is much less than 1 mg and inexperienced laboratories can sometimes produce aberrant results.

The mechanism of over-absorption of copper is not fully known but successful treatment has been based on the elimination of excess copper from the body. This can be done most effectively by prolonged treatment with 1–2 g of penicillamine a day by mouth. If this is instituted before irreparable damage has occurred there may be an astonishing reversal of incapacitating neurological symptoms and even improvement in liver function. The loss of copper can be measured by the great increase in urinary excretion and more directly observed in the fading of the green pigment of the corneal ring.

In this remarkable instance the concept of a reversible biochemical lesion has therefore superseded that of inherited neuronal degeneration.

In Wilson's disease the combination of liver and brain disease had always suggested a metabolic or toxic cause, but in *phenylketonuria* there was no such indication, and the syndrome was discovered by testing the urine of mentally defective children. It is known to be transmitted by a single autosomal recessive gene, and the essential metabolic defect is identified as a failure to convert phenylalanine into tyrosine because of lack of specific enzyme activity. The metabolic needs of the developing brain are different from those of the adult, and cerebral damage results from the greatly excessive concentration of phenylalanine caused by the metabolic block. Some of the phenylalanine is converted into phenylpyruvic acid, which appears in the urine. The disease can therefore be detected during the first few weeks after birth by the green colour produced by this substance when the urine is tested with ferric chloride, conveniently used as Phenistix applied to a wet napkin. This has not proved sufficiently reliable and is being replaced by microbiological and biochemical estimations of phenylalanine blood levels.

Mental retardation is obvious at six months and most affected children are idiots, although rarely intelligence is normal. The disease is not usually progressive beyond infancy, though epilepsy and disorders of movement may appear. As a side-effect of the metabolic defect the children are blonde and have blue eyes. Phenylketonuria is an uncommon disease but is said to account for 1% of mental defectives in institutions.

A concerted attempt has been made to detect all cases as soon as possible and to institute treatment before brain damage has occurred. This is based on altering the environment by removing phenylalanine from the diet. This is arduous and expensive but the results, if not as good as was first hoped, clearly show that the clinical effects of the metabolic error can be diminished. If treatment is begun before the age of ten weeks, preferably earlier, and is steadfastly maintained, intelligence can be expected to be normal.

The much less frequent inborn errors of *galactosaemia* and *homocysteinuria* can also be treated by withdrawing from the environment the normal metabolites that become 'toxic' when they are present in concentrations uncontrolled by the normal enzymatic chains.

The clinical features of *acute intermittent porphyria* are described in Chapter 6. This metabolic error is often transmitted as a dominant characteristic and although it may be lethal, it does not declare itself until adult life. An enzyme dysfunction is certainly present in the liver, involving the chain of conversion of delta-aminolaevulinic acid and porphobilinogen into porphyrins and leading to excessive production of the former, but these metabolites, which accumulate in excess, have not been shown to damage the nervous system directly, and the precise cause of the clinical syndrome is obscure.

The *lipidoses* are rare genetically determined diseases in which a metabolic disorder is evident in the accumulation of intracellular lipids. Investigation has identified a large number of enzyme deficiencies each leading to the accumulation of a specific lipid. In Tay-Sachs disease (amaurotic family idiocy) the impact is primarily on the nervous system. Ninety per cent of cases of this infantile form occur in Jewish families, but other varieties occur later in life without any racial predilection. In all forms of cerebromacular degeneration there is progressive dementia and often major and myoclonic epilepsy. Blindness is associated with a 'cherry-red' spot at the macula, where the blood vessels can be seen through the degenerated nervous tissue of the retina. The disease is progressive and fatal. The metabolic disorder is recognizable only by observing the deposition of intracellular gangliosides in the nervous system at autopsy or on cortical biopsy, although vacuolated circulating leucocytes are sometimes seen.

In other forms of lipidosis the nervous system is less prominently involved, but a progressive dementia may occur in Gaucher's disease, which is characterized by accumulation of a gluco-cerebroside in the liver and spleen.

It is usual to consider the leucodystrophies as a distinct group of rare and little understood diseases in which the formation or maintenance of myelin is disordered. Of this heterogeneous collection the condition of *metachromatic leucodystrophy* probably qualifies as an inborn error of metabolism. In the infantile form there is progressive motor and mental defect from a very early age, but there are also later forms in which spastic paraplegia is a prominent feature. In addition to the loss of myelin or failure of normal myelin formation there is an accumulation of sulphatide lipids in the brain, peripheral nervous system, and kidneys. The metachromatic material from which the condition derives its name can be detected in the urine. The infantile form is recessively inherited. Knowledge of the underlying metabolic defect has not advanced to the point where any treatment is available.

Periodic paralysis is a rare but dramatic condition, usually genetically determined. The classical form is transmitted by dominant inheritance. The patients are often extremely muscular, and symptoms do not develop until early adult life. Attacks of paralysis frequently occur on awakening in the morning, after a heavy meal, or during rest after exertion. The severity varies from slight weakness to almost complete paralysis of the limbs and trunk, with sparing of the bulbar muscles. The duration of attacks is also highly variable but they often last for several hours. In this form the serum potassium level during an attack is low, but usually above the very low levels needed to produce paralysis in other forms of hypokalaemia. The potassium is not lost in the urine, since the output is reduced, but it is taken up by the muscles: biopsies taken during an attack contain numerous vesicles. Sodium is retained prior to an attack. The underlying cause of the disorder has not been determined, but there is an obvious resemblance to the effects of an aldosterone-secreting tumour of the adrenal, and biochemical evidence indicates that attacks are preceded by, or associated with, increased adrenal activity.

Diagnosis can usually be established by estimating serum potassium during an attack, if necessary induced by a carbohydrate meal and insulin, which increase muscle potassium. Paralysis can be cut short by 2–4 g of potassium chloride by mouth. Prophylactic treatment with 100 mg of spironolactone four times a day may be completely successful, and treatment can sometimes be stopped after a year without subsequent relapse.

A rarer form of periodic paralysis, labelled *adynamia episodica hereditaria* represents in some ways the obverse of this metabolic disorder, since the serum potassium is high during attacks, which can be prevented by diuretics that increase potassium excretion. The attacks are seldom as severe as in the classical form. A third variety occurs in which the serum potassium is normal during attacks.

McArdle's disease is described in Chapter 7.

SYSTEMIC METABOLIC DISEASE

The effects on the nervous system of generalized metabolic disease comprise a third category. Of these the most obvious is the failure of oxygen supply to the brain. A minor degree of hypoxia plays a part in the intermittent nocturnal confusion, sometimes amounting to delirium in cardiac failure. In the elderly patient persistent mental changes may be the presenting sign of heart failure.

Cardiac arrest, ventricular asystole, or ventricular fibrillation cause almost immediate loss of consciousness. In Stokes–Adams attacks due to heart block the ventricular contraction begins again within a few seconds, and no cerebral damage results, though the risk of sudden death is of course constantly present. Reversible cardiac arrest is now commonplace, but the time available for effective action to protect the brain is brief. Exactly how brief it is impossible to gauge, since patients sometimes emerge intact from periods of apparently complete cerebral anoxia that are theoretically intolerable. Clinical evidence of neuronal loss in brain-damaged survivors usually suggests widespread involvement of the cerebral cortex, with particular emphasis on the parietal and temporal lobes. Aphasia accompanied by varying disorders of spatial orientation is often seen and a particularly distressing sequel is uncontrollable jerking of the limbs during attempted voluntary movement—action myoclonus.

In *pulmonary disease* both anoxia and carbon dioxide retention affect cerebral function. In obstructive airway disease the latter factor is certainly the more important, particularly during acute exacerbations. Brief lapses of posture of the outstretched fingers and hands at intervals of from one to several seconds are often seen in these patients. Consciousness is disturbed to a degree that varies from mild confusion to coma, the latter sometimes precipitated by the administration of oxygen leading to increased retention of carbon dioxide. In patients permanently short of breath at rest from pulmonary disease there may be persistent intellectual defect accompanied by marked changes in the electroencephalogram.

Severe *hepatic failure* is also regularly accompanied by neurological signs. In early decompensation the intellect is blunted and there is coarse tremor of the outstretched hands. In more advanced stages consciousness is severely impaired and death in coma is common. When jaundice is clinically obvious diagnosis should present no difficulty, but in its absence the metabolic origin of chronic fluctuating clouding of consciousness may not be recognized. The precise cause of the cerebral symptoms is not known, but is clearly related to failure of the liver to deal with some product of protein derived from the gut. The level of ammonia in the blood is often raised but its relationship to the clinical condition is not exact. Porto-caval anastomosis, which allows products absorbed from the gut to reach the brain before passing through the liver, may precipitate neurological complications. The benefits of restricting protein in the diet are often remarkable. In severe relapse no protein whatever is given, and bacterial activity in the gut is inhibited with neomycin. If improvement follows, a level of dietary protein must be found that will keep the patient alert. This is often in the region of 30 g a day. The electroencephalogram is useful in judging the effect because slowing of the record is an early sign of neurological involvement.

In *renal failure* it is again usually impossible to attribute neurological symptoms to a specific metabolic defect. Disturbances of ionic concentration are certainly more important than those of organic compounds. Major epileptic fits are not uncommon in uraemia, and more localized myoclonus is also frequent. The survival of many patients with chronic renal failure treated by dialysis has revealed progressive and often intractable polyneuritis as a serious complication. A further unpleasant complication known as dialysis dementia or encephalopathy has also recently appeared in some centres. The onset may be insidious or rapid and declares itself with speech disturbance, curiously enough usually stuttering. This is followed by aphasia, dementia, hallucinations and myoclonus. The EEG contains much slow activity. There is much evidence to suggest that the condition is due to aluminium intoxication introduced during dialysis.

When respiratory, hepatic or renal function fails there are certain similarities between the effects on the nervous system: disturbance of consciousness and involuntary movement are the prominent features.

This reflects the diffuse nature of the neuronal disorder in all three conditions, but there are considerable differences in the prominence of individual symptoms and in the tempo of development.

Ionic concentrations exert a considerable effect on the function of the neurone, on axonal conduction, and on neuromuscular conduction and muscle fibre contraction. In clinical practice only gross deviations from the normal can be recognized. The influence of the potassium ion in familial periodic paralysis has already been mentioned, but the association is more commonly seen in potassium depletion. Despite advances in the management of fluid and electrolyte imbalance this type of depletion has increased in frequency because of the injudicious use of oral diuretics. These powerful agents used in continuous high dosage without potassium replacement may reduce the serum level to dangerous levels. Such levels cause severe paralysis of the muscles of the trunk and limbs, though those supplied by the cranial nerves are spared. Treatment is hazardous and not invariably successful. The serum potassium may also be reduced to the point of producing paralysis in the rare condition of Conn's syndrome due to an aldosterone-secreting tumour of the adrenal.

The calcium ion is intimately concerned with the excitability of nervous and muscular tissue. Hypocalcaemia is one of the causes of *tetany*. In mild spontaneous attacks of tetany the hands alone are involved, the digits being extended and closely adducted to form the *main d'accoucheur*. In more severe attacks the muscles of the feet also go into spasm which may spread to proximal segments of the limbs and to the trunk, causing difficulty in breathing. Sensory symptoms, tingling and pain, are common. Overt tetany occurs when too much parathyroid tissue has been removed at thyroidectomy and in idiopathic hypoparathyroidism. The detection of latent tetany is difficult. Chvostek's sign, a contraction of the facial muscles on tapping the facial nerve as it crosses the mandible, is positive but is also present in many normal people. Trousseau's sign is elicited by inflating a sphygmomanometer cuff above the systolic pressure for two minutes: if the test is positive this will result in the hand adopting a tetanic posture. By far the commonest cause of tetany is reduction of the P_{CO_2} by overbreathing. This dramatic but essentially benign syndrome is usually found in adolescent subjects, but is also encountered in adults. Some are clearly unstable and emotionally disturbed, but in many the condition seems to be of superficial origin and rapidly resolves with reassurance. Lesser degrees of over-ventilation may not be easy to detect and will nearly always be denied by the patient, though she may admit to 'shortness of breath' during his panic attacks.

The hyperexcitability of nervous tissue produced by hypocalcaemia

METABOLIC DISEASE 245

may also show itself in generalized epileptic fits, but these are distinctly rare.

Disorders of calcium and phosphorus metabolism of quite different nature may be associated with weakness of the proximal muscles of the legs and sometimes of other muscles. Osteomalacia from any cause as well as hyperparathyroidism due to an adenoma may produce this condition. Beyond the fact that it is muscular and not neurogenic, little is known of its mode of production. The weakness is fully reversible by correction of the biochemical disturbance.

Depletion of serum magnesium due to loss from the gastrointestinal tract or repeated dialysis causes a remarkable state of hyperexcitability distinct from tetany. The patient is usually confused or delirious and has exceedingly rapid involuntary movements including both tremor and myoclonus: Trousseau's sign is negative.

Disorders of glucose metabolism frequently affect the nervous system, as might be expected in view of the almost total dependence of nervous tissue on glucose as a metabolic substrate. Diabetic neuropathy is described in Chapter 6. Most diabetics on insulin are familiar with the effects of hypoglycaemia: lack of motor control leads rapidly to confusion and unconsciousness. This can be prevented or corrected with sugar and is inconvenient but seldom dangerous. Massive overdosage with insulin, usually during unskilled treatment of diabetic coma, can cause irreversible diffuse brain damage unless it is recognized and vigorously treated.

Spontaneous hypoglycaemia is difficult to diagnose. A harmless form in which the blood sugar swings too high after a carbohydrate meal and then falls too low is common and of little importance. Reactive hypoglycaemia of this type occurs after partial gastrectomy and also in some tense and anxious subjects. This form can be diagnosed by a glucose tolerance curve. The symptoms are faintness and sweating about an hour after a meal, and treatment consists in reducing the amount of carbohydrate at any one meal.

Hypoglycaemia due to an insulin-producing adenoma is rare and cannot be diagnosed by a glucose tolerance test because the hypoglycaemia is not reactive. The symptoms are closely related to prolonged abstention from food particularly when associated with muscular exertion. The minor manifestations are indeed difficult to distinguish from those of vertebrobasilar insufficiency—transient diplopia and paraesthesiae around the lips and in the mouth. In more severe attacks consciousness is disturbed, and prolonged confusion resembling temporal lobe epilepsy may occur or even major fits. Many patients notice an increase in appetite and a rapid gain in weight. Occasionally the symptoms are predominantly psychiatric comprising a fluctuating confusional state without loss of consciousness.

If the patient is seen in an attack the diagnosis can be established by examining the blood sugar and this opportunity should not be missed. Levels well below 20 mg/100 ml (1 mmol/l) have been found. The patient can be rapidly restored with glucose by any convenient route. If the diagnosis is suspected from the history an attempt must be made to produce an attack by prolonged starvation in hospital. An overnight fast is seldom sufficient, though the blood sugar may fall unduly low. Fasting may have to be protracted to the limit of tolerance, and may even then fail to provoke an attack in a patient subsequently found to have a pancreatic adenoma. Success is much more likely if the patient is exercised. The use of more dangerous provocative tests such as the response to tolbutamide is unnecessary. In many centres it is possible to obtain a measurement of plasma insulin which should put the diagnosis beyond doubt. If a single adenoma is present its removal results in complete cure.

Further reading

Arieff A.I., Llach F. & Massey S.G. (1976) Neurological manifestations and morbidity of hyponatraemia. *Medicine*, **55,** 121.

Strickland G.T. & Leu Mei-Ling (1975) Wilson's disease. *Medicine* **54,** 113.

Walshe J.M. (1970) Wilson's disease. *Brit. J. Hosp. Med.* **4,** 91.

CHAPTER 15
Developmental Diseases

The developing nervous system is vulnerable to many noxious agents, and the effects of genetically transmitted defects, of structural chromosomal abnormalities and of external influences cannot always be distinguished one from another. The neuronal damage caused by abnormal concentrations of metabolites in phenylketonuria is clearly of a different order from the effects of haemorrhage into the brain as a result of birth injury. However, gross structural defects can result from both intrinsic and external causes and may also have important secondary effects on development. There are many factors of which we are ignorant, notably the metabolic needs of the neurones at different sites and at different stages of development.

The embryology of the nervous system is necessarily complicated in detail, but consists in essence of the formation of a simple tube of neural tissue at an early stage of embryonic life. Its elaboration into the daunting complexities of the brain and spinal cord allows almost unlimited opportunities for maldevelopment. Many of the most severe, including virtual absence of the forebrain, are incompatible with life. Lesser defects are often found in combination and are therefore difficult to identify clinically. Thus, absence of the corpus callosum may be found with severe distortion of the gyral pattern of the cerebral cortex. Such children are nearly always mentally retarded, but in rare cases where agenesis of the corpus callosum or even absence of a large part of the cerebellar hemisphere occur in isolation, clinical abnormalities may be minimal.

CONGENITAL HYDROCEPHALUS

This important and relatively common disorder epitomizes the difficulties of distinguishing inherent defects of development from the effects of external agents. Cerebrospinal fluid is formed by the choroid plexus in the lateral, third and fourth ventricles and if its escape is partially or completely blocked the ventricles dilate. Obstructive hydrocephalus of this type is common in adult life as the result of any expanding lesion impeding the free flow of spinal fluid, but in the infant other causes operate. The aqueduct of Sylvius may be narrowed due to malformation or, judging by the presence of inflammatory cells, as a result of infection. Sometimes stenosis of the aqueduct, apparently present since birth, produces no symptoms until adult life, but it is also one cause of hydrocephalus in the infant. The flow of spinal fluid may be obstructed at the point of exit from the foramina in the roof of the fourth ventricle. This may result from subacute or chronic inflammatory changes in the adult, but in infancy a severe degree of obstruction rapidly produces hydrocephalus.

In communicating hydrocephalus there is no obstruction to the flow from the ventricles to the subarachnoid space but either the fluid cannot reach the convexity of the brain, or normal absorption does not take place through the arachnoid villi into the venous sinuses. Again the relative contributions of congenital malformation of the arachnoid membrane and the effects of intrauterine infection are debatable.

Hydrocephalus and enlargement of the head may develop *in utero* to such a degree that survival is impossible. However, the head is usually normal in size or only slightly enlarged at birth but expands rapidly within the first few weeks or months. The mean normal head circumference at birth is approximately 35 cm (13.5 inches), increasing to 40 cm (15.7 inches) at three months and 43 cm (17 inches) at six months. It is the rate of growth that is important, and an increase of 5 cm in a month is not uncommon in hydrocephalus. The expanded cranial vault, tense fontanelles, depression of the orbits and dilated scalp veins are obvious enough in severe cases but lesser degrees may be overlooked or ignored particularly if the baby otherwise seems to be developing normally. If hydrocephalus is allowed to advance unchecked mental retardation, optic atrophy, ocular palsies and spastic weakness of the limbs are almost inevitable even if other developmental abnormalities do not add to the disability. In a few children hydrocephalus becomes arrested and symptoms are minimal or limited to slight enlargement of the head.

Many cases of infantile hydrocephalus are associated with *meningomyelocoele*. This consists of partial failure of fusion of the spinal canal—spina bifida—with protrusion through the defect of a sac of meninges and normal or abnormal nervous tissue. The common site is the lumbar spine and more rarely the cervical region. Surgical treatment of the meningocoele may be followed by great aggravation of the hydrocephalus.

In a high proportion of cases hydrocephalus is accompanied or caused by the congenital malformations of the kind first described by Chiari. In these the medulla lies in the upper cervical canal and is surrounded by tongues of abnormal cerebellar tissue. The cisterna magna is obliterated and the flow of spinal fluid from the foramina of the fourth ventricle is obstructed.

Early diagnosis of congenital hydrocephalus is important because, while intellectual function is sometimes remarkably preserved in children in whom the width of the cortex has been drastically reduced by the enlargement of the ventricles, the risk of irreversible brain damage is constantly present unless pressure is relieved. Investigation may show the site of the obstruction, but the distinction between communicating and non-communicating hydrocephalus is now less important. CT scan shows that the lateral ventricles are enormously dilated. The third ventricle, but not the fourth, will be dilated if the aqueduct is stenosed. Once it has been established that hydrocephalus is present, and is not due to any lesion directly amenable to surgery, treatment consists in the insertion of a valve between the lateral ventricles and the jugular vein. This allows the escape of spinal fluid from the ventricular system whatever the cause of obstruction. The operation is not without hazards, disappointments and complications, especially bacterial infection of the valve, but it has notably reduced the mortality and morbidity of congenital hydrocephalus.

The rare condition of craniostenosis, in which there is premature fusion of many of the cranial sutures, produces a dome-shaped head with a superficial resemblance to hydrocephalus. The condition must be recognized since it causes raised intracranial pressure and blindness which can be prevented by radical surgery to open out the sutures.

The commonest evidence of failure of complete closure of the neural tube or of its coverings is *spina bifida occulta*. This is usually an entirely harmless condition in which the posterior arches of one or more vertebrae are incomplete, usually in the lumbar region, the sacrum or the cervical spine. There is evidence of multifactorial genetic transmission. It is tempting to attribute various symptoms to a hypothetical accompanying neurological defect, but usually unjustified. The condition is detected only on radiological examination, but may be suspected by the absence of one or more lumbar spinous processes. When a depression of the skin or a tuft of hair is present at the same site the condition is no longer described as occult and the possibility of an accompanying neural defect is much increased. In such children continued observation is essential: if a dermoid cyst or lipoma is present the cauda equina may be compressed or the normal development of the spinal cord prevented.

Loss of the ankle jerks and development of pes cavus are indications for myelography since any operation that is needed should be undertaken before sphincter control is impaired.

The spinal cord may be unnaturally elongated and tethered in the lower lumbar region or it may even be split by a bony spur—diastematomyelia. The symptoms are similar to those of spina bifida except that spasticity may be present and disability may be progressive owing to continued growth of the spinal column relative to the tethered spinal cord. Diagnosis can be established by myelography, and removal of the spur prevents deterioration. Over-enthusiastic attribution of banal symptoms such as nocturnal enuresis to spina bifida occulta must be resisted, but the importance of partially curable malformations in the production of pes cavus, spastic weakness of the legs and diurnal incontinence has been underestimated.

Meningo-myelocoele presents an important problem. It is immediately diagnosable at birth since in the usual form there is an obvious swelling over the lower spine or less commonly in the neck. Without treatment ulceration and fatal infection of the enlarging sac is almost inevitable, and if removal of a meningeal diverticulum were all that was involved no great problem would arise. In many such infants, however, the spinal cord is also abnormal and is partially or wholly included in the sac. The legs are partially or wholly paralysed and control of the sphincters may never be achieved. There is some evidence that immediate removal of the sac may improve the prognosis for useful movement of the legs and one school of thought vehemently advocates immediate operation in every case. Other surgeons are more cautious and operate only where either the absence of paralysis or its presence in minimal degree allow some hope of a reasonable functional result. The prevention of meningitis by immediate operation certainly saves lives in the short term and surgeons are faced with the unenviable task of deciding immediately and in an emotionally charged atmosphere whether or not to perform an operation that may result in the survival of a child paralysed below the waist and at risk to hydrocephalus and all its complications.

The *Chiari malformation* has already been mentioned as an important cause of congenital or infantile hydrocephalus, but it is becoming increasingly evident that congenital lesions of this type may also produce symptoms in adult life. The malformation of the cerebellum and consequent compression of the brain stem may result in focal symptoms such as cerebellar ataxia, but of much greater importance is the obstruction of the normal flow of spinal fluid. It now seems highly probable that syringomyelia, long regarded as a degenerative disease, is often due to mechanical factors of this kind.

SYRINGOMYELIA

The symptoms of syringomyelia usually begin between the ages of 20 and 40. Both sexes are affected and there is no obvious genetic factor. In most patients the onset is gradual, the initial symptoms being sensory loss, pain or weakness in one hand. Loss of pain and thermal sensation is often so profound that quite severe burns of the fingers may be entirely painless, only the smell of burning flesh drawing attention to the forgotten cigarette. In contrast, diffuse spontaneous pain in the arm may be severe. Examination at this time will show wasting of the hand muscles and appropriate weakness, absent tendon jerks in the arm and dissociated sensory loss; that is to say, loss of pain, tickle and thermal sensation with preservation of light touch, vibration sense and postural sense, over the whole limb. Mild scoliosis is usual.

If the disease progresses there is increasing evidence of destruction of the lower motor neurones supplying the arms and of bilateral long tract involvement. The arms are wasted and the legs become spastic. Sensory loss spreads and may lose its dissociated character in some areas. The lower cranial nerves often become involved, producing dysphagia and vocal cord paralysis. The loss of sensation spreads to the face, sparing the central area. Less common signs are a Horner's syndrome or sometimes excessive sweating on one side of the face. Painless swelling and destruction of a shoulder or elbow joint exactly comparable to the Charcot joints of tabes dorsalis is relatively common and may even be the first symptom. Progression is by no means inevitable and in some patients relatively mild disability may persist unchanged for many years. In such cases the onset has often been relatively or absolutely sudden and may have followed exertion or even sneezing.

The spinal cord contains an elongated fluid-filled cavity, a syrinx (Fig. 29, following p. 152), more or less centrally situated when fully developed but often asymmetrical. It extends over many segments, always including the cervical spinal cord. The cause of the symptoms and signs can easily be recognized from the structures within the cord that are compressed or destroyed by this expanding cavity. The fibres serving pain and thermal sensation are involved early as they cross in the centre of the cord. The anterior horn cells in the cervical region and later the descending corticospinal tracts and ascending spinothalamic fibres are affected, but the dorsal columns are usually spared. In a few cases, however, there may be marked proprioceptive loss of sensation in the upper limbs with relative sparing of the lower—a curious finding also encountered in other lesions in the region of the foramen magnum. The loss of sensation on the face is explained by involvement of the spinal root of the trigeminal nerve.

It is only recently that persistent assaults on the degenerative theory of the causation of this disease have achieved any success. The fundamental lesion appears to be obstruction to the flow of cerebrospinal fluid between the cisterna magna and the spinal subarachnoid space, either because of a congenital abnormality or because arachnoid adhesions have formed following some known or forgotten episode of meningitis. The commonest anomaly found is the Chiari malformation in which abnormal cerebellar tissue extends through the foramen magnum and down the spinal canal for a variable distance. In some patients there is also obstruction to the escape of cerebrospinal fluid through the foramina in the roof of the fourth ventricle. These obstructions lead either to cerebrospinal fluid being forced from the fourth ventricle down the central canal of the spinal cord, or on an alternative theory, distending perivascular spaces within the spinal cord. The initial syrinx may later rupture into the substance of the cord or extend upwards into the medulla. The sudden onset or worsening of symptoms in some patients following sneezing suggests that a sudden rise in venous pressure may be the effective force. The nature of the obstruction can usually be demonstrated by myelography.

The results of surgical treatment based on these findings cannot yet be fully assessed but there is no doubt that allowing free escape of fluid from the fourth ventricle and preventing further dilatation of the syrinx can be followed by remarkable improvement, though long-standing destructive changes are naturally irreversible.

Syringomyelia also occurs in *primary basilar impression* and probably for similar reasons. This is a genetically determined anomaly of the base of the skull in which the basilar and condylar portions of the occipital bone are displaced upwards. Externally this produces a short neck and low hair line, while internally the posterior fossa is constricted. Both syringomyelia and hydrocephalus may result, with onset in adult life. The diagnosis can be made by radiological demonstration which shows the anterior part of the atlas vertebra sharply tilted upwards. Decompression of the posterior fossa relieves most of the symptoms, particularly headache and papilloedema due to hydrocephalus. Secondary basilar impression is the result of bone disease such as rickets, osteomalacia or Paget's disease, and occasionally causes similar symptoms.

CEREBRAL PALSY

The term cerebral palsy is obviously imprecise but is generally used to describe the effects of maldevelopment of the brain or of damage sustained during the first three years of life. Progressive disease is therefore excluded. The pathology is naturally varied and clinical terminology sometimes confusing.

In all forms of congenital cerebral palsy motor activity is retarded, and it is usual to distinguish three main groups entirely on related clinical findings: the spastic, ataxic and athetoid forms. This classification is of little real value and reflects no consistent difference in cause or pathology. The common spastic variety is subdivided into diplegia, in which the legs are more affected than the arms; paraplegia, where the legs alone are affected; and hemiplegia, often bilateral, where the upper limb is the more affected. While hemiplegia clearly differs from paraplegia the distinction of diplegia from double hemiplegia is arguable and in any case of little value.

Spastic diplegia, or *Little's disease*, is the commonest form of cerebral palsy. The causative lesion varies from malformation of the cerebral cortex to more centrally placed lesions in the internal capsules, probably due to birth trauma. Motor development, particularly of walking, is delayed to a degree depending on the severity of the defect. If the child is held up the spastic legs are extended and adducted and the feet strongly plantar-flexed. Spasticity in the sense of increased resistance to passive movement becomes increasingly obvious as the child grows. The use of the hands may be virtually normal but there is usually some evidence that the upper limbs are involved. Intelligence is sometimes normal, but as in any form of cerebral palsy mental deficiency is common. Hemiplegia and double hemiplegia is more often due to birth injury than malformation and a history of transient intrauterine hypoxia or of difficult labour is very common. Mental impairment is more frequent and more severe. Hemiplegic cerebral palsy is usually accompanied by failure of normal development of the affected limbs. Even in the relatively common variety where symptoms and signs are minimal the congenital nature of a mild spastic weakness of one leg may be revealed by measurable shortening or obvious lack of muscular development.

The ataxic form is comparatively rare and less easy to recognize. Development is slow but neither hypotonia nor ataxia can be easily recognized in early life. Developmental defects of the cerebellum are usually responsible. The athetoid form is also difficult to diagnose early. The characteristic writhing movements usually develop only during childhood and the condition may first be suggested by abnormal postures often complicating an accompanying congenital hemiplegia. A frequent but not invariable pathological finding is status marmoratus of the striatum in which the grey matter is divided by strands of white myelinated fibres. Many children who survived kernicterus due to erythroblastosis foetalis had an athetoid form of cerebal palsy, often accompanied by deafness.

Hemiplegia may be acquired in infancy as a disastrous complication of apparently banal infection such as tonsillitis, or following injury or operation to the head or neck. The onset is usually heralded by a major convulsion and some cases are probably due to embolism from a clot in the carotid artery. Meningitis in infancy may cause hemiplegia or any form of spastic cerebral palsy.

Epilepsy is common in all forms of cerebral palsy, particularly in hemiplegia, where temper tantrums are also often a sore trial to the family. Anticonvulsants must be used to control the fits but unfortunately their use is sometimes accompanied by deterioration in temper and behaviour.

The prognosis of cerebral palsy depends more on the severity of the mental and physical disability than on the cause or the method of treatment. No improvement can be hoped for in a paralysed microcephalic child and attention must be centred on humane care of the patient and the family. As soon as the diagnosis and probable outcome are known a full explanation must be sympathetically given to the parents. The risk of a second spastic child is small in the absence of any known genetic defect, but where this is in any doubt expert help must be sought from a genetic counselling service.

If the child seems educable to any degree, training in elementary motor skills must be energetically pursued. Even to sit upright is a major gain, and to learn to walk at the age of eight is a notable advance towards independence. Spasticity is often a major component of the disability, particularly when the legs cross or 'scissor' on standing and the feet are held in plantar flexion. Vigorous passive movement can probably prevent or delay the onset of contractures in the calf muscles, but physiotherapy has only the most transient effect on spasticity. Judicious surgery is often helpful, particularly lengthening the Achilles tendon to allow the heel to touch the ground, and operations to overcome adductor spasm. Drugs have so far proved of little value. The necessity for education is now well recognized and many of the more fortunate spastic children can be trained for a useful and enjoyable life.

A few particular points deserve mention. Congenital pseudobulbar palsy with dysarthria and dysphagia and dribbling may occur with little or no disability in the limbs. High-frequency deafness especially is often overlooked and may be mistaken for mental deficiency. In hemiplegia epilepsy and behaviour disorder may be so severe that the operation of hemispherectomy may be considered. In some such patients removal of the damaged hemisphere, sparing the basal ganglia, may not only control these symptoms but may paradoxically be followed by improvement in function of the paretic limbs.

In the *Sturge–Weber syndrome* a port-wine naevus of the face is accompanied by an extensive capillary angioma of the cerebral cortex with underlying atrophy, hemiparesis, epilepsy and mental deficiency. X-ray commonly reveals a characteristic pattern of calcification in the underlying cortex. Fragments of this syndrome, which does not appear to be inherited, are common and most patients with the facial naevus have no nervous disorder.

Increasing attention is being paid to what may be regarded as a minimal form of cerebral palsy, although there is no direct evidence of brain damage or maldevelopment. Progress is only a little delayed but all movements are clumsily performed. The ungainly walk, shambling run and sprawling handwriting are not accompanied by any signs of spasticity or cerebellar ataxia and these children, often of superior intelligence, have been called 'congenitally maladroit'. Many mentally defective children have physical defects, sometimes obvious cerebral palsy, but more often microcephaly and poor motor control. During infancy differentiation between mental and physical disabilities due to cerebral defect presents obvious difficulties but it is likely that few educable children are now overlooked.

Investigation for possible chromosomal abnormalities is rarely helpful in developmental neurological disorders. No structural abnormality of the chromosomes has been detected in the well-recognized inherited diseases. In many of the rare chromosomal abnormalities mental deficiency has been present but the only common form is mongolism, where there is an extra chromosome 21. These children develop slowly but rarely have specific neurological abnormalities apart from mental defect due to a deficiency of cortical neurones. Motor control is clumsy. The facial resemblance to the Oriental is seldom striking and the condition is immediately recognizable in Chinese or Japanese children. These children are usually tractable and docile, often fascinated by music, but seldom capable of absorbing any useful training.

CONGENITAL DYSLEXIA

Congenital dyslexia is now recognized with increasing frequency. In the fully developed condition the child, most often a boy, is quite unable to form any association between the written or printed word and the sound and meaning of which it is a symbol. Reading and writing are therefore impossible. Lesser degrees result in delayed reading or persistent inability to spell common words but are not important. Dyslexia was formerly often mistaken for laziness or mental deficiency, but these children are normally intelligent and cooperate in strenuous training. Specialized education is required and there is also an undoubted tendency to spontaneous improvement. Failure to acquire this peculiarly human cerebral function has not been explained on an anatomical basis but the condition is often hereditary. Invincible illiteracy is sometimes surprisingly encountered in highly successful men.

CRANIAL NERVE ANOMALIES

Many developmental defects affecting the cranial nerves have been described and only the most important can be mentioned here. Congenital nystagmus takes many forms. When vision is defective, pendular as opposed to jerking nystagmus is common, but congenital jerking nystagmus with a quick and slow phase may occur with normal vision. This can cause confusion if the patient is complaining of headache or giddiness, and for clarity of diagnosis and the avoidance of radical investigations at the hands of neurosurgeons, congenital nystagmus should always be clearly noted in the patient's record as soon as it is recognized.

Congenital unilateral Horner's syndrome or isolated ptosis is also common and is transmitted in some families by dominant inheritance. Its effect is cosmetic only, though again it may be misinterpreted as due to an acquired lesion.

Bilateral facial weakness, *Moebius' syndrome*, is rare but may be a source of diagnostic difficulty. The child may cry without any distortion of the face and the eyes are never closed. If the buccal muscles are also affected feeding is difficult.

No comprehensive account of the innumerable congenital defects of the nervous system can be attempted here but certain principles may be firmly stated. Parents must be fully informed and expert genetic advice sought when necessary. No educable child must be overlooked, and unremitting efforts must be made to treat symptoms such as spasticity or contractures. Finally it must be remembered that the major disability is sometimes secondary to a remediable obstruction to the flow of spinal fluid rather than to irrevocable degeneration.

Further reading

Barnett H.J.M., Foster J.B. & Hodgson P. (1973) *Syringomyelia*. Saunders, London.
Stark C.D. (1977) *Spina Bifida*. Blackwell Scientific Publications, Oxford.

CHAPTER 16
Degenerative Diseases of Genetic or Unknown Origin

The formidable task of bringing order to the confused mass of chronic neurological disease was one of the triumphs of the classical method of relating accurate clinical observations to necropsy findings. The method carries the inherent temptation to regard the diagnosis of an eponymous hereditary palsy, or of some systematized degeneration, as an end in itself. In most specialties it is no longer permissible to speak of 'degenerative' disease, and either some hint of causation has been discovered or ignorance is more subtly concealed. Neurones do not degenerate without reason, nor do they suffer from lack of vital force, the 'abiotrophy' still solemnly proposed as a satisfying explanation of many diseases. The discovery of a metabolic abnormality may allow the trail of causation to be followed to the point where rational treatment can be devised, and a number of diseases formerly classified simply as degenerative already fall into this category. Unfortunately there are still many where no such advance has been achieved.

Present evidence suggests that many such diseases will ultimately be classified as inborn errors of metabolism. There are many reasons why the biochemical defect transmitted by the genetic code may escape detection. It may be confined to the central nervous system, it may be effective only during a limited period of development, or it may involve metabolic pathways that we have no means of investigating. As a result there are important genetically determined diseases of which only a descriptive account can be given.

THE SPINOCEREBELLAR ATAXIAS

This is a group of diseases, overlapping in both clinical and pathological features but presenting as 'classical' forms sufficiently often to allow recognition of certain main varieties. Of these the commonest is *Friedreich's ataxia*. Transmitted by recessive autosomal inheritance, the onset of neurological symptoms is usually in the second decade but the common accompaniments of pes cavus and scoliosis may present earlier.

Cerebellar ataxia affecting gait, manual dexterity and often speech is commonly the initial and predominant symptom. Progression is slow, but walking becomes increasingly impeded and eventually impossible. In addition to ataxia, dysarthria and sometimes nystagmus there is evidence of more widespread disease since the plantar reflexes are extensor and the tendon jerks paradoxically absent. Postural sense is often lost in the toes. Many additional features occur less constantly: dementia, optic atrophy and nerve deafness, for example, tend to be specific for a single family. Dorsal scoliosis and pes cavus are usually present. The course of the disease is highly variable, but few patients survive the fourth decade. Death often follows insidious coma, the cause of which is quite unknown. The cerebrospinal fluid provides no help in diagnosis, being normal throughout the disease.

Abnormalities outside the nervous system are frequent, particularly diabetes mellitus of early onset and heart disease. The latter is seldom clinically obvious, but electrocardiographic abnormalities may be detected. Occasionally disorders of cardiac rhythm such as intractable paroxysmal tachycardia may dominate the clinical picture and even prove fatal. The search for an inherited metabolic defect in Friedreich's ataxia has been unrewarding but some evidence of failure of incorporation of linoleic acid into cell membranes has recently been found.

Apparently distinct variants, which may nevertheless occur in the same family as cases of Friedreich's ataxia, are characterized by a later age of onset, preservation of the tendon jerks, or pure cerebellar ataxia. In some forms heredity may be dominant or may appear to play no part at all. The minute description of these variations is at present of little value, particularly since definitive diagnosis can be made only at necropsy and not always then. It is, however, important to be aware that systematized degeneration of the cerebellum and its connections, with or without spinal cord disease, may occur on a genetic basis or sporadically and over a wide range of ages. When causation is better understood the clinical distinction between such conditions as olivo-ponto-cerebellar atrophy and late cortical cerebellar atrophy will assume greater importance.

In classical Friedreich's ataxia the atrophy affects mainly the spino-cerebellar tracts and posterior columns, and to a lesser degree the cortico-spinal tracts within the spinal cord. Involvement of the dorsal roots accounts for the loss of tendon jerks, and the cerebellar nuclei also degenerate.

In the presence of a clear family history the diagnosis of Friedreich's ataxia should present no difficulty. Even in sporadic cases the combination of ataxia, absent tendon jerks and extensor plantar reflexes in a young person is sufficiently distinctive. In the rarer forms in which tendon jerks are preserved or increased differentiation from multiple sclerosis is obviously difficult. In the pure cerebellar ataxias, which are usually sporadic and affect older people, cerebellar tumour or degeneration in association with a remote carcinoma must be considered. Drug intoxication is also important. Phenytoin and alcohol may have both temporary and permanent effects on the cerebellum, while barbiturates and chlordiazepoxide (Librium) are not uncommon causes of ataxia, the former being almost an occupational hazard in nurses.

Hereditary spastic paraplegia shows some genetic overlap with other forms, but is usually distinctive in being a dominant trait. Spasticity of the legs without sensory loss may develop at any age and is only slowly progressive. It is sometimes accompanied by wasting of the hand muscles. Without clear evidence of a family history it may be mistaken for other causes of progressive paraplegia such as multiple sclerosis or spinal cord compression.

PERONEAL MUSCULAR ATROPHY

Peroneal muscular atrophy is comparatively common and is much less crippling. It is usually transmitted by dominant inheritance. The age of onset is variable but is often in childhood. Pes cavus is common and probably precedes the wasting of the intrinsic muscles of the feet that later becomes obvious. The dorsiflexors of the feet and toes, the anterior tibial group of muscles, are nearly always the most severely affected, resulting in the gradual onset of foot drop. As the other distal muscles waste the ankles become increasingly unstable but the gait remains remarkably effective. Over a period of many years the muscles of the lower part of the thighs may be involved, producing the 'inverted champagne bottle' appearance, and the intrinsic hand muscles also atrophy. The condition is not completely stereotyped and there is a well-recognized variant in which the hand muscles are first affected. Despite severe muscle atrophy disability is characteristically slight.

Other signs are usually present. The ankle jerks are absent and there is loss of vibration sense at the ankles.

This disease is not primarily one of muscle, at least in the great majority of cases, because nerve conduction as measured electrically may be greatly slowed. Pathologically there is either predominantly loss of axons or of myelin in peripheral nerves, depending on the genetic type, with an excess of connective tissue, and muscle atrophy of neurogenic type. In some families of typical peroneal muscular atrophy the peripheral nerves are obviously thickened. This is a different condition from the *hypertrophic polyneuritis of Déjérine and Sottas*. As originally described

DEGENERATIVE DISEASES

this was a severely crippling form of polyneuritis, recessively inherited and progressive from childhood. The main nerve trunks are enormously thickened. As with many hereditary nervous diseases scoliosis and pes cavus are common, and there may be features suggesting cerebellar involvement. An occasional curiosity is the Argyll Robertson pupil. When the nerve roots are also greatly thickened the cerebrospinal fluid protein may be raised and there may even be compression of the spinal cord. In less severe forms the clinical picture may be that of peroneal muscular atrophy with thickened nerves, or it may be impossible to determine whether they are thickened or not. In the first case described nerve hypertrophy was not detected during life.

Histologically, in addition to loss of axons and segmental demyelination, there is an excess of amorphous mucoid material within the nerves and many fibres are surrounded by thick sheaths of Schwann cell processes and collagen, the 'onion-bulbs'. These appearances are not, however, pathognomonic of the hereditary form of hypertrophic neuropathy.

Although there is no treatment that can modify the course of any of these hereditary palsies symptomatic treatment must not be neglected. In particular orthopaedic measures to improve the stability of the ankles in peroneal muscular atrophy are often useful.

HUNTINGTON'S CHOREA

This is a much more clearly defined entity than the spinocerebellar and cerebellar ataxias and is transmitted by dominant inheritance. The cardinal symptoms are dementia and involuntary movements and although there is some variation in the mode of presentation and speed of progress the end result is distinctive.

Symptoms most commonly begin in the fifth decade, that is to say after the next generation has been born, and it is therefore sometimes possible to trace affected families through many generations. It is extremely unusual not to find a positive or strongly suggestive family history. The first symptom is usually a reduction of activity and restriction of interest, at first thought to be unimportant or merely the result of eccentricity. In other cases clumsiness leads to injury, and until the disease is recognized restlessness and involuntary movements may be attributed to post-traumatic hysteria. Involuntary movements usually appear within a year of the onset of psychiatric symptoms. Sometimes dementia may predominate and chorea can only doubtfully be detected, but when the presenting symptom is chorea dementia is nearly always detectable. The movements are at first slight and amount to little more than continuous fidgeting, but they slowly increase until they are almost incessant. They are unmistakably choreic (see Chapter 13) consisting of brief movement of a limb or segment of a limb or of the face and trunk, never affecting single muscles. They are quite irregular and follow no set pattern of distribution. Sustained muscle contraction is interrupted, so that the grip fluctuates and the tongue cannot be held protruded, a most reliable sign. As the disease advances the patient becomes helplessly demented and totally disabled, the final state being one of severe cachexia. Insight is often lost early in the disease so that even if the family disease is well known to the patient he may not realize that he is developing it himself.

When dementia is present alone, the differential diagnosis is from other forms of progressive mental deterioration at this age, in particular Alzheimer's disease. Careful observation will usually detect slight or suggestive abnormal movements. Other forms of chorea must also be considered but rheumatic chorea is very rare in the adult and senile chorea is probably a form of Huntington's disease.

In children, in whom the disease is rare, and occasionally in adults, chorea may not occur, but rigidity of the limbs with dysarthria and dysphagia are the presenting symptoms.

Pathologically there is loss of neurones, predominantly from the caudate nucleus, pallidum and cerebral cortex, with less constant changes in other areas.

A child of a patient with Huntington's chorea has a 50% chance of developing the disease and will have had the experience of observing its development in the parent. The risk naturally diminishes with advancing age and if symptoms have not appeared by the age of 50 it is no more than 5%. If affected members could be detected before the onset of symptoms they could be advised not to have children and the disease largely eradicated. Unfortunately abnormalities of GABA metabolism detected appear to be the result of the disease and not the cause and in contrast to Parkinson's disease no effective symptomatic treatment has been derived from this finding. There is at present no means of diagnosing the disease before symptoms have appeared.

Many drugs have been claimed to reduce the involuntary movements, but it is difficult to obtain prolonged improvement without intolerable side-effects. Tetrabenazine (Nitoman) is by far the most effective agent, the usual dose being around 75 mg a day, but has the disadvantage of sometimes producing deep depression. The management of the patient and of the family, both those involved in daily care of the patient and those at risk for the disease, demands, but seldom receives, the utmost skill of the physician.

TUBEROSE SCLEROSIS

Tuberose sclerosis is an uncommon condition also transmitted by dominant inheritance. The clinical expression is varied, since many organs are involved to differing degrees. The most common presentation is that of a mentally retarded child with epilepsy and a rash (adenoma sebaceum) on the cheeks. This consists of small raised pink nodules which in milder cases may be mistaken for acne, especially as it usually appears around puberty. In the younger child depigmented patches are commonly found. Severe mental defect may occur but in some families there are *formes frustes* with only slight evidence of the defect. Phakomas, or developmental tumours of glial tissue, are often found in the retina.

Pathologically the obvious lesion is the presence of fibrocellular nodules, the tubers, in many organs, principally the brain where they may be calcified, but also in the heart and kidneys. Congenital malformations of the brain are also found, especially absence of the corpus callosum.

The cause is unknown and there is no treatment apart from that of the epilepsy.

NEUROFIBROMATOSIS

Neurofibromatosis is a much commoner dominantly inherited defect, mainly affecting the skin and the nervous system. The changes in the skin often occur in isolation and may be trivial or extremely disfiguring. Brown pigmentation on the trunk and proximal segments of the limbs occurs in sharply defined patches, the café-au-lait spots. Cutaneous fibromas are soft painless swellings, but neurofibromas on cutaneous nerve twigs are firm and often tender. The plexiform neuroma is fortunately rare as it causes grotesque hypertrophy of the affected part.

These lesions, while often distressing, do not affect the function of the nervous system. A neurofibroma on a main nerve trunk can present as an isolated palsy, the cause of which may be suspected if characteristic skin lesions are also present. More centrally a neurofibroma on a nerve root may compress the spinal cord and present with root pain at the level of the lesion and progressive weakness and sensory loss below this level. Spinal neurofibromata often occur without evidence of diffuse neurofibromatosis, and the acoustic neurofibroma (see Chapter 10) which is histologically identical, more often than not develops in isolation. Bilateral acoustic neurofibromata occasionally complicate neurofibromatosis in children, and small tumours may grow on other cranial nerves.

Bone changes are often seen, particularly severe kyphoscoliosis. The posterior aspects of the lumbar vertebrae sometimes appear concave on X-rays and may falsely suggest the presence of an expanding lesion within the spinal cord.

Neurofibromata are benign tumours arising from the Schwann cells of the peripheral nerves. Sarcomatous change is rare. In the central nervous system malignant tumours may occur, of which the commonest is glioma of the optic nerve.

MOTOR NEURONE DISEASE

It is now customary to group *progressive muscular atrophy, progressive bulbar palsy* and *amyotrophic lateral sclerosis* together under this title, since they are all different modes of expression of a progressive degenerative disease. The symptoms and physical signs are almost entirely those due to loss of upper and lower motor neurone function in varying proportions, but histologically less conspicuous degenerative changes are found in other pathways. The main lesion, however, and certainly the cause of the symptoms, is degeneration of anterior horn cells, of equivalent motor cells in the cranial nuclei, and of neurones in the frontal and precentral cortex.

The corticospinal tracts show secondary loss of myelin and axons. The process is seldom absolutely symmetrical, and seems to be somewhat less systemized than the degeneration seen in the hereditary ataxias. Histology provides no hint of the cause of the neuronal loss.

The disease usually occurs in middle life or later, but very occasionally begins as early as the second or third decade. The mode of onset varies according to the site of impact of the disease. When the initial symptoms are those due to loss of lower motor neurones in the spinal cord the first complaint is nearly always of weakness in one hand or arm. Pain is uncommon, but cramp or 'locking' in the finger flexors is often complained of. A little later wasting of the hand muscles may become obvious to the patient. When examined at this stage there will probably already be wasting of all the intrinsic hand muscles, thus excluding a lesion of the ulnar or median nerve as a cause. Weakness will be present in the flexors and extensors of the wrist and perhaps more widely. A lesion of the brachial plexus or nerve roots may be suspected but there is no sensory loss, and in spite of the obvious clinical signs of lower motor neurone damage the tendon jerks are nearly always preserved and often remarkably increased. This is a sign that upper motor neurones are also involved. Careful scrutiny of the muscles of the shoulder girdle will often reveal *fasciculation* in muscles that are not apparently weak, and this may be present on both sides. Fasciculation, as its name implies, consists of contractions of muscle bundles, occurring irregularly and at very varying frequencies. When it is severe it produces a restless flickering contraction that the patient finds unpleasant. These signs are almost conclusive evidence of motor neurone disease but may occasionally be caused by other forms of spinal cord disease, in particular cervical myelopathy due to spondylosis. The diagnosis will usually declare itself before long by obvious spread to muscles that could not be involved by a lesion of the cervical cord. In rare cases where the lumbar enlargement of the spinal cord is first involved, the diagnosis may be in doubt for longer, and causes of root compression or of peripheral nerve disease must be excluded.

If the medulla is first affected the symptoms are those of bulbar palsy, with difficulty in speaking and swallowing. In the early stages it may not be possible to detect anything beyond a slight change in the quality of the voice, but by the time swallowing is affected the tongue is usually wasted, wrinkled and fasciculating. The normal tongue may appear to fasciculate even when lying on the floor of the mouth, and a gloomy prognosis should certainly not be given unless there are confirmatory signs. The paralysis may remain confined to the bulbar muscles throughout the disease, but often some wasting and fasciculation round the shoulders can be seen. Advanced bulbar palsy abolishes speech, and meals become a torment with food entering the larynx. The facial muscles are often involved as well as those of the pharynx and palate, but the ocular muscles are never affected.

Amyotrophic lateral sclerosis implies muscle wasting combined with signs of damage to the corticospinal tracts in the lateral columns of the spinal cord. It is common for wasting of the arms to be followed by spasticity of the legs, but rarely the latter may be the presenting feature. There is no sensory loss, which is a point of distinction from many other causes of progressive spastic paraparesis, and a careful search will usually show unmistakably abnormal fasciculation. Sometimes the condition of *pseudobulbar palsy* is produced by bilateral loss of motor neurones from the frontal cortex. The tongue is not wasted but is slow and 'spastic' and there is marked emotional lability and some dementia.

Investigation is needed only to exclude other conditions. A similar clinical picture may sometimes occur with carcinoma of the lung, and the chest should be X-rayed. The cerebrospinal fluid is usually normal but occasionally the protein level is moderately raised.

However it presents, motor neurone disease is progressive. The speed of deterioration varies greatly but few patients live more than three years from the first symptom, bulbar paralysis being obviously the most dangerous as it immediately threatens life. No cause has been found or reasonably conjectured. Usually no genetic factor can be identified, but in a few families nearly every member may be affected by an apparently identical disease. A somewhat different form is endemic in the island of Guam, but intensive investigation has thrown no further light on causation. Sometimes the association of local injury, particularly electric shock, and the site and time of onset of the wasting is remarkable, but clearly injury to a hand is an unlikely cause of diffuse progressive neuronal disease. The fasciculation so commonly seen is not diagnostic since it occurs in other conditions in which lower motor neurones are gradually lost. The surviving motor units expand and supply fibres to the denervated muscle fibres previously supplied by the dead units. The resulting giant units are in some way unstable and discharge spontaneously in an irregular manner. Normal units may sometimes behave in the same way, and an unfounded fear of having developed motor neurone disease is by no means uncommon in the medical profession.

Only symptomatic treatment can be attempted, and even this is seldom helpful. It is usual to try to maintain morale by the use of a placebo. Whether to tell the patient the prognosis can only be judged individually but clearly this is sometimes necessary. Tube feeding or gastrostomy must occasionally be used in bulbar palsy but usually by this stage the inhalation of secretions rapidly and mercifully leads to pneumonia.

Progressive degeneration of motor neurones also occurs in *infantile spinal muscular atrophy* or Werdnig–Hoffman's disease. This is transmitted by autosomal recessive inheritance. The disease shows itself at birth or in the succeeding few months. The baby is hypotonic and becomes increasingly feeble. It is difficult to detect wasting in the early stages, but fasciculation of the tongue is an important sign. There are many causes for hypotonia and failure to thrive in infancy, and unless there is a clear family history or obvious widespread muscle atrophy of lower motor neurone type, such cases as benign hypotonia and cerebral palsy must be considered. The disease is progressive and fatal. Benign spinal muscular atrophy, or Kugelberg–Wielander disease, has been recognized more recently. It usually presents in the second decade with symmetrical proximal weakness and wasting of the limbs. Although the symptoms indisputably arise from degeneration of anterior horn cells the resemblance to limb-girdle muscular dystrophy (Chapter 7) is so close, even extending to pseudohypertrophy of the calf muscles, that even the greatest experts are not always able to draw a dividing line, and indeed perhaps none exists. The disease is genetically determined, being transmitted by recessive inheritance. It is only 'benign' in comparison with motor neurone disease and usually progresses slowly to moderately severe disability.

PRESENILE DEMENTIA

This is merely a descriptive title with somewhat vague connotations. It is generally accepted that in extreme old age even the most fortunate do not escape some decline in mental ability. Memory for recent events becomes uncertain and apprehension of new material less rapid. There is, however, a great difference between these trivial disabilities of the nonagenarian and the mindless incapacity of the many who become gravely demented in the seventies. Both may, however, be regarded as suffering to different degrees from the effects of senility. The point where the presenium merges into senility is necessarily imprecise and the distinction between the expected failings of old age and dementia is similarly hard to define.

The common form of progressive dementia beginning in the fifth or sixth decade is *Alzheimer's disease*. In this condition there is widespread cortical neuronal degeneration producing a characteristic appearance within the cell body known as the neurofibrillary tangle. In addition there are numerous plaques containing amyloid and presumably indicating the site of destroyed nerve cells. Minor degrees of these changes, particularly the plaques, have been found on routine examination of the brain even in young adults and are almost invariably present in the aged. Exactly when the changes can be said to indicate the presence of disease is difficult to decide but there is no such difficulty concerning the clinical evidence in middle-aged patients. Alzheimer's disease is a common and tragic condition. There is undoubtedly a genetic element in some families but details are often difficult to obtain. The common mode of onset is with memory failure. This is such a common complaint, whether justified or not, that in the early case its importance may be hard to estimate but within a few months or even weeks it becomes plain that this is no mere absentmindedness or distraction. Failure of memory is followed by defect in reasoning, often aggravated by aphasia. Loss of topographical memory, due to parietal lobe damage, is also common. Neglect of personal hygiene is not usually an early sign or may be concealed by relatives.

In a typical moderately advanced case the patient will have difficulty in understanding speech but will be able to converse in commonplace phrases and platitudes that may for a time conceal the severity of the aphasia. Memory for recent events is certainly affected, leading to repetitive questioning, but remote memory is also soon impaired. Vision is not affected but reading is impossible because of aphasia and intellectual defect. Some interest in television may be preserved, providing some relief for the unfortunate family. There are no abnormal signs in the limbs but the patient may become virtually helpless, needing assistance with all the semiautomatic activities of everyday life. The course of the disease is progressive but often prolonged, patients dying of the complications of the helpless state after five or more years.

A second form of cortical degeneration, Pick's lobar atrophy, is relatively much more rare in this country. The degenerative process is different and is localized to the frontal and temporal lobes to varying degrees. The differentiation from Alzheimer's disease in life could be made by an expert but at present serves no practical purpose.

It is only comparatively recently that much attention has been paid to the possible cause of these devastating diseases which have been dismissed as degenerative and not further explained. Biochemical investigation has indicated some promising leads but has not advanced to the point where effective treatment can be given.

The differential diagnosis of dementia in a patient of fifty is a most important and difficult task and it is vital that no treatable cause must be missed. Chronic intoxication with bromide, chloral, barbiturates or alcohol is easily overlooked, but nystagmus and slurred speech commonly accompany the mental slowing. Myxoedema should be recognized at once provided it is considered at all. General paralysis now usually presents with simple dementia, often without the classical pupillary changes and tremor. Hepatic encephalopathy may also present with dementia and little or no clinical evidence of liver disease. A cerebral tumour, particularly a meningioma of the convexity or in the frontal region, or any tumour blocking the free flow of cerebrospinal fluid can cause dementia with no other signs. Deficiency of vitamin B_{12} is another important and completely reversible cause. Finally it must be remembered that failure of memory, lack of concentration, and slow thinking are extremely common in depression.

Recently there has been much interest in the condition labelled *normal pressure hydrocephalus*. The precise limits of this condition are not yet defined, but dilatation of the lateral ventricles may be the result, not of atrophy, but of obstruction to the flow of cerebrospinal fluid. This is obvious when a tumour constricts the aqueduct, but more subtle forms of block may occur, in particular prevention of flow of cerebrospinal fluid upwards through the opening in the tentorium cerebelli to its main source of absorption on the convexity of the cerebral hemispheres. Such a block may result from arachnoidal adhesions following infection, or subarachnoid haemorrhage, or for no definable reason. As the connection between the ventricles and the subarachnoid space is not obstructed this condition is known as communicating hydrocephalus. The characteristic triad of symptoms consists of dementia, ataxia in walking and incontinence of urine. In such patients the CT scan may show dilated ventricles without cortical atrophy, although these appearances are not diagnostic and the distinction from Alzheimer's disease can be difficult (Fig. 30, following page 152). Improvement in walking following lumbar puncture and the removal of CSF on three successive days is regarded by some surgeons as an indication that a valved shunt between the lateral ventricle the left atrium is worth attempting.

In a disappointingly small proportion of these patients a remarkable degree of improvement can be achieved. Whether the hydrocephalus can really be produced with no rise in pressure is open to question, but certainly the pressure measured at lumbar puncture in these patients is not raised.

PROGRESSIVE SUPRANUCLEAR PALSY

This condition has only recently been recognized but is probably not uncommon. It begins in middle life, the first symptom usually being unexplained falls. The highly characteristic feature is the appearance of progressive paralysis of conjugate movements of the eyes, always beginning with vertical movements. Eventually the eyes become immobile and at this stage there is usually the dysarthria and dysphagia of pseudobulbar palsy and a striking tonic extension of the neck on standing up, also probably the result of loss of upper motor neurone function. The cause is unknown and treatment unavailing.

IDIOPATHIC ORTHOSTATIC HYPOTENSION

This is also a new addition to the list of degenerative diseases. In its pure form it occurs around the age of 50, much more commonly in men. The presenting symptom is of fainting on standing up or walking a short distance, and it is easy to verify that the blood pressure drops immediately the patient stands or even sits upright. Often many years before these presenting symptoms there may have been impotence and loss of sweating. This may follow a bizarre pattern initially, but eventualy there may be no sweating in response to heat. In other patients there may be additional features of Parkinson's disease or cerebellar ataxia. Remarkably noisy snoring at night with periods of apnoea is another common feature.

The lesion responsible for this severe autonomic disturbance is degeneration of the sympathetic system, but opinion is still divided as to whether this is entirely central or peripheral.

Symptomatic treatment of the idiopathic form of orthostatic hypotension is surprisingly effective. Up to 0.1 mg thrice daily of 9-alphafluorohydrocortisone acts as a plasma expander and is most effective in preventing syncope. Combined with elastic stockings and an abdominal binder this treatment may permit a full round of golf instead of unconsciousness after walking 20 yards, but because of the loss of sweating, constricting binders cannot be tolerated in summer. Sleeping with the head of the bed raised about one foot reduces the loss of fluid during the night and helps to maintain the arterial tension. The cause is unknown and curative treatment is impracticable.

Further reading

Heathfield K.G.W. (1973) Huntington's chorea: a centenary review. *Postgrad. Med. J.* **49**, 32.

Hughes R.C., Cartlidge N.E.F. & Millag P. (1970) Primary neurogenic orthostatic hypotension. *J. Neurol. Neurosurg. Psychiat.* **33**, 363.

Konigsmark B.W. & Weiner L.P. (1970) The olivo-ponto-cerebellar atrophies. *Medicine*, **49**, 227.

Pearce J. & Miller E. (1973) *Clinical Aspects of Dementia*. Baillière, London.

Pratt R.T.C. (1967) *The Genetics of Neurological Disorders*. Oxford University Press, London.

Smith J.S. & Kiloh L.G. (1981) The investigation of dementia. *Lancet*, **1**, 824.

Steele J.C. (1972) Progressive supranuclear palsy. *Brain* **95**, 693.

CHAPTER 17
Epilepsy, Syncope and Narcolepsy

EPILEPSY

Since our ideas of epilepsy are based on an uneasy medley of keenly observed clinical events and ill-understood physiological concepts, no definition of the epileptic fit is wholly satisfactory. The essential clinical feature is a paroxysmal or episodic disorder of cerebral function, but this in itself is not a satisfactory definition because it would include several varieties of transient cerebral ischaemic attack as well as many reversible metabolic disorders. An abnormal excessive discharge of cerebral neurones is probably another essential feature, though it is usually presumed rather than observed; such discharges can, however, be recorded in people entirely free from symptoms. An epileptic fit does not consist of abnormal brain waves alone, and cerebral dysrhythmia, once seriously suggested as a definition, is now no more than a useful expression when we wish to discuss a patient's symptoms in front of him without using the emotive word epilepsy. Despite these considerations, and despite the fact that there exists a borderland where no sharp boundaries can be drawn, most epileptic fits can be recognized immediately for what they are when they are observed or described by witnesses.

A patient who has had repeated epileptic fits may justifiably be said to be suffering from epilepsy, but the concept of epilepsy as a disease and the categorization of patients as epileptic must be approached with more caution than the use of such descriptive labels as diabetic or myasthenic. Epileptic fits result from a variety of causes, and indeed a fit can be induced in anyone by an electric shock applied to the brain. The pattern of the fit depends not on the cause but on the site of the abnormal cerebral discharge. An epileptic fit is therefore always epileptic: the word epileptiform is meaningless and should be abandoned.

The *major fit* or grand mal is the commonest and most easily recognized form of epilepsy. Consciousness is lost, usually abruptly, and the patient falls to the ground, sometimes with a hoarse cry as air is driven from the chest. The limbs are rigid, the legs extended and the arms flexed. All the muscles of the trunk and limbs are in strong contraction simultaneously.

Breathing is arrested and the face is suffused, cyanosed and contorted. This tonic stage must necessarily be brief and is succeeded by the clonic stage, in which the generalized contraction is interrupted by short periods of relaxation. The effect is that of violent jerking as the muscles contract again at progressively longer intervals. If this phase is prolonged for more than a few minutes the clonic movements may become more conspicuous on one or other side, or in one limb. In these convulsive stages of the fit the tongue may be bitten and the bladder emptied. As the jerking stops the patient is flaccid and deeply comatose, with stertorous breathing and a flushed face. Reflex activity is retained but the plantar reflexes are often extensor. The coma is of variable duration but commonly lasts for 15 minutes or longer. Even the most painful stimuli produce no response, and shockingly severe burns may result. On recovery of consciousness the patient is confused and drowsy, has a headache, and may vomit. He may fall into a deep sleep, from which he can be roused. The following day the severe exertion of the convulsion may show itself by widespread muscular pain, the familiar stiffness. Minor variations are common and in particular it may not be possible to recognize a tonic stage.

In the past the term *petit mal* has often been regarded as synonymous with minor epilepsy, and has been used to describe any epileptic phenomenon short of a major convulsion. Today its use is more restricted to a specific form of minor epilepsy, occurring in childhood, and characterized during the attack by three-per-second generalized wave and spike wave activity in the electroencephalogram (EEG). In this specific sense petit mal is as distinctive as grand mal, though much less dramatic. The essential feature is sudden loss of consciousness just as in major epilepsy, but without falling and with only the smallest suggestion of convulsive movement. The face may flush or go pale, the eyes frequently blink, and occasionally there is slight twitching of the hands, but commonly enough the only abnormality observed is sudden blankness of expression—the so-called 'absence'—and a momentary arrest of activity. Incontinence is rare and objects held are seldom dropped. The attack lasts only for a few seconds and ends as abruptly as it began. Sometimes conversation is resumed immediately and the patient is unaware that anything has happened. More commonly the train of thought is broken and the fit is followed by brief bewilderment.

Myoclonic epilepsy occurs most commonly as sudden jerking of one or both arms, soon after rising in the morning, flinging objects from the hand. Such jerks may herald a major fit. In severe cases where the whole body is involved by a jerk of this kind the patient may fall without losing consciousness. Most often, however, these attacks occur in patients who are also subject to major fits at other times.

These three types of fit are those encountered in *primary generalized epilepsy*, otherwise known as idiopathic epilepsy. Primary refers to the absence of anatomical brain damage. Generalized indicates that the abnormal cortical discharges are universal and simultaneous resulting in immediate loss of consciousness without focal features. The less common myoclonic attacks result from less widely spreading discharges, also originating in the central structures. Neither the nature of the underlying abnormality nor the nature of the trigger or triggers that fire off an attack in a patient with this susceptibility are known, though the tendency for epileptic fits to follow awakening or overbreathing, and to occur premenstrually, suggests that such triggers may be both physiological and biochemical.

Since there is no focal brain damage in idiopathic epilepsy, there are no signs of localized cerebral dysfunction in the fit. Grand mal with unheralded loss of consciousness may also result from a localized lesion, but when certain areas are involved symptoms of local cerebral dysfunction often precede the loss of consciousness as a warning or aura. Sometimes the aura arises in isolation, constituting the only evidence of the fit. The most easily recognized form of focal epilepsy is the *Jacksonian fit*, in which movements begin on one side of the body. Clonic jerking begins most often at the angle of the mouth, in the thumb or in the great toe, and spreads with increasing amplitude. Sometimes it is possible to recognize that the spread or 'march' of the fit successively involves structures controlled by contiguous areas of the motor cortex, suggesting an orderly progression of abnormal excitation. The jerking may stop at any stage, or it may spread until consciousness is lost in a major convulsion. Such a fit is still described as Jacksonian because it began unilaterally. A focal onset has a much greater clinical significance than the asymmetrical clonic movements sometimes seen in the later stages of a major fit.

The transient unilateral weakness known as Todd's paralysis is seen particularly after a focal motor fit. It has been attributed to exhaustion of the affected neurones, but it is probably a manifestation of continued abnormal neuronal discharge. Todd's paralysis is often seen in children following major convulsions without any focal features, and does not necessarily indicate an anatomical lesion.

Epilepsy originating in the sensory cortex causes crude sensations of tingling, coldness or even pain in the opposite side of the body, again beginning locally and spreading, either as an aura or constituting the entire fit. Focal fits from the occipital cortex cause unformed visual hallucinations such as bright colours or flashing lights. More complex organized visual phenomena such as formed hallucinations result from lesions further forward in the occipito-parietal region.

It will be obvious that most of these phenomena not only point clearly to a certain area of the brain but also indicate the side of the discharging focus. The commonest form of focal fit originates in one or other temporal lobe, with focal features that are highly variable and seldom lateralizing. The simplest is an unpleasant sensation or 'sinking feeling' in the epigastrium, rising to the head and followed by a major convulsion. Formed visual, auditory and olfactory hallucinations of extraordinary complexity may occur, usually stereotyped for each patient, and often accompanied by emotional disturbances that are usually unpleasant and frightening. The patient may have great difficulty in describing or remembering these experiences, but can always recognize the onset of an attack. The *déja vu* sensation is so common in normal people that in itself it cannot be regarded as epileptic, but in the patient with epilepsy it is accompanied either by other hallucinatory sensations or by more frankly epileptic phenomena.

In *temporal lobe epilepsy* these sensory or mental phenomena either precede a major fit or are accompanied by motor activity much less easily recognizable as epileptic. Consciousness is clouded rather than lost, and the patient responds vaguely when spoken to. The picture is very variable, but the essential feature is the performance of complex and coordinated but inappropriate movements, quite distinct from disorganized clonic jerking. Smacking the lips, muttering unintelligibly, rubbing the hands together, shuffling papers, or searching the contents of the handbag are typical activities, but there are many more including undressing, micturating, and other acts liable to misinterpretation. Temporal lobe fits of this kind, sometimes known as complex partial seizures, last for several minutes, and are often followed by a more prolonged period of less severe confusion and amnesia. Misdiagnosis as petit mal should rarely occur if the duration of the fit and the nature of the movements can be established.

The precise place of the phenomenon of *automatism* in the epileptic context is not easy to define. It implies that for a more or less prolonged period the patient carries out normal or at least coordinated activities without knowing what he is doing and without subsequent recollection of the events. This is, of course, exactly what happens in many temporal lobe fits, where in most cases it must be regarded as a part of the fit itself and not as a peculiar post-epileptic state. The automatism that sometimes follows a major fit is clinically indistinguishable from that seen as part of temporal lobe epilepsy, and requires no separate description. Claims that criminal acts have been committed during epileptic automatism should be treated with the greatest reserve.

Many other forms of partial or minor epilepsy occur, especially in patients with chronic brain damage. These are hard to classify and sometimes even to recognize, but they are mostly characterized by brief loss of consciousness and clonic jerking, with or without falling and incontinence of urine. Again the distinction from true petit mal may be difficult, but it is important both in relation to treatment and prognosis.

Diagnosis of epilepsy

If an attack is witnessed it is always possible to recognize grand mal, petit mal and Jacksonian motor fits. The epileptic nature of a typical temporal lobe fit once seen can always be recognized. A hysterical imitation of grand mal is easily distinguishable by the nature of the movements, the absence of deep unconsciousness, and the circumstances of the attack; but more sophisticated hysterical phenomena may closely resemble one or other of the many atypical forms of temporal lobe epilepsy. It is, however, unusual for the physician to see a fit, and diagnosis usually depends on the account given by the patient and by witnesses. The nature of premonitory symptoms may furnish an important clue, but they are sometimes lacking, and the patient may be unable to contribute more than a description of his condition after recovery of consciousness and a statement as to whether or not he had bitten his tongue or been incontinent. Perhaps the most important single feature in the patient's history is that in contrast with a syncopal attack he does not feel completely well for a matter of hours. Sensible eyewitnesses can usually furnish a description of the fit which permits a reasonably reliable diagnosis, but witnesses may not have been present or may not be sensible. A fit is frightening to the uninstructed, and a distraught relative may be excused an incoherent account. Description is often coloured by popular misconceptions about epilepsy and patients are exasperatingly described as 'fighting'—a term that might signify clonic jerking, the more coordinated movements of a temporal lobe attack, or merely a hysterical display. At second hand distinction is impossible.

Brief rigidity may occur at the onset of a syncopal attack, particularly in those prone to faint on slight trauma or at the sight of blood. The very rare occurrence of urinary incontinence in these circumstances is a further possible source of confusion.

Whatever the difficulties, the decision as to whether the patient has had one or more epileptic fits depends on clinical evidence since investigation can add little. Few patients with symptoms even remotely resembling any form of epilepsy now escape an EEG. There is some merit in this practice, though it does not lie in establishing or excluding the diagnosis of epilepsy. The proportion of abnormal records in adult patients known to have epilepsy is not significantly higher than in the general population, and many of the abnormalities so painstakingly described are in no way specific for epilepsy. When there is clinical doubt about the diagnosis of epilepsy the EEG is very unlikely to resolve it. Nevertheless, the EEG has added greatly to our knowledge of epilepsy and may provide valuable information as to why an individual patient has fits. The only diagnostic EEG abnormality that may be found in the record of a patient with idiopathic epilepsy between his attacks (the interseizure record) is a diffuse, paroxysmal disturbance beginning and ending abruptly, in the form of more or less regular slow waves and spikes at a frequency of three per second. Similar discharges are seen during attacks of petit mal, but they may be present in the interseizure records of other patients with a history of major fits alone. The finding of such an abnormality is very strong though not absolutely conclusive evidence that the epilepsy is idiopathic and not due to focal brain damage.

In patients with focal epilepsy it may be possible to detect abnormal discharges from the neighbourhood of the damaged area of cortex in the form of spikes or slow waves. This is important in the search for a lesion possibly amenable to surgery. A pathological diagnosis can never be made on EEG evidence, but generally speaking focal spikes are more commonly found in the vicinity of atrophic lesions such as scars, while very slow focal 'delta' waves may indicate a tumour or some other comparatively large and recent destructive lesion. This distinction is not entirely reliable.

In epileptic patients with other evidence of chronic brain damage such as spastic cerebral palsy or mental deficiency the EEG is often diffusely and continuously abnormal, and may show a variety of paroxysmal discharges, but these can hardly be regarded as of diagnostic value.

Diagnosis of the cause

Epileptic fits occur in many types of acute metabolic disorders or infections, where the cause is usually obvious. It is the patient who has had one or more undoubted fits but has no other complaints who presents a formidable and often insoluble problem. Idiopathic epilepsy normally presents in childhood but not in infancy, and its diagnosis becomes increasingly improbable when the fits occur for the first time over the age of 20. The natural history of idiopathic epilepsy is not stereotyped. One common pattern comprises the onset of petit mal about the age of eight. Such attacks are sometimes very frequent, especially in the early morning, and may occur 50 times or more each day. This situation may be complicated at any time by the occurrence of a major convulsion, but in some children the condition remains one of petit mal alone. In others there is no petit mal, and epilepsy is manifest in major convulsions from the start, mostly nocturnal or in the mornings. Whether or not it is complicated by grand mal, petit mal often ceases in adolescence and continues into adult life in only a small minority of cases. Patients with idiopathic epilepsy may become morose and eccentric in later life, partly no doubt as a result of their handicap, but there is no initial question of associated mental disorder. A case of this type with no abnormal signs and with three-per-second wave and spike discharges in the EEG can confidently be diagnosed as primary generalized epilepsy.

Chronic epilepsy beginning in the first two years of life is often due to brain damage sustained at birth and occasionally to progressive disease. Young children with a high fever are particularly liable to isolated major fits during the infection. The possibility of meningitis must be remembered and if there is the slightest cause for suspicion lumbar puncture must be done: indeed some authorities would regard it as obligatory. For the most part these *febrile convulsions* indicate no more than a low convulsive threshold which rises with maturity, and seldom develop into chronic epilepsy. However, prognosis must be more guarded when a slight fever is recorded after a fit in a child previously completely well.

Repeated and, particularly, prolonged febrile convulsions must not be ignored as there is some evidence that brain damage sustained during such fits may cause temporal lobe epilepsy in later life. Some children have fits almost every time they have a fever, but unfortunately there is no oral anticonvulsant that could act quickly enough if given when the child becomes ill. The alternatives are to give phenobarbitone regularly up to the age of 5 in children known to have this tendency, or where there is a family history of epilepsy, or to concentrate on preventive treatment during febrile illness. This must include tepid sponging and aspirin but opinion is divided on whether drugs are useful. It is impossible to reach adequate blood levels with oral anticonvulsants in time to be effective. Alternatives suggested have included intramuscular amytal or rectal paraldehyde, 1 ml per year up to 5 ml, administered by the mother at the onset of fever. There are obvious objections to regular medication for several years in young children and these have not been fully overcome.

A benign form of epilepsy has been recognized in children. The fits are brief and entirely nocturnal with complete and lasting remission after a year or two.

It is, however, the patient who develops epilepsy in adult life who forms the heart of the problem. Petit mal does not occur for the first time in the adult, but there is a regrettable tendency to refer to any fit not obviously major as petit mal, perhaps with the notion of softening the blow by a less alarming label. In most of these patients no cause for major or temporal lobe epilepsy can be found or reasonably conjectured, no matter how thorough the investigation. Few such patients, and none whose fits reveal any focal features, can be regarded as suffering from idiopathic epilepsy in the sense used here, and such attacks are better described as cryptogenic. A very careful history must be taken with a special search for focal features, for evidence of possible fits in the past, and for other neurological symptoms or signs of any kind. It is vital to question witnesses of any attacks that have been observed, since patients have no idea of their behaviour during temporal lobe attacks and may neglect to mention or fail to recall even a motor Jacksonian onset. A comparatively common event is a single major fit occurring after the withdrawal of no more than moderate doses of barbiturates, and this may be revealed only by close questioning. A prolonged alcoholic orgy may precipitate fits which can also follow reduction of a heavy regular intake. The possible relationship of epilepsy to hypoglycaemia must also be remembered, but the common occurrence of epileptic fits during the interval between rising and breakfast is more probably connected with the radical alteration in cerebral activity between sleep and waking. Banal head injuries are proffered as a cause of epilepsy by many patients, but injuries that have not produced loss of consciousness are almost certainly irrelevant: epilepsy rarely follows even severe closed head injuries, and the penetrating wounds that are a potent cause of traumatic epilepsy are unlikely to escape notice.

Examination must be thorough but is usually normal. X-rays of the chest and skull should be obtained and, if available, a CT scan. How far a normal scan can be taken to exclude a cerebral tumour in a patient without physical signs is not yet known but almost certainly an operable meningioma would be detected and there is no great advantage in the early diagnosis of gliomas. If CT scan is not available an EEG should be done as a delta focus must be regarded as a physical sign. In these circumstances the EEG abnormality should be followed up by carotid angiography on the appropriate side. The patient should be seen at regular intervals both to ensure proper control of treatment and to observe indications for further investigations.

If no cause can be found in most patients with fits, why do they have epilepsy? In this connection valid evidence is scanty, and the situation is confused by the probability that frequent severe fits may themselves cause structural damage to the brain through anoxia. In temporal lobe epilepsy the characteristic pathological finding is scarring, plausibly attributed to birth injury. Angiomatous malformations and scars due to head injury or cerebral infarction may be clinically undetectable, and indeed many would escape exhaustive investigations even if these were indicated. The rigid distinction between idiopathic and symptomatic epilepsy implied in the present text is almost certainly an over-simplification, but better understanding and control of epilepsy probably depend more on advances in normal and abnormal cerebral biochemistry than on histopathological studies.

Mental changes

Although most patients with epilepsy remain mentally normal throughout their lives, the chronic wards of mental hospitals contain many epileptic patients. This is not because of the patient's fits or because epilepsy has affected their reason, but because structural brain damage has caused both fits and behaviour disorders. The latter may be particularly striking in patients with temporal lobe epilepsy, and here the relation between abnormal behaviour and fits may be much closer. Indeed chronic and longstanding abnormal discharges from one or other temporal lobe are not infrequently associated with prolonged but intermittent truculence and aggression.

Another familiar problem is presented by the epileptic child whose mental ability declines, often drastically, over the course of a year or two. The explanation of this phenomenon is obscure, but in most cases the epilepsy is a manifestation of brain damage and the patient's deterioration is caused by the underlying cerebral condition rather than by the epilepsy itself. There is suggestive but inconclusive evidence that prolonged anticonvulsant therapy may adversely affect cerebral function by interfering with the normal action of folic acid.

Treatment

Even if an obvious cause such as a cerebral tumour has been found, preventive treatment of epilepsy consists in the regular administration of drugs. We know remarkably little about their mode of action, and they have been developed by trial and error in patients and in experimental animals. The drugs that are effective in grand mal, temporal lobe epilepsy and other focal fits are rarely helpful in petit mal, while a second group that prevent petit mal may even increase the number of major fits.

Amongst the first group phenobarbitone is still a useful drug, although its reputation has unjustifiably suffered from the laudable reluctance to prescribe barbiturates in other conditions. The average adult dose is 30 mg two or three times a day but many patients can tolerate more, especially if dosage is gradually increased. Overdosage causes drowsiness, but the patient's attribution of fatigue and depression to this drug is seldom justified.

Phenytoin in an average adult dose of 100 mg thrice daily, or in a single 300 mg dose, is a very effective anticonvulsant. Toxic effects are, however, relatively common and remarkable. For most patients there is a critical dosage above which they will develop severe cerebellar ataxia with nystagmus, slurred speech and inability to walk. Fortunately these alarming signs melt away within a week of reducing dosage to a tolerated level. It is best to reduce dosage, since the complete withdrawal of the drug's powerful anticonvulsant effect may provoke an attack of status epilepticus. Occasional effects of chronic therapeutic doses are hirsutism, hypertrophy of the gums, sometimes requiring gingivectomy, and an acute lymphadenopathy.

Primidone (Mysoline) is closely chemically related to phenobarbitone, but is more effective in certain patients. The average dose is 250 mg thrice daily, but some patients cannot tolerate more than a minute dose when treatment is started. The results of this intolerance are extremely unpleasant, amounting to ataxia, drowsiness and even stupor. It is therefore best to begin with only a fragment of a tablet at bedtime for a few days, after which nearly all patients rapidly acquire the normal tolerance.

Like many drugs these anticonvulsants may cause a skin rash and very rarely damage the bone marrow. A much commoner haematological effect, especially with primidone, is a megaloblastic anaemia that may be so trivial as to be detectable only by blood examination, or may be clinically severe. It is rapidly relieved by folic acid, but in some patients this unfortunately also antagonizes the anticonvulsant effect.

Sulthiame (Ospolot) has been claimed to be effective in resistant temporal lobe epilepsy but it is a relatively toxic drug producing dizziness and tachypnoea. Carbamazepine (Tegretol) is highly regarded by some authorities, particularly in children with temporal lobe epilepsy, but most would not regard it as a drug of first choice. It must not be given as a single daily dose as this does not maintain adequate blood levels.

The more recently introduced sodium valproate (Epilim) is often highly successful in the treatment of primary generalized epilepsy, being active against both major fits and petit mal. The dose is relatively large, up to 2 g a day in divided doses but, apart from transitory dyspepsia, at first there appeared to be a few side-effects. This was too good to last and hepatic damage is now being reported, although infrequently.

Sodium valproate is probably the drug of first choice in petit mal because its action against grand mal avoids the necessity of giving two drugs. Ethosuximide, in a dose building up to 250 mg three times a day is effective for petit mal but does not influence major fits. Toxic effects are rare. Acetazolamide (Diamox) in a dosage of 250 mg two or three times a day, or even more, sometimes stops petit mal attacks, especially where there is an association with overbreathing. It is also occasionally helpful in major epilepsy, but in either case the drug is apt to lose its effect, sometimes rapidly. Toxic effects from electrolyte disturbance are hardly ever encountered, but paraesthesiae in the extremities are an indication to withdraw treatment.

The principles of anticonvulsant treatment are simple, but the details require considerable experience. In major or focal fits it has been claimed that control using the single drug phenytoin, provided that this is monitored by blood levels, can be as effective as any combination but this is not general experience. Certainly treatment should be started with either phenobarbitone or phenytoin and the other drug only introduced if control cannot be obtained in spite of adequate blood levels. Combined tablets should never be used as they render alteration of dose difficult. The addition of a second agent is often beneficial but multiple drugs should certainly be avoided. If control is not achieved primidone can be substituted for the phenobarbitone in the combined treatment, the change being made gradually. There is no safe and effective substitute for phenytoin. Effective and relatively non-toxic levels of phenytoin are 35–70 μmol/l and of phenobarbitone 40–100 μmol/l. With both drugs this is roughly equivalent to 1–2 mg/100 ml. Whether efficient monitoring is possible from random out-patient levels is not established. It is certainly possible to detect the patient who is not taking the drugs at all.

It is clearly impossible to attempt to control epilepsy without prolonged regular administration of anticonvulsants but there is increasing disquiet about our ignorance of what we are really doing and about the growing list of previously unsuspected adverse effects. In addition to the known hazards it has recently been found that anticonvulsants can cause osteomalacia. Far more potentially serious is their probable teratogenic effect, particularly that of phenytoin. The implications of the reported findings have not been fully explored but it would seem unwise to begin treatment with any drug other than phenobarbitone in a patient who might become pregnant. On the other hand, to withdraw anticonvulsants from a woman with epilepsy when pregnancy is suspected or confirmed is to expose her to an unacceptable risk. The increased frequency of fits sometimes observed in patients with drug-induced folate deficiency when this is treated with folic acid has been interpreted as meaning that anticonvulsants prevent fits by interfering with folate metabolism. The explanation, however, appears to be the reverse, that folic acid lowers the blood level of phenytoin, thus accounting for the failure to control the fits.

The response to treatment can never be predicted in an individual patient, and when fits are infrequently spaced the assessment of treatment takes time. The physician should resist the tendency to change the routine at every visit, and since much the commonest cause of a recurrence of attacks in a patient previously well controlled is a simple failure to take the tablets regularly, such an event is not in itself an indication for a modification of treatment. Modern anticonvulsants are very effective, and in a proportion of patients the fits can be completely controlled, while in many others they can be made no more than occasional occurrences. Epilepsy in patients with diffuse brain damage sustained in infancy is frequently uninfluenced by treatment and cannot often be completely controlled. Always uncertainty about the natural history of epilepsy increases the difficulties of therapeutic assessment. Most neurologists institute treatment only after a second fit, but once introduced it should be maintained until control is as complete as can be achieved. If complete control is obtained gradual withdrawal of therapy after a traditional period of three years' freedom from attacks can be attempted if strongly desired by the patient. In fact, however, the fits recur in so large a proportion of chronic cases that there is a good deal to be said for maintaining treatment indefinitely: a recurrence of fits is a serious blow to the patient's morale, and although the majority of patients are anxious to manage without drugs, most return to them. In many patients treatment must be life-long, since the best we are able to achieve is some reduction in the frequency of attacks.

Petit mal tends to respond to treatment either completely or not at all. When treatment is successful the fits stop completely and treatment can often be withdrawn after a year or so with no return of symptoms. In other cases it is possible to achieve a worthwhile reduction in the number of fits, but totally resistant cases are distressingly common. Many children are grossly over-treated and are less incapacitated by frequent 'absences' than by the effect of massive dosage with a large variety of drugs. The unusual instances where petit mal persists into adult life are quite intractable.

Temporal lobe epilepsy resistant to drugs can sometimes be treated with dramatic success by amputation of the temporal lobe, after elaborate EEG and radiological studies to identify the side and site of origin of the abnormal electrical activity. The trouble with this form of treatment is that its results are highly unpredictable, and it is impossible to forecast which patients are likely to benefit and which may be made considerably worse. For this reason the method is not widely practised.

Treatment of an epileptic fit consists solely in preventing the patient from harming himself by suffocation, drowning or other hazards. The commonest cause of death is suffocation in bed, and the patient who sleeps alone should leave his bedroom door open. The conventional loosening of the collar during an attack is little more than a helpful gesture, and attempts to prevent the patient biting his tongue are apt to lead to bitten fingers.

Status epilepticus

This is a grave complication of epilepsy, consisting of repeated major fits without recovery of consciousness in between them. A patient in status is therefore by definition in coma. In some patients with chronic epilepsy the clinical course is punctuated by repeated episodes of status. In others it arises only after a careless lapse of treatment. In a few patients a single bout or repeated episodes of status represent the only manifestation of epilepsy. Most patients are spared this complication. Treatment is urgent since the patient will die if the fits are not stopped. The most effective treatment is the intravenous injection of 10 mg of diazepam (Valium), repeated if necessary. If only a transient effect is produced an intravenous drip containing 100 mg of diazepam per 500 ml of saline may be set up. This drug is not always effective, and paraldehyde by intramuscular injection still retains its usefulness. The dose is 10 ml into the upper and outer quadrant of the buttock, repeated as necessary. The buttocks may be sore when the patient regains consciousness but this is a small price to pay. Intramuscular phenobarbitone is not an adequate measure for the treatment of status. Intravenous phenytoin is effective but dangerous because of its cardiac action. Frequent monitoring of blood levels is essential but not usually available. Chlormethiazole is not adequate treatment for status and should not be used. In desperate emergencies where fits occur in rapid succession intravenous thiopentone must be used, a loading dose followed by 100 mg an hour by drip. Assisted respiration will certainly be needed and an endotracheal tube must be passed at once. Normal doses of conventional anticonvulsants must be continued via a nasogastric tube. One method that has attained popularity during the current enthusiasm for intensive care units is the prevention of the motor phenomena of the fit by means of paralysing drugs, on the assumption that it is the anoxia during the fit that is fatal. This is not so. It is the repeated and long-term disruption of cerebral function from the epileptic process itself that is the danger, and curare without adequate anticonvulsants is lethal no matter how well the airway is maintained.

Flicker-induced epilepsy

Exposure to a bright light flickering at about 14 flashes a second will induce EEG abnormalities in many people who have never had a fit. In established epilepsy the proportion and severity of such abnormalities is higher and in such patients a history may be obtained that some fits are induced by exposure to flicker. Those whose fits occur exclusively in response to this stimulus are in a separate category. Flicker may occasionally result from the sun shining through a row of trees or railings while the patient drives or walks past, but can very seldom cause a fit, the common source being television. The normal projection flickers when it is viewed in the peripheral visual field or with the eyes close to the screen, when the power of flicker fusion is much reduced. Coarser flickering occurs when the set requires adjustment. The common history is therefore that the picture begins to flicker, the patient stoops to adjust it with the face close to the screen and then has a fit. In some children the trait is marked and yields some obscure pleasure. Such a child cannot be left alone with the television set since he immediately applies his face to the screen to induce a fit. Exhortation is useless, but fortunately anticonvulsants are often effective. In the more usual case where there is no such compulsion anticonvulsants should not be prescribed as it is sufficient to view the television from a safe distance or not at all.

Infantile spasms

This inadequate title is used to describe an extremely serious progressive disorder of infancy. At the age of a few months to a year these children develop curious attacks in which they flex suddenly at the waist, the so-called 'salaam attack'. These are frequent, and major fits soon occur. The child's development is arrested and mental deficiency and blindness commonly result. Attempts have been made to link this syndrome with failure of pyridoxine activity, but with inconclusive results. In some children the disease follows inoculation, particularly against pertussis. The fits are resistant to anticonvulsants but can sometimes be controlled with corticotrophin. Whether they are controlled or not the outcome is rapidly fatal in about half these children and most of the remainder suffer from severe brain damage. The EEG is extremely abnormal, often showing the complete disorganization known as hypsarrhythmia.

Management

Epilepsy is common and probably affects one in 200 of the population in one form or another. In addition to the individual misery it causes it presents a massive social problem. The treatment of epilepsy is not with drugs alone, and meticulous explanation in terms that the patient and his relatives can understand is equally important. There are many popular beliefs to be dispelled, in particular the common assumption that epilepsy is a form of insanity and that recovery is impossible.

Advice is sought on many problems. Obviously work where a fit would endanger the patient or others cannot be advised, and in these mechanized times this severely limits the possibilities for the manual worker. The law has been modified to permit driving after 2 years without a fit or after 3 years of fits occurring only in sleep. Sympathy for the patient must be tempered by consideration for others and in our view these provisions are too lax, a view supported by the total prohibition on driving heavy goods vehicle with even a very remote history of epilepsy. Every patient who has had epileptic attacks is liable to recurrence. Cases within personal experience include one man with only two fits in ten years who drove for 200 yards along a footpath while unconscious, another with nocturnal fits only who drove off the road at high speed while 'asleep' in broad daylight, and a third who killed another motorist in a second attack of very minor temporal lobe epilepsy. If any patient with a history of epileptic attacks is to be allowed to drive, a five-year interval of freedom would be a better safeguard, but it is sensible that continued treatment is now permitted.

The question of marriage and heredity is often raised. Epilepsy is no bar to marriage but the unaffected spouse must be fully informed. There is no denying that in certain families epilepsy occurs in succeeding generations or in several siblings, and it is not always the same type of epilepsy. On the other hand, the parents of the large majority of epileptic patients are not affected. When only one parent has epilepsy the increased risk to the children is negligible, but two epileptic subjects should be discouraged from having a family. Carrying out an EEG on the prospective partner of an epileptic is non-contributory.

Most epileptic mothers pass through pregnancy without any notable increase in the frequency of their fits but sometimes there is a considerable exacerbation. This rarely reaches the point at which the epilepsy is a threat to life, and termination of pregnancy on these grounds is infrequent. Clearly no patient with frequent fits can be encouraged to have a large family since there are serious problems in caring for young children when unconsciousness may occur at any moment without warning. It has been unconvincingly claimed that the contraceptive pill aggravates epilepsy. The effect is certainly not pronounced.

The epileptic life is hedged with restrictions. Work is difficult to obtain or to keep. The dread of further fits arouses fear in onlookers. Restrictions should be as few as possible, particularly in children. Swimming unaccompanied by an adult aware of the diagnosis is obviously unwise, and riding a bicycle when petit mal is frequent can be dangerous. In the adult, apart from the restrictions on working conditions immediately imposed by the community, it is probably wise to warn against alcohol. Some patients can drink with impunity, but in many even moderate indulgence precipitates a fit. Patients with epilepsy do not always accept advice and may perhaps excusably go to great lengths to conceal their disability.

SYNCOPE

Simple fainting is uncommon in adults and is characteristically seen in tall, gangling adolescents. Girls who want to attract attention may also indulge in faked or hysterical swooning. Generally, however, the circumstances of an attack render the diagnosis of a genuine faint fairly reliable. Common factors are an upright posture, a hot room, no breakfast, and dysmenorrhea. The postural factor is especially important in habitual fainters, who practically always give a history of postural dizziness or syncope on standing up suddenly after sitting or lying for a period. A history of fainting while standing in morning prayers at school is also common. Postural fainting of this kind is of no serious significance, and passes with adolescence.

Some patients have a more obstinate tendency to syncope provoked by slight injury, the sight of blood, an injection, or hearing conversations on medical matters. While this tendency does not carry the serious implications of epilepsy it can be almost equally troublesome, and it is very resistant to treatment. A source of some confusion is that such patients often have a brief anoxic convulsion with rigidity and occasionally even incontinence of urine. The patient should sit down at the slightest warning, and should not receive injections or have wounds dressed except when lying down. The trait is often familial.

Micturition syncope is virtually confined to middle-aged men. The patient leaves his bed to pass water and faints suddenly while doing so. He is already somewhat hypotensive because of postural and skin vasodilatation, and the reduction of intra-abdominal pressure caused by emptying the bladder is the last straw. The patient seldom experiences this on more than two or three occasions, and avoids it by sitting down to pass water. The extreme pain of *proctalgia fugax* is commonly accompanied by sudden unconsciousness, and is sometimes mistaken for epilepsy, but is in fact syncopal.

Cough syncope is an uncommon complication of obstructive airway disease in middle-aged men. A bout of coughing, not always severe, is immediately followed by unconsciousness. The rise in pressure in the thorax during coughing prevents the return of venous blood to the heart and the cardiac output is drastically but briefly reduced. Treatment must be that of the chest condition. The Stokes–Adams attack characteristic of partial heart block is also syncopal, though here of course there is an important basis of structural myocardial disease. The resemblance to epilepsy may be close, and indeed convulsive movements are sometimes seen, as in any severe syncope.

A second cause of syncope of grave significance in adult life is now recognized with increasing frequency. Idiopathic orthostatic hypotension (see Chapter 16) is due to degeneration of the central and probably also the peripheral sympathetic autonomic nervous system.

Orthostatic hypotension with syncope also occurs in tabes dorsalis and diabetic neuropathy, and is quite common in patients receiving hypotensive therapy. It is an occasional side-effect of treatment with other drugs, particularly imipramine and chlordiazepoxide.

The *carotid sinus syndrome* is one of those disorders diagnosed frequently by a small group of physicians but never recognized by most. Its basis is an extreme sensitivity of one or both carotid sinuses to external pressure in arteriosclerotic subjects. Turning the head so that the sinus is compressed by the collar causes slowing of the pulse and giddiness or syncope. The condition is said to respond to treatment with atropine by mouth or to operative denervation of the carotid sinus. It is claimed that this syndrome can be detected by massaging the vulnerable carotid sinus while listening to the apex beat, but as a routine manoeuvre in patients with attacks of unconsciousness is very seldom rewarding.

NARCOLEPSY

This strange disorder of sleep develops in adult life without obvious cause. The cardinal symptom is an irresistible urge to sleep. It is intermittent and quite distinct from the chronic fatigue of debilitating physical disease or 'neurasthenia', or the blunting of alertness typical of chronically raised intracranial pressure. At first the attacks occur mainly at rest and especially in circumstances where relaxation and some drowsiness can be regarded as normal. Falling asleep in public transport, in the cinema, or even on the hard benches of the outpatient department can be described as little more than an exaggeration of normal behaviour, but in severe cases of narcolepsy sleep overcomes the patient between the courses of a meal or even between one mouthful and the next. When the need presents, the patient may fall asleep while standing if he tries to fight it off. He is easily rousable, but left alone will sleep for minutes or even a few hours. The condition may be very disabling.

Some disorder of the alerting mechanisms of the reticular formation can be presumed, but structural disease is not found. In the fully developed case other features are present, notably *cataplexy*. This is an even more remarkable symptom, in which sudden weakness occurs following certain emotional stimuli. These vary from one patient to another but laughter, suspense, excitement or mounting frustration are typical examples. The weakness may be localized, amounting to no more than a sudden dropping of the head or jaw, but all grades of severity are encountered including falling helpless to the ground. Consciousness is always retained.

Other features of the syndrome are hypnagogic hallucinations—vivid visual dreams, usually terrifying, at the moment of dropping off to sleep—and sleep paralysis. This may occur quite apart from narcolepsy in the form of so-called 'night-nurses' paralysis', and consists of complete inability to move immediately after waking. It is frightening but momentary. Patients with narcolepsy combined with cataplexy have an abnormal nocturnal sleep pattern. Instead of the normal first hour of deep dreamless sleep these patients pass immediately into the phase of rapid eye movements during which dreams occur.

The treatment of narcolepsy is difficult. Dextramphetamine has long been the standard agent and is undoubtedly effective symptomatic treatment, but increasing doses may be needed with unpleasant toxic effects. Drugs introduced originally for the treatment of depression have been found to be useful. Protryptyline may be effective in narcolepsy and clomipramine in cataplexy. In severe narcolepsy relief can seldom be achieved without unpleasant dose-related side-effects.

Further reading

Laidlaw J. & Richens A. (eds.) (1976) *A Textbook of Epilepsy*. Churchill Livingstone, Edinburgh and London.
Matthews W.B. (1973) The clinical value of routine electroencephalography. *J. R. Coll. of Phys. Lond.* **7**, 207.
Guilleminault G. & Dement W.C. (1977) 235 cases of excessive daytime sleepiness. *J. Neurol. Sci.* **31**, 13.

CHAPTER 18
Migraine

Migraine is a common and distressing paroxysmal disorder of function, one of many everyday non-lethal ailments where there are wide gaps in our knowledge of causation and treatment.

The sexes are affected approximately equally. The onset is usually between the age of 15 and 30, with some scatter beyond this range, and recognizable migraine may be preceded by paroxysmal vomiting in the young child, or by travel sickness. Difficulties of definition render estimates of prevalence unreliable, but some surveys have found 10% or more of the population to be affected, though severe migraine is much less frequent. In many families the incidence is considerably higher, and genetic factors are important, inheritance following the pattern of dominant transmission.

Clinical features

There are innumerable variants, but the classical attack of migraine follows a recognizable sequence. A warning signal may be a sensation of unusual well-being, followed by vague uneasiness. The commonest prodromal symptom is a shimmering 'heat haze' disturbance of vision in one half of the visual field. Coloured zig-zag lines may spread over the whole field, followed by patchy loss of vision or by hemianopia, or by loss of both peripheral fields, producing tunnel vision. Tingling and numbness begins in one or other hand and spreads slowly up the arm to the lips and tongue, where both sides are affected. The arm feels heavy and perhaps weak, but can be moved. Sometimes, disturbingly, speech is disordered, so that words are mispronounced or cannot be expressed at all. As one symptom appears and develops, so the others fade, and after about 20 minutes vision returns to normal and the pain begins. Headache is often unilateral, the hemicrania from which the word migraine is said to be derived, but can also be occipital, or involve one or both eyes or the whole of the head. It increases rapidly and becomes incapacitatingly severe, aggravated intolerably by bright light or noise. Wretchedness is completed by waves of nausea, followed by incessant vomiting. The victim lies in a darkened room, having ejected his ineffective remedies, and relief comes only from sleep after some hours of misery. On waking, the severe attack is over but some headache may persist even for a day or two. Fortunately not all patients have attacks of such severity, and those who do also have less prostrating paroxysms. Prodromal symptoms may be absent or entirely visual. It may be possible to continue work throughout the headache and many patients never vomit. It also occurs in a much less definitive form, in which headache is the only symptom but is recognizably of the same type as in the classical syndrome. Throbbing or continuous pain in one temple, in one eye, or at the back of the head may be an almost daily event, either in those who have seldom or never had a full attack, or following a series of severe attacks in any migraine sufferer. Even in such cases, however, the elements of classical migraine are recognizable and the condition may be authenticated by an occasional disabling attack. Migraine often follows a set pattern in a particular patient, at least for many years; at the best a mild nuisance, and at the worst a dreaded enemy.

Attacks begin at any time of day, and occasionally awaken the patient in the early morning. In one form, the headache is already fully developed on waking and no prodromata are ever experienced. The frequency varies from once a year to several times a week, but is often about once a month, with more frequent minor episodes. Week-end migraine is common and peculiarly annoying, as these often industrious people find their leisure ruined. A premenstrual incidence is also common, but hardly ever exclusive. Classical migraine nearly always remits during pregnancy, but often increases temporarily at the menopause. Beyond the age of 55 migraine nearly always becomes less frequent and eventually ceases.

Clinical variants

Hemiplegic migraine is a rare and sometimes alarming variation, quite distinct from the relatively common unilateral paraesthesiae. The onset is often in childhood and the first attack causes justifiable concern. Headache and rapidly advancing hemiparesis can give rise to fears of cerebral abscess, aneurysm, or tumour, and unless the brevity of the attack is recognized as the signature of migraine it may lead to investigation in a neurosurgical unit. Carotid angiography may be undertaken, a procedure which greatly aggravates and prolongs hemiplegic migraine. The angiogram is normal and even the most severe attack subsides in two or three days without residual signs. There is often a strong family history of florid migraine, and together with a tendency of subsequent attacks to affect alternate sides this should lay the ghost of structural cerebral disease.

The diagnosis of *ophthalmoplegic migraine* is often made but seldom justified. Patients may describe visual prodromata as 'double vision', but in this context the term is nearly always found to mean distortion of the visual fields, and true diplopia is rare. A patient with an aneurysm on the internal carotid artery may have one or more attacks of unilateral pain behind the eye, accompanied by a partial third nerve palsy, but the resemblance to migraine is seldom close. Occasionally, however, otherwise classical migraine may be repeatedly accompanied by transient unilateral ptosis or ocular palsy, but even where this persists angiography is normal.

Causation

The importance of genetic factors has already been mentioned, but precisely what is inherited apart from a tendency to headache is unknown. Attempts to identify a specific psychological type are unhelpful. Certainly there is a high incidence among successful over-conscientious obsessionals, but the classical syndrome is also encountered amongst the feckless or mentally defective. An attack of classical migraine is an astonishingly severe disturbance of function and it is remarkable that so little should be known about its causation. It is generally accepted, on slender evidence, that there is an instability of vasomotor control, the prodromal symptoms being due to constriction of cerebral arteries causing transient cortical ischaemia, and the headache to dilatation chiefly of extracranial vessels. The vascular origin of the pain is easy to verify, since the superficial temporal arteries are often obviously dilated and tender during an attack, while compression of one carotid artery often relieves the headache immediately but temporarily on that side. Within the skull, the arteries and the meninges in their vicinity are sensitive to pain, and undoubtedly contribute to that of migraine. The immediate cause of these vascular responses is unknown and the only consistent pattern of abnormality of humoral agents is a fall in circulating 5-hydroxytryptamine (serotonin) at the onset of the headache. Serotonin may by liberated from platelets and taken up by the arterial wall, causing vasoconstriction and the prodromal symptoms. Histamine produced locally may be responsible for vasodilatation and pain. How these events might be triggered and how they could cause symptoms on one side of the head is unknown. Water retention plays an ill-defined part in the acute attack, to the extent that some patients actually increase in girth and their attack is followed by diuresis. Articles of diet have been incriminated, either as a cause of allergy or as a source of amino-acids that might act in the same way as tyramine in cheese provokes headache and hypertension in those taking monoamine oxidase inhibiting drugs. Certainly cheese, chocolate and onions precipitate attacks in some patients, but there is no accompanying hypertension and the elimination of these foods from the diet does not abolish migraine. Emotional strain and overwork have an inconstant effect and often it is relaxation of the stress that acts as the trigger.

The effect of oral contraceptives is inconsistent, but if there is any change, it is usually an increase in frequency and severity of the attacks. Occasionally, and for no clear reason, the effect is to produce remission.

Alcoholic excess aggravates migraine and even moderate indulgence will precipitate an attack in some patients, though it may prove beneficial in others. A low blood sugar due to inadequate infrequent meals is another potent factor.

Diagnosis

Migraine may sometimes be confused with less specific chronic recurrent forms of headache and indeed is often combined with chronic tension headache due to contraction of the scalp muscles (Chapter 3). It is, however, the prodromal symptoms that more often lead to diagnostic error. The unilateral paraesthesiae bear a superficial resemblance to focal sensory epilepsy, but the speed of spread over minutes rather than seconds is so much slower in migraine that the distinction should not prove difficult. An attack of migraine, sometimes the first, may be triggered by a blow on the head, giving rise to a suspicion of cerebral damage, particularly if the sensory or visual symptoms are more prominent than the headache. The injury is usually trivial, often no more than heading a football, and the symptoms are transient, so that again no serious diagnostic difficulty should arise. More important are the exaggerated notions commonly held on the subject of symptomatic migraine—migraine secondary to structural intracranial disease. It is often found that patients presenting with subarachnoid haemorrhage due to a ruptured aneurysm or arteriovenous malformation have a history of migraine, and it is indeed possible that the vascular anomaly has in some way been a contributing factor. This has led to the elaborate and quite unjustified investigation of migraine sufferers in the expectation of finding such anomalies. Patients with headache always on the same side, paraesthesiae always in the same arm, or dysphasia in all attacks are submitted to carotid angiography, even by experienced neurologists apparently undeterred by invariably normal results. Migraine alone, however bizarre, is never an indication for angiography, which will invariably prove negative in the absence of persisting physical signs. Additional features, such as focal epilepsy or a cranial bruit, must obviously be considered on their own merits.

Typical prodromal symptoms not followed by headache are relatively common in chronic migraine sufferers, but when these occur for the first time in middle age they are probably due to permanent structural arterial narrowing. When similar symptoms develop in women taking oral contraceptives, these should be stopped at once.

Treatment

There is no wholly effective treatment for migraine and the response is highly individual. It is reasonable to explore the patient's environment for causes of stress, but the results of relieving even the most crushing burdens of overwork or responsibility are nearly always disappointing. Most patients who have recognized that their symptoms are aggravated by alcohol or diet will already have made sensible adjustments. The urging of prolonged holidays on those who would rather be at work is a tempting but ineffective form of preventive medicine.

Drug treatment may be prophylactic or directed to the acute attacks, but if these are infrequent any form of continuous treatment is unnecessary. Simple analgesics such as soluble aspirin are always the first choice and are effective in mild attacks. In severe migraine, the headaches may be rendered tolerable provided the tablets are not vomited. Ergotamine tartrate is a popular remedy, its use being based on its vasoconstrictor action. It may be given by mouth, by inhalation or by suppository. The oral dose is 1 mg either swallowed or dissolved beneath the tongue, repeated in 30 minutes if necessary, and again for one further dose. Absorption is improved if metoclopramide is given simultaneously. If vomiting prevents absorption, a convenient inhaler is marketed (Medihaler), or often more effective, a suppository which also contains caffeine (Cafergot). There are many proprietary oral preparations combined with anti-emetic drugs. If these remedies are to be of any use, they must be taken as soon as an attack is suspected. If used correctly, ergotamine tartrate will cut attacks short in some patients, but in many others it has no beneficial action at all. Despite its evil reputation, toxic effects from peripheral vasoconstriction are extremely rare. The main difficulty in the chronic use of ergotamine is the production of ergotamine-dependent headache only relieved by further doses of the drug. The effect of prophylactic drugs is hard to assess, as any good placebo will reduce the frequency of migraine in at least half the patients. Phenobarbitone 30 mg twice or thrice daily is sometimes helpful, but phenytoin is not. Antihistamine drugs are sometimes very effective, particularly in patients who awaken with migraine. Here attacks can often be entirely prevented by 10 to 25 mg of promethazine at bedtime. Ergotamine should not be used continuously. The most effective agent so far produced is methysergide, a drug with complex properties including an antiserotonin action. It is given as 1 mg three times daily, increasing to double this dose if necessary, but no higher. Migraine is abolished in some patients, but in others it is scarcely modified. Toxic effects include immediate giddiness and severe pains in the legs without obvious vasoconstriction. The drug should not be given if there is a history of ischaemic heart disease. Long-term side-effects include retroperitoneal fibrosis causing pain in the groin and urinary symptoms. This can be avoided by interrupting the treatment every six months for a period of a month. Unfortunately, many patients who initially respond well to methysergide later relapse. This drug should obviously only be used when prostrating migraine is occurring once a week or even more frequently. Newer antiserotonin agents are being introduced which it is hoped will prove more effective and less toxic. Pizotifen is often effective but may cause troublesome weight gain. Another introduction in the prophylaxis of migraine is clonidine in small doses. One tablet of 0.025 mg is given twice a day, increasing if necessary at fortnightly intervals to three times this dose. The response is variable and severe migraine may not respond at all but toxic effects are gratifyingly slight. Propranolol is also an effective preventive treatment in some patients. Many doctors and many patients have individual prescriptions for migraine which mitigate its full rigours, but lack of a reliable universal remedy suggests that our ideas of causation are insufficiently precise.

MIGRAINOUS NEURALGIA

This condition, also known as cluster headaches or histamine headache, is certainly related to migraine but has a different natural history. It is much more common in men and often begins in the third decade. There are no prodromal symptoms and the pain is in one frontal region or around the eye. It rapidly increases to a frightening intensity, but usually begins to subside after twenty minutes. At the height of the attack the eye waters and is often bloodshot, and the nostril on that side is blocked. The eyelids may be reddened and oedematous. Attacks occur up to three or four times in 24 hours, often in the middle of the night, for a period of about six weeks. The patient is then entirely free of headache for from one to three years, when a similar bout develops on the same side for no discoverable reason.

An extensive acquaintance with this syndrome reveals variations in the site of the pain and its periodicity, but the classical condition should be immediately recognizable. This expectation is not fulfilled, because the initial diagnosis is always either sinusitis or trigeminal neuralgia. The cause is unknown and the suggested link with histamine is based on similarity with the effect of this substance rather than with any confirmed disorder of histamine release. The association with migraine is not immediately obvious since most of these patients are free of classical migraine, but it is emphasized by its response to prophylactic treatment. Methysergide in full doses is completely effective in most cases, but if it fails, then dihydroergotamine may be given by injection. The maximum dose is 0.5 mg night and morning, and many patients manage well on 0.25 mg at night only. They must inject themselves and it is essential to omit treatment one day a week to see if the bout has ended. Prophylaxis, although troublesome, is effective and eagerly adopted by the patient but treatment of such attacks as breakthrough is unavailing. In some unfortunate patients attacks continue with no suggestion of clustering and may prove resistant to the usual prophylactic measures. A short course of prednisolone may break the sequence and prolonged treatments with lithium carbonate is also often successful.

COUGH HEADACHE

A relatively common and disturbing symptom unrelated to migraine is headache on coughing. The patient is usually an adult and fortunately not commonly the subject of chronic chest disease. The complaint is of sudden sharp pain in the head on coughing, followed by prolonged dull aching. Sometimes other similar activities, such as sneezing, laughing or straining, produce the same pain, and a bizarre variant is headache only on laughing. These manoeuvres have in common a sudden increase in intracranial venous pressure, and this history arouses suspicion of some cause of raised intracranial pressure briefly exacerbated by coughing. In fact a cerebral tumour is hardly ever present in these patients, but the symptoms are so persistent that in spite of the complete absence of physical signs, investigation by CT scan is sometimes inescapable. Curiously enough, cough headache is sometimes relieved for several weeks by the unpleasant procedure of air encephalography. This can scarcely be regarded as a rational or effective form of treatment but the condition may eventually remit.

Further reading

Caviness V.S. & O'Brien P. (1980) Headache. *New Engl. J. Med.* **302**, 446.
Lance J.W. (1978) *Mechanism and Management of Headache*, 3rd edn. Butterworth, London.

CHAPTER 19
Neurological Aspects of Psychiatry

All doctors are consulted by many patients whose symptoms do not appear to be due to organic disease and the neurologist probably sees more than most. Symptoms of psychiatric and neurological disease undoubtedly overlap and many examples immediately come to mind. Failure of concentration or memory, restriction of the content of speech, sensations of disorientation, visual and auditory hallucinations, delusions and many abnormal bodily sensations can all arise from such gross organic lesions as a brain tumour or from disease for which no structural or biochemical cause has yet been disovered. Even the most ardent exponents of the psychodynamic basis of schizophrenia and depression must, or at least should, accept that psychological causes act through the physical agency of the brain and most forms of successful treatment of these diseases are based on this assumption. There is therefore a grain of truth in the saying that psychiatry is 'neurology without physical signs'. The neurologist has a complex role in the disputed territory between the two disciplines.

DEPRESSION

Depression frequently presents with somatic symptoms, of which headache is one of the most common. This may cause some diagnostic anxiety when it follows the pattern of many depressive symptoms in being at its worst on waking in the morning, superficially resembling the headache of raised intracranial pressure. The distress of depression may often be interpreted by the patient as 'dizziness', quite unlike any form of vertigo but regrettably often treated with such powerful and inappropriate agents as prochlorperazine (Stemetil). Of all the varied sensory symptoms encountered perhaps the most consistent is that of pain in the face. This is virtually confined to women, often young, and may be unilateral or bilateral. It is never paroxysmal although nearly always treated unavailingly with carbamazepine (Tegretol). In this condition and in many others, there are none of the classical signs of severe depression, and indeed any disturbance of mood may be indignantly denied or attributed to the pain. Particularly in younger patients with unilateral pain there is often an excellent response to imipramine, although whether this is solely due to its antidepressant action is not clear. In contrast, patients with headache, if not too chronic, are frequently greatly relieved to be asked whether they are depressed and do not reply that they have nothing to be depressed about and are eager to accept treatment.

The neurologist encounters depression in another aspect; not the cause but the result of symptoms. Most patients with Parkinson's disease are depressed, no doubt because of a biochemical disorder related to the disease process. Depression induced by chronic progressive disease is also common, although relatively less so in multiple sclerosis. The fortitude of many of those affected by motor neurone disease is remarkable, but, particularly when respiration begins to be affected, the symptoms are terrifying and their steady increase demoralizing. There is a high incidence of suicide in patients with epilepsy, partly no doubt due to the ready accessibility of lethal drugs, and also in Huntington's chorea, both in the early stages of the disease and in unaffected members of families with the disease. Antidepressants are effective in Parkinson's disease but not in depression from loss of hope.

The early symptoms of raised intracranial pressure, particularly when this arises from a frontal lobe tumour, have often been misinterpreted as the loss of interest and concentration characteristic of depression and the clinical distinction can be very difficult.

ANXIETY

As with many psychiatric diagnostic categories the precise boundary between depression and anxiety is not easy to define. Both are, in any case, normal responses to stress and the point at which they become pathological may also be debatable. Many people are recognized by themselves and their families as chronic worriers and others willingly and indeed sometimes proudly acknowledge that they have always suffered from 'nerves'. They do not make popular patients partly because their symptoms are usually intractable and partly because of recurrent misgivings lest the headache, dizziness, tingling or pain in the arms, to use familiar examples, might after all be due to some cause needing quite different management. It is this that leads to unnecessary, expensive and occasionally harmful investigations.

The symptoms of tension headache and of the common forms of non-vertiginous dizziness are described in Chapter 3. Investigations should include a blood count and ESR and, with persistent symptoms, X-rays of the skull are almost unavoidable and are reassuring to the patient. It may well be that certain forms of dizziness at present thought to be psychogenic may eventually be found to be due to subtle disturbances of vestibular or oculomotor functions, but the imposing battery of tests available in modern audiolgy departments is quite inappropriate in such cases. An accurate and painstaking history is far more informative. In the other common neurological complaint where no abnormal signs are found, pain and tingling in the arms, X-rays of the neck should be obtained, not to exclude cervical spondylosis which is almost invariably present after the age of 40, but to ensure that no other cause of root or brachial plexus compression has been overlooked. The carpal tunnel syndrome in one of its more unusual presentations should also be carefully considered as a possible cause for protracted symptoms.

Treatment of these patients presents formidable problems. Reassurance and detailed explanation of how symptoms can result from muscular tension, in turn due to mental tension, should always be attempted but is seldom successful. If relief of one symptom is obtained it may be succeeded by chest pain, backache or indigestion, leading to a further round of investigations. These patients are reluctant to accept that their symptoms are not due to organic disease and resist referral to psychiatrists who, in any case, do not appear to have any effective treatment. The temptation is to prescribe tranquillizing drugs and it is difficult to resist. It is unlikely that the beneficial effects in this particular group of patients much exceed those of a sufficiently impressive placebo but adverse effects and disproportionate cost should be avoided. Barbiturates, in particular sodium amytal, that were formerly prescribed in large quantities, should not be given. Vitamins are harmless but expensive. Diazepam is currently the favourite agent and if it has harmful effects these are less pronounced than those of other drugs formerly in common use. Withdrawal symptoms can, however, occur in the course of the day, leading to higher doses. Prolonged treatment must be avoided. Major tranquillizing drugs should never be used in this context as all have potentially grave toxic effects particularly in chronic use. In a substantial proportion of those with persistent tension headache there is an underlying mild chronic depression which will yield to tricyclic antidepressant drugs.

The patient with more acute symptoms of anxiety presents a more tractable problem. Sometimes there is an obvious immediate cause of distress, one commonly encountered being the death of a friend or relative from a brain tumour or subarachnoid haemorrhage. The complaint may be of severe headache or of attacks of panic. These are accompanied by overbreathing which can result in a wide variety of unpleasant sensations including paraesthesiae, tetany, dizziness and faintness and even, it is claimed, loss of consciousness. Less drastic overbreathing may be responsible for minor unexplained symptoms in the head and limbs. These patients are in real need of reassurance that they do not have a tumour in the head or are about to burst an aneurysm, and some explanation of how panic can cause their symptoms. Large doses of minor tranquillizers, but in short courses only, are helpful. The advice to hold the breath for as long as possible at the onset of an acute episode will prevent the alarming symptoms of hypocapnoea resulting from overbreathing, and rebreathing into a paper bag held over the nose and mouth is even more effective. It must be remembered that panic attacks also occur in the serious condition of agitated depression requiring quite different management.

DELIRIUM AND CONFUSIONAL STATES

The keynote of these conditions is clouding of consciousness, and with this is associated failure of attention and of recent memory. These lead to the patient's disorientation both in time and space, to violent emotional disturbance usually of a fearful kind, to misinterpretation of his environment, and to hallucinations which are often visual. It is characteristic that these symptoms are worst during the hours of darkness, when some degree of brief disorientation is within the range of normal experience. The delirious and confused patient is often excited, terrified, and difficult to control.

The causes of such a syndrome are innumerable. Amongst those most commonly encountered must be numbered hypoxia due to cardiac or respiratory disease; cerebral infarction; severe general infections; hypoglycaemia; uraemia; liver failure; poisoning with drugs of the atropine or amphetamine groups; and alcohol. Crises of Graves' disease or myxoedema, bromide intoxication, and post-operative hypoxia, are amongst other well-recognized causes. Many patients recovering from significant closed head injury pass through a stage of noisy traumatic delirium, which is usually a favourable prognostic sign indicating progress towards recovery of consciousness.

Syndromes of this kind often develop in patients already in hospital, where the nature of the underlying illness is already known. This is, however, not invariable and where the illness develops at home the patient may be admitted to an acute psychiatric unit rather than a general medical ward. This happens, for example, in every epidemic of meningococcal meningitis and from time to time to patients with drug intoxication or withdrawal, acute alcoholism, encephalitis, or cerebral metastases, to mention but a few familiar examples. Such cases underline the impossibility of separating neurological from psychiatric illness and the need for the psychiatrist to be well grounded in internal medicine.

The delirious or acutely confused patient requires constant attendance and skilled and sympathetic handling, but the onset of such a syndrome in a medical or surgical ward is emphatically not a signal for transfer to a psychiatric unit. Most cases respond to medical treatment within a few days. Hypoxia must be obviated by appropriate treatment with adequate ventilation and often oxygen. Dehydration must be relieved and intravenous high-potency Parentrovite (containing Vitamin B complex and vitamin C) given initially each day and later on alternate days. Sedation presents important problems. Chlorpromazine is the drug of choice, and 50 mg or more should be given intramuscularly every four hours. A useful alternative is chlormethiazole (Heminevrin) tyhat can be given by intravenous drip.

HYSTERIA

The widely held impression that conversion hysteria as witnessed and induced by Charcot is no longer seen is far from true. Hysterical paralysis, sensory loss, muscular spasm and fits are still frequently encountered and the ability to recognize them for what they are can save time, effort and expense. Conversely, many conditions, particularly involuntary movements, are mistakenly thought to be hysterical, resulting in inappropriate management.

Weakness of hysterical origin is fluctuating and contradictory. A patient unable to lift the heel from the bed while lying supine will have no difficulty in walking. A patient who cannot plantar flex his foot against resistance can stand on tiptoe. There will be no alteration in reflexes but wasting may occur in a limb that has not been used for a long time. An experienced observer will usually have no difficulty in making the distinction from organic weakness but it must be remembered that an upper motor neurone lesion may result in loss of use rather than paralysis and this may also result in inconsistent findings on examination, although not closely resembling those of hysteria. There is also the well-known diagnostic trap set by truncal ataxia. A patient with a midline cerebellar lesion may be unable to walk, stand or even sit upright although no ataxia or weakness of the limbs can be found when examined individually.

Hysterical sensory loss is usually of glove and stocking distribution or affects the whole of one side of the body. Both these patterns can result from organic disease, the former from polyneuritis and the latter most commonly in brain stem infarction, but the nature of the loss is usually distinctive. Glove or stocking loss will have an absolutely sharp upper limit but this limit can be made to shift by altering the position of the patient's sleeve or trouser leg. Hemisensory loss can sometimes be induced to change sides by turning the patient over to examine the back. The psychological processes resulting in sensory loss on the side nearest the window, for example, baffle understanding. Other anomalies can be found. Loss of postural sense extending to the large joints is incompatible with normal use of the limbs. Vibration sense, which is extensively conducted through bone, can be shown to be present on one side of the forehead and absent on the other side 2 cm away.

Hysterical muscle spasm is much less common and much more difficult to diagnose with confidence. Usually seen in children it results in severe deformity of one limb with permanent joint changes. It is these patients who may have a series of corrective orthopaedic operations completely without success. Hysterical fits were described in Chapter 17. Hysterical blindness now seems to be a great rarity.

Many of the manifestations of hysteria described above are evanescent features found on one examination and, if ignored, do not persist. It is tempting to interpret them as an attempt to make sure that the doctor takes their symptoms seriously. The method of management of persistent disabling hysteria must depend on the view taken of the psychological basis of the condition. Psychiatric teaching still seems to be rigidly devoted to the theory of unconscious motivation. In general, referral of a patient with hysterical paraplegia to a psychiatrist is not rewarding as the report is all too often that the patient does not have an hysterical personality with the implication that the diagnosis is therefore wrong. Unconscious motivation is difficult to accept, particularly in members of the nursing and other medical professions who, when they develop hysterical symptoms, may go to astonishing extremes. Features that can be accepted as hysterical, such as repeatedly falling down an iron stairway, may be combined with actions that could scarcely be unconscious, as, for example, squeezing raw fish in a handkerchief into a specimen of urine to produce albuminuria. Whatever the underlying mechanism it is usually clear enough that the patient does not wish to be cured and all attempts will fail. Hypnosis may indeed sometimes be dramatically successful and should certainly be attempted. Patients do not always relapse, perhaps because the 'gain' demanded by many authorities as essential for the diagnosis, is merely the attention of the doctors, certainly achieved by a miraculous cure.

Conditions often mistakenly diagnosed as hysterical include facial hemispasm, spasmodic torticollis, torsion dystonia, writer's cramp,

Wilson's disease and dyskinesia due to drugs. Unfamiliar involuntary movements are nearly always organic.

EPILEPSY

Epilepsy is not, of course, a mental disease but was formerly often treated by incarceration in a lunatic asylum. This unjustified link between epilepsy and madness has, to some extent, persisted in popular imagination. Patients with epilepsy due to brain damage may certainly have mental symptoms also arising from the same cause, but not from the epilepsy. Two aspects should be mentioned. A small proportion of patients with temporal lobe epilepsy develop a condition closely resembling schizophrenia and there appears to be no way of predicting this outcome. The question is often raised as to whether violent crimes can be committed during an epileptic fit followed by amnesia for the event. This almost certainly does not occur. Brief episodes of irrational violence may, however, be an epileptic phenomenon although this is certainly not the only cause and there is no question of subsequent amnesia. A trial of anticonvulsants is justified even in the absence of overt epilepsy.

Index

Abducent nerve (VIth cranial)
    functions 16
    lesions 65–66
Abscess, cerebral 182–183
    staphylococcal, acute epidural 188
    treatment 183
Acalculia 175
Accessory nerve (XIth cranial)
    distribution 15
    involvement 80
Acetylcholine in myasthenia gravis 129
    and preganglionic fibres 27
    role in transmission 4
Acetazolamide in epilepsy 281
Acoustic nerve, syndromes 75–79
    tumours 178
ACTH in Guillain–Barré syndrome 120
    in multiple sclerosis 216
Acyclovir 201
Adenoma, insulin-producing 245
    pituitary 172, 176–177, 178, 181
Adenosine arabinoside 201
Adynamia episodica hereditaria 242
Afferent system, form and function 6–11
Akathisia 230
Alcohol, and peripheral neuropathy 110–112
Alcoholic myopathy 135
Alphafluorohydrocortisone in idiopathic orthostatic hypotension 270
Alzheimer's disease and presenile dementia 267–268
Amantadine, in Parkinson's disease 224
Amblyopia, tobacco 59
Amino-acids, metabolism in nervous system 5
Amnesia, post-traumatic 138–139
    retrograde 138
    transient global 150–151
Ampicillin in meningitis 193, 194
Amputation neuroma 93
Amyloidosis 117
Amyotonia congenita 133
Amyotrophic lateral sclerosis 264
Amyotrophy, diabetic 115
    neuralgic 121
Anaemia, pernicious 236–237

Aneurin, *see* Vitamin B_1
Aneurysms 163
    unruptured 165–166
Angiography, carotid, in cerebral abscess 183
    in cerebral tumours 180
    in cerebrovascular disease 160
    in migraine 290, 292
Angioma, cerebral 163–165
Anosmia, ammonia test 36
    clinical features 58–59
    following head injury 58, 143
Anticholinesterase drugs in myasthenia gravis 130
Anticoagulant therapy in cerebrovascular disease 161
Antihistamines for migraine 294
Anxiety 298–300
Aphasia 25
    tests 43
    see also Speech
Apraxia 155
    constructional 175
    test 43
    see also Speech
Arachnoid membrane 32
Arms, examination 38–40
Arteritis, cranial 167
    giant-cell 166–167
Astereognosis 174
Astrocytes 3
Astrocytoma 171, 173, 177, 178, 181, 185
Ataxia, Friedreich's 258–260
    in hysteria 301
    spinocerebellar 258–260
Atheroma, pathology in ischaemic vascular disease 148–149
Atherosclerosis, in ischaemic vascular disease 149
Athetosis 227–228
Atrophy, benign spinal muscular 266
    infantile spinal muscular 266
    optic, *see* Optic atrophy
    peroneal muscular 260–261
    Pick's lobar 268
    progressive muscular 264
Audiometry, for assessing deafness 75

INDEX

Autonomic system, form and functions 27–29
Axon, motor 14–15
  sensory 2
Azathioprine 128

Babcock sentence 44
Babinski reflex 19, 41
Barbiturates, in anxiety 299
  causing ataxia 260
Basal ganglia 23
  chorea and athetosis 227–228
  diseases 221–234
  neuroanatomy 221
  Parkinson's disease 221–227
  syndromes, nature 232–234
    stereotaxic surgery 234
Basilar artery, occlusion 157
Basilar impression, primary and secondary 252
Bell's palsy, characteristics, course and treatment 52, 72–73
Benzhexol, in Parkinson's disease 224
Benztropine, in Parkinson's disease 224
Beriberi 235
Betahistone 76
Blackouts 56–57
Bladder, control 28–29
  in spinal cord damage 101, 104–105
  see also Micturition
Blood pressure, nerve control 29
Blood supply, of nervous system 29–31
Brachial plexus injuries 93–94
Brain, blood supply 29–31
  abscess *see* Abscess
  death 45
  metastases 172
  stem, infarction 156
  tumour, causing raised intracranial pressure 169–182
    and headache 51, 52
    see also Cerebral and individual headings
  venous drainage 31
Brown–Séquard syndrome 100

Cafergot in migraine 293
Calcium, disorders of metabolism 244–245
  and muscle weakness 135
Canals, semicircular, and vestibular nerves, investigations 78
Canicola fever 197
Carbachol in urine retention 104
Carbamazepine in epilepsy 280
  in neuralgia 71

Carbon dioxide in ischaemic vascular disease 161
Carcinoma, and myasthenic syndrome 135–136
Carcinoma, peripheral neuropathy and 115–116
  in polymyositis 127
Cardiac arrest 242
Carotid artery occlusion 155–156
  sinus syndrome 151, 287
Carpal tunnel syndrome 89–91
Cataplexy 288
Catheterization in spinal cord injury 104
Cauda equina 249
  claudication 97
  tumours 188
Causalgia 93
Central motor pathway 17
Cerebellum, form and functions 22
Cerebral, abscess 182–183
  cortex, form and functions 23–25
  palsy 253–255
    clinical features 253–254
    management 254
    minimal form 255
    prognosis 254
  tumour, cerebellar hemisphere 177
    cerebello-pontine angle 178
    diagnosis 178–181
    frontal lobe 173–174
    midline cerebellar 177–178
    parietal lobe 174–175
    pathology 171–172
    pons 178
    temporal lobe 175–177
    treatment 181–182
Cerebrospinal fluid, *see* Fluid, cerebrospinal
Cerebrovascular dementia 157–158
Cerebrovascular disease 147–168
  differential diagnosis 150
  investigation 159–162
  palsy, pseudobulbar 157
  treatment 159–162
  surgical 160
Cervical cord injury 102
  myelopathy 105
  ribs, management 94
  root compression 97–98
    chronic 97–98
Chiari malformation 249, 250, 252
Chiasma, lesions 62
Chloramphenicol in meningitis 193, 194
Chlordiazepoxide causing ataxia 260
  causing hypotension 287
Chlorpromazine in tetanus 209

INDEX

in vomiting in vertigo 76
Chordoma 172
Chorea 227–228
  gravidarum 228
  Huntington's 227, 261–262
  rheumatic 227, 228
    in pregnancy 228
  Sydenham's 227
Circle of Willis, form and functions 30
  in occlusive vascular disease 147–148
  in subarachnoid haemorrhage 163
Circumflex nerve, injury 88
Cisternal puncture 49
Clomipramine, in cataplexy 288
Clonazepam, and restless legs 122
Clonidine, in migraine 294
Clumsiness 54–55, 155
Cochlear branch of VIIIth nerve, distribution 13
Collagen-vascular diseases, and peripheral neuropathy 116–117
Coma, deep, and death, distinction 45–46
  examination in 45–46
  in subarachnoid haemorrhage 163–164
  traumatic 139
Compression, acute, of spinal cord 187–188
  chronic 185–187
Computerized axial tomography *see* CT scan
Concussion 137, 138
  post-concussional syndrome 142
Confusional states 300–301
Conn's syndrome 244
Consciousness 26–27
  loss of 45–46, 242
    after head injury 137–138
Contraceptives, oral, and epilepsy 285
  and migraine 292
  and ischaemic cerebrovascular disease 149
Convulsions, febrile, in childhood 277
see also Epilepsy
Copper in Wilson's disease 239
Corneal reflex 18, 37
Corticospinal (pyramidal) tract, chronic compression 186
  distribution 16
  dysfunction 99
Corticosteroids, in herpes zoster 202
  in giant-cell arteritis 166
  in Guillain–Barré syndrome 120
  in multiple sclerosis 216
  in myasthenia gravis 131
  in polymyalgia rheumatica 129
  in polymyositis 128

in post-herpetic neuralgia 202
Costoclavicular compression syndrome 94
Cough headache 295–296
Cough syncope 287
Cramp 52, 54
Cranial arteritis, clinical features and treatment 166
Cranial nerve anomalies 256
  examination 35–38
  sensory, distribution 9
  syndromes 58–80
Craniopharyngioma 172, 177, 178, 179, 181
Craniostenosis 249
Creutzfeldt-Jakob disease 204
Cryptococcus neoformans 208
CT scan in benign intracranial hypertension 184
  in cerebral abscess 183
  in cerebral tumour 161, 179
  in differential diagnosis from subdural haematoma 161
  in epilepsy 278
  in head injuries 139, 140, 141
Cystogram, micturating 105
Cytosine arabinoside 201

Deafness, causes 75
  following head injury 144
  nerve, causes 75
see also Hearing
Death, and deep coma, distinction 45–46
Deficiency diseases 235–238
Degenerative diseases of genetic or unknown origin 258–270
Delirium 300–301
Dementia, cerebrovascular 157–158
  dialysis 243
  differential diagnosis 268
  neurosyphilis 206
  presenile 267–269
Demyelinating diseases 210–220
  acute disseminated encephalomyelitis 217–219
  multiple sclerosis 210–217
  neuromyelitis optica 219–220
  Schilder's disease 220
Depolarization of cell membrane 2–3
Depression 297–298
  treatment 298
Dermatomes 7, 8
Dermatomyositis, acute 127
Developmental diseases 247–256
Devic's syndrome 219
Dexamethasone, use in cerebral tumour 182

Dextramphetamine in narcolepsy 288
Diabetes, hypoglycaemia in 245
Diabetic amyotrophy 115
  neuropathy 114–115
Dialysis dementia 243
Diamox, *see* Acetazolamide
Diazepam, in anxiety 299
  in epilepsy 283
  in status epilepticus 283
Dilator muscle, pupil, nerve supply 28
Dimenhydrinate in vertigo 76
Diplopia 36
  clinical features 66
Dixarit, *see* Clonidine
Dizziness, in depression 297
  diagnosis 53–54
  duration 53
  postural 77
  in post-concussional syndrome 142
  sensations 53–54
Dopamine, in Parkinson's disease 225
  role in transmission 4
Double vision 55–56
Dramamine, *see* Dimenhydrinate
Drug-induced ataxia 260
  involuntary movements 230
  Parkinson's disease 224
Duchenne muscular dystrophy 123–125
Dura mater 32
Dysarthria 43
Dyslexia, congenital 255–256
Dysphasia 26
Dystonia, torsion 229–230
Dystrophia myotonica 126

Echoencephalography, in cerebral
    tumour 180
Edrophonium chloride and myasthenia
    gravis 130
  and myasthenic crisis 131
Ekbom's syndrome 122
Elbow, injury and ulnar nerve palsy 87
Electroencephalography in cerebral
    abscess 183
  in cerebral tumour 179–180
  in encephalitis 203
  in epilepsy 272, 275–276, 278
Electrolytes, role in metabolism of NS 5
Embolism, cerebral 147, 152
Encephalitis, herpes simplex 200–201
  lethargica 198, 223
  subacute inclusion body 203
  viral 198–199
Encephalomyelitis 198–199
  acute disseminated 217–219
  benign myalgic 203

experimental allergic 217
Encephalopathy, hypertensive 159
  progressive multifocal 203
  Wernicke's 111–112
Endocrine myopathies 133–135
Ependymoma 172, 185
Ephedrine, in micturition problems 104
Epilepsy 271–286
  automatism 274
  causing loss of consciousness 56
  in cerebral palsy 254
  in children 276–277
  definition 271
  diagnosis 275–276
  diagnosis of cause 276–279
  familial tendencies 285
  flicker-induced 284
  focal fit 52, 273, 276
  grand mal 271, 273
  and hypocalcaemia 245
  idiopathic 273, 276
  infantile spasms 284
  investigations 278–279
  Jacksonian fit 273
  management 284–286
  mental changes 279
  myoclonic 272
  paraesthesiae 53
  petit mal 272, 274, 276–277, 281, 282
  pregnancy 281, 285
  primary generalized 273
  psychiatric symptoms 303
  status epilepticus 283
  temporal lobe 274, 277, 278, 282
  temporal lobe, removal 282
  Todd's paralysis 273
  traumatic 145–146
  treatment 279–283
    effects 281
    response 282–283
  tumours and 173
Epilim *see* Sodium valproate
Equilibrium, neuro-anatomy 14
Erb's paralysis 94
Ergotamine, in migraine 293, 294
  in migrainous neuralgia 295
Escherichia coli, meningitis 193, 194
Ethambutol 196
Ethopropazide, in Parkinson's disease 224
Ethosuximide in epilepsy 281
Examination, nervous system 35–49
  adult 35–49
  infant 46–47
Extrapyramidal system diseases 221–234
  form and functions 22–23

interconnections 221
Eyelids, examination 37
Eyes, movements, examination 36–37
  peripheral visual fields, examination 36
  and reflex activity 21
  visual activity, examination 36

Face, examination 37
  nerve supply 9
Facial nerve (VIIth cranial) function 16
  hemispasm 74
  paralysis, after head injury 143
    bilateral 74
  pain in depression 297
  syndromes 72–75
  weakness, bilateral 256
  see also Palsy, facial; Trigeminal nerve
Fasciculation 264, 265
Femoral nerve, involvement in pelvic
  malignant disease 88
Fibres, afferent, form and function 6–11
  fusimotor 7
Fits, epileptic, see Epilepsy
  febrile in childhood 277
Flicker-induced epilepsy 284
Floppy baby and congenital myopathy
  132–133
Fluid, cerebrospinal in brain abscess 183
  chemical composition 32–33
  circulation 33
  in lumbar puncture 48
  in meningitis 193, 195
  in multiple sclerosis 214
  in tumour 169, 180
  reduction 182
Folic acid deficiency 237, 281
Foster Kennedy syndrome 174
Friedreich's ataxia 258–260

Gamma-aminobutyric acid, role in
  transmission 4, 236
Gait, in examination 35
Galactosaemia 240
Gaucher's disease 241
General paralysis of the insane 205, 206
  treatment 207
Genetically determined diseases,
  see also Inborn errors of metabolism
  peripheral neuropathy 118–119
Glial cells 3
Glioblastoma multiforme 171, 181
Glioma, infiltrating, of pons 178
Glossopharyngeal nerve, distribution 11
  involvement 79
  neuralgia 71
Glucose metabolism, disorders 245

nervous system 3
  see also Hypoglycaemia
Glutamic acid, role in metabolism 5
Glycine, role in transmission 4
Glycogen, disordered metabolism 133
Glycolysis 3–4
Graves' disease 134
Guanidine in myasthenic syndrome 136
Guillain–Barré syndrome 119–121
  pathology 120
  treatment 120
Gyrus, post-central, function 11

Haemangioblastoma 172, 177
Haematocrit, moderately raised, and risk of
  infarction 149
Haematoma, acute subdural 141
  chronic subdural 140–141
  extradural 140
Haemophilus influenzae 193, 194
Haemorrhage, acute pontine, effect on
  pupils 68
  cerebral 158–162
  extradural, after head injury 139, 140
  in head injury 138
  investigation and treatment 159–162
  pathology and clinical features
    158–159
  subarachnoid 163–165, 191
    clinical features 163–165
    coma 164
    diagnosis 164
    surgery 164–165
  surgical treatment 160
Hartnup disease 238
Head, circumference, in infants 47
Head injury 137–146
  acute, management 139–140
  causing anosmia 58
  closed 137–140
  intracerebral haemorrhage 139
  open 137
  sequelae 142–145
Headache 50–52
  chronic 50
  cluster 294
  complication of lumbar puncture 49,
    51
  cough 295–296
  cranial arteritis 51
  in depression 298
  histamine 294
  hypertension 51
  lumbar puncture 49, 51
  in meningitis 190
  migraine 51, 289–296

INDEX

pituitary tumour 52
  of raised intracranial pressure 51
  site of pain 51
  in subarachnoid haemorrhage 163
  as symptom 50–52
  tension 51
  tumour 51, 52
Hearing, examination 37–38
  neuro-anatomy 13
  see also Deafness
Heavy metals and peripheral neuropathy 113
Hemiballismus 228
Hemiparesis, after head injury 143
Hemiplegia in cerebral palsy 253, 254
  clinical features 153–154
Hemispasm, facial 74
Hepatic failure, and cerebral symptoms 243
Hepato-lenticular degeneration 238
Herpes simplex encephalitis 200–201
  zoster 201–202
    clinical features 201
    and facial palsy 73
Holmes–Adie syndrome 68–69
Homocysteinuria 240
Horner's syndrome 68, 156
  congenital unilateral 256
Huntington's chorea 227, 261–262
  characteristic 261–262
  treatment 262
Hydrocephalus, congenital 247–250
  clinical features 247–249
  diagnosis 249
  infantile 248
  meningo-myelocele 248, 250
  normal pressure 268–269
  otitic 162
  spina bifida 248–250
  spina bifida occulta 249–250
Hypertension in cerebrovascular disease 149
  headache 51
  intracranial, benign 184
Hypertensive encephalopathy 159
Hypnosis in hysteria 302
Hypocalcaemia 244
Hypoglossal nerve involvement 80
  nucleus, XIIth cranial 15
Hypoglycaemia 245
  spontaneous 245
  causing loss of consciousness 57
Hypotension, idiopathic orthostatic 269–270, 287
  with syncope 287
Hypothalamus, form and functions 29

Hypoxia 242–243
Hysteria 301–303
  clinical features 301
  diagnosis 302
  fit 56–57, 301
  sensory loss 301–302

Idoxuridine in herpes simplex encephalitis 201
Imipramine, causing hypotension 287
  in depression 298
Impulse, nerve, propagation 1–3
Inborn errors of metabolism 238–242
Incontinence, in spinal cord injury 101
  management 104–105
Industrial hazards and peripheral neuropathy 113
Infarction, cerebral 148, 152–158
  spinal cord 167–168
Infections 189–209
Insulin neuritis 115
Intellectual functions, testing 44
Intracranial pressure, effect of abscess 183
  effect of tumour 169–182
  in benign intracranial hypertension 184
  in cough headache 295
  in depression 297
  in meningitis 191–192
  raised, in headache 51
  reduction 182
Involuntary movements 222–224
Ischaemia, cerebral, transient, symptoms and management 149–152
Ischaemic vascular disease 148–158
Isoniazid and optic atrophy 59
  and peripheral neuropathy 113
  in tuberculous meningitis 196

Jargon aphasia 26
Jerks, tendon, in examination of NS 38–40

Kanamycin causing deafness 75
Kayser–Fleischer ring 238
Kernig's sign 45, 190
Klumpke's paralysis 94
Knee jerks 40
Korsakow's psychosis 112
Kugelberg–Wielander disease 266
Kuru 203–204

Laminectomy in cervical myelopathy 107
Lead, and peripheral neuropathy 113
Legs, examination 40–41
  restless 122

Lentiform nucleus, neuro-anatomy 23
Leucodystrophies 241
Leucoencephalitis, acute
    haemorrhagic 219
Levodopa, in Parkinson's disease
    225–226
Lhermitte's sign 213
Limbs, lower, in examination of NS
    40–41
  upper, examination 38–40
Lipidoses 240–241
Lipids, role in metabolism 5, 59
Listeria monocytogenes 192, 194
Little's disease 253
Locked-in syndrome 157
Lumbar puncture, complications 49
  contraindication in cerebral
    tumour 180
  headache 49
  indications 48
  measurement of pressure 48
  in meningitis 193, 196
  method 47

McArdle's disease 133
Magnesium, disorders of metabolism 245
Median nerve, carpal tunnel
    syndrome 89–91
  lesion 88
Medulloblastoma 172, 177, 178
Ménière's disease, clinical features 76
  treatment 76–77
Meningeal artery, middle, in head
    injury 140
Meninges, form and functions 32
Meningioma 58, 172, 173, 174, 181, 185
  clinical features 174
  olfactory groove 174
  parasagittal 174
Meningism 191
Meningitis 189–198
  aseptic 197–198
  clinical features 190-192
  cryptococcal 208
  E. coli 193, 194
  Haemophilus influenzae 193, 194
  irritation 190, 198
  Listeria monocytogenes, and
    immunosuppressant
    therapy 192, 194
  Neisseria meningitidis 192
  pathology 189–190
  pneumococcal 192
  Pseudomonas pycocyaneus 192, 194
  purulent 192–194
    treatment 193–194
  tuberculous 195–197
    cerebrospinal fluid 195
    clinical features 195
    diagnosis 195–196
    treatment 196–197
  viral 189, 198
Meningo-myelocele 248, 250
Mental changes after head injury 144
Meralgia paraesthetica 88–89
Metabolic disease 235–246
  deficiency diseases 235–238
  inborn errors of metabolism 238–242
  and peripheral neuropathy 117–118
  systemic 242–246
Metabolic myopathies 133
Metabolism of nervous system 3–6
  amino acids 5
  electrolytes 5
  glucose 4
  lipids 5
  sodium 5
  vitamin B_1 3
Metachromatic leucodystrophy 241
Metastases, cerebral 172
Methysergide, in migraine and migrainous
    neuralgia 294, 295
Metoclopramide, in migraine 293
Metrizamide 187
Micturition, control 28–29
  in spinal cord injury 101
  management 104–105
  syncope 286
Migraine 151, 289–296
  alcohol 292
  causation 291–292
  clinical features 289–290
  clinical variants 290–291
  diagnosis 292–293
  diet 292
  headache 51
  hemiplegic 290
  ophthalmoplegic 291
  treatment 293–294
Migrainous neuralgia 294–295
Moebius' syndrome 256
Mononeuritis multiplex 108, 109, 114,
    116–117
Motor neurone disease 264–266
  characteristics 264–265
  diagnosis 265
  management 266
  prognosis 265
Motor system, form and functions 14–18
Multiple sclerosis 210–217
  clinical features 211–212
  course 212–214

INDEX 311

diagnosis 214–215
and infection 217
management 216–217
optic atrophy 59
pathogenesis 215–216
pregnancy 217
prevalence 215
treatment 216–217
Muscle spindles, form and function 6, 7
Muscular dystrophy, biochemical
    abnormality 124
    Duchenne 123–125
    dystrophia myotonica 126
    facio-scapulo-humeral 125
    limb-girdle 125
    ocular 125–126
    progressive 123–127
    sex-linked recessive transmission 123–127
Musculo-cutaneous nerve, injury 88
Myasthenia gravis 129–132
    cholinergic crisis 131
    clinical features 129–130
    diagnosis 130
    treatment 130–131
        surgical 131–132
Myelitis, acute transverse 217–218
    subacute necrotic 218
Myelography 187
    in cervical myelopathy 107
    in spinal cord compression 187
Myelopathy due to spondylosis 105–107
    cervical 106
Myoclonus, 232
Myopathy, carcinoma 135–136
    congenital, and the floppy baby 132–133
    endocrine 133–135
    metabolic 133
    non-dystrophic 132–136
    toxic 135
Myotonia congenita 126–127
Mysoline *see* Primidone
Myxoedema, muscle weakness 134

Narcolepsy 287–288
Neisseria meningitidis 192
Neomycin causing deafness 75
Neostigmine in myasthenia gravis 130
Nervous system, examination 35–49
Neuralgia, dental 70
    glossopharyngeal 71
    migrainous 294–295
    post-herpetic 202
    trigeminal, characteristics and treatment 69–71

pain 70–71
Neuralgic amyotrophy 121
Neuritis, diabetic peripheral 114–115
    lead 113
    optic 61, 211
Neurofibroma 172, 185, 187
    acoustic 172, 178, 181
    causing root compression 98
Neurofibromatosis 263–264
Neuroglia, form and function 3
Neuroma, amputation 93
Neuromyelitis optica 219–220
Neurones 1–3
    cortical 24–25
    lower motor, lesions 82
    lower sensory, lesions 82
    upper motor, and hemiplegia 153–154
    trauma 99–100
Neuronitis, vestibular 77
Neuropathy, peripheral 108–122
    alcoholic 110–112
    amyloidosis 117
    carcinoma 115–116
    collagen-vascular diseases 116
    demyelination 110
    diabetes 114–115
    drugs and 112–113
    external toxins and 110–114
    genetically determined 118–119
    Guillain–Barré syndrome 119–121
    heavy metals and 113
    industrial hazards and 113
    intrinsic disease 114–118
    isoniazide 113
    lead 113
    metabolic diseases 117–118
    neuralgic amyotrophy 121
    nutritional causes 114
    pathogenesis 109–110
    porphyria 118
    restless legs 122
    of unknown cause 121
Neurosyphilis 204–208
    congenital 207–208
    effect on optic nerve 59, 206
    treatment 207
Nicotinamide, deficiency 237–238
Nissl granules 2
Noradrenaline, action 27
    role in transmission 4
Numbness, clinical features 52–53
Nystagmus 36–37
    clinical features 66–67
    congenital 67, 256
    induced 78–79
    'jelly' 67

Ocular movements, examination 36–37
   paralysis 64, 65
Oculomotor nerve (IIIrd cranial) effect of
   lesions 64–69
   functions 16
Olfactory nerve, anosmia 58–59
   injury 58–59
Oligodendroglioma 172, 179
Ophthalmoplegia, in thyroid disease 134
   internuclear 156
Optic atrophy, causes 59
   degenerative disease 62
   Foster Kennedy syndrome 174
   Leber's hereditary 59, 61
   primary, clinical features 59
   secondary 60
   fundi, examination 36
   nerve, form and distribution 12–13
   syndromes 59, 64
   neuritis 61, 211
   neurosyphilis 206
   pernicious anaemia 237
   tract, lesions 62–64
   tumours 59
Orphenadrine, in Parkinson's disease 224
Ospolot, see Sulthiame
Osteomalacia 135
Otorrhoea, cerebrospinal, traumatic 146
Over-breathing 244

Pain, paraesthesiae 53
   root 185
Palatal myoclonus 232
Palsy, abducent nerve 65
   Bell's 52, 72–73
   brachial plexus 93–94
   bulbar 79–80
   in motor neurone disease 264
   in myasthenia gravis 130
   supranuclear 157
   cerebral 253–255
   facial, bilateral 74
   and herpes zoster 73
   supranuclear 74
   ocular 64–66
   pressure, of peripheral nerves 86–88
   progressive supranuclear 269
   pseudo-bulbar 80, 157
   in amyotrophic lateral sclerosis 265
   radial nerve 86
   'Saturday night' 86
   ulnar nerve 86–87
   see also Paralysis
Panencephalitis, subacute sclerosing 203
Papilloedema, clinical features 60–61

Para-aminosalicylic acid in tuberculous
   meningitis 196
Paraesthesia, origin 53
   pain 53
   symptoms 53
Paralysis agitans 221
   Erb's 94
   Klumpke's 94
   periodic 241–242
   in spinal cord injury 101–103
   management 103–105
   Todd's 273
   see also Palsy
Paraplegia, hereditary spastic 260
   hysterical 301
Parkinson's disease 221–227
   arteriosclerotic 223–224
   clinical features 222–223
   depression 298
   drug-induced 224
   post-encephalitic 223
   treatment 224–227
   surgical 226
Pathways, central motor 16–17
   central nervous, integration 18
   central sensory 9–10
Pellagra 238
Pelvic girdle, and myopathy 136
Penicillin, in meningitis 193, 194
   in neurosyphilis 207
Periodic paralysis 241–242
Peripheral nerves, acute trauma 83–86
   innervation 84
   irritative and entrapment
   syndromes 88–93
Peroneal muscular atrophy 260–261
Peroneal nerve palsy 86
Phenobarbitone in epilepsy 277,
   279–280, 281
   in migraine 294
Phenothiazine, side-effects 230
Phenylketonuria 239–240
Phenytoin, in epilepsy 280, 281
   in trigeminal neuralgia 71
Phosphorus, disorders of metabolism 245
Phytanic acid 119
Pia mater 32
Pick's lobar atrophy 268
'Pins and needles' 52, 236
Pituitary tumours 172, 176–177, 178
Pizotifen in migraine 294
Plantar reflex 19, 40
Poliomyelitis 199–200
Polyarteritis nodosa 110, 116–117, 128,
   167

INDEX

Polymyalgia rheumatica 129
Polymyositis 127–129
  clinical features 127–128
  diagnosis 128
  prognosis and treatment 128
Polyneuritis, acute infective 119
  hypertrophic, of Déjérine and
    Sottas 260–261
  post-diphtheritic 120–121
  see also Neuropathy, peripheral
Polyradiculitis, see Guillain–Barré
  syndrome
Porphyria, clinical features 118–119
  metabolism 240
Post-concussional syndrome 142
Post-traumatic amnesia 138–139
Postural dizziness 77
Postural sense 41
Potassium, depletion 244
  in periodic paralysis 241–242
  role in metabolism 5
Prednisolone in polymyalgia
  rheumatica 129
Prednisone in giant-cell arteritis 166
Preganglionic fibres, form and
  functions 27–28
Presenile dementia 267–269
Primidone, in epilepsy 280, 281
Prochlorperazine in depression 297
Proctalgia fugax 286
Protein synthesis in brain 4
Protryptyline in narcolepsy 288
Pseudo-bulbar palsy see Palsy,
  pseudo-bulbar
Pseudo-hypertrophy 124
Psychiatric disorders 297–303
  see also individual headings
Ptosis, congenital 256
Pulmonary disease and anoxia 242
Pupil, Argyll Robertson 68, 205
  defects 67–69
  Horner's syndrome 68
  pin-point, in acute pontine
    haemorrhage 68
  tonic 68–69
Pyramidal tract, see Corticospinal tract
Pyridostigmine in myasthenia gravis 130
Pyridoxine, deficiency 236
Pyruvate 236

Queckenstedt's test 186

Rabies 199
Radial nerve palsy 86
Radiotherapy, for cerebral tumours 181
Receptor organs, form and functions 6
Reflex, activity 18–21
  Babinski 19
  gag 18
  grasp, in infants 46
  integrative action 21
  phasic 20
  plantar 19
    during stupor 45
    in examination of NS 40
    in infants 46
  stretch 19
  sucking 46
  tendon, during stupor 45
    in examination of NS 40
  tonic neck, in infants 46
Refsum's syndrome 119
Renal failure, and cerebral symptoms 243
  chronic, peripheral neuropathy in
    117–118
Restless legs 122
Retrograde amnesia 138
Rhinorrhoea, cerebrospinal,
  traumatic 146
Rifampicin causing liver damage 196
Romberg's test 35, 206
Roots, nerve, lesions 95–98
  pain 185

Saint Vitus' dance 227
Salaam attack 284
Scan, CT see CT scan
Schilder's disease 220
Sciatic nerve, trauma 88
Sciatica, bilateral 97
  chronic, diagnosis and treatment
    96–97
  clinical features and management
    95–97
Semicircular canals, function 78
Sensation, measurement 41–43
  see also Numbness
Senses, special 12–14
Sensory loss, hysterical 301–302
Sensory nerves, facial supply 9–11
Sensory tracts in spinal cord injury 100
Serotonin, role in transmission 4
Skull, examination 38
Sleep, see Narcolepsy
Smell, sense, examination 35–36
  loss, see Anosmia
  neuro-anatomy 12
Snellen's types 36
Sodium pump 2
  role in metabolism of the CNS 5
  valproate 280

Space-occupying lesions of the CNS 169–188
Spastic diplegia 253
Speech 25–26, 43
  loss, see Aphasia
Sphincters, in spinal lesions 100–101
  management 104
Spina bifida 248–250
Spina bifida occulta 249–250
Spinal cord, acute compression 187–188
  blood supply 31
  central sensory pathway 9, 10
  chronic compression 185–187
  in hydrocephalus 250
  injury to 101–105
  subacute combined degeneration 236–237
  traumatic lesions 98–107
  tumours of 184–185
  vascular disease 167–168
Spinal shock 99
Spine, examination 38
Spinocerebellar ataxias 258–260
Spironolactone, in periodic paralysis 242
Spondylosis causing myelopathy 105–107
  clinical features 105–106
  diagnosis 106–107
  treatment 107
Status epilepticus 283
Stemetil, see prochlorperazine
Stereognosis 42, 174
Steroids in myasthenia gravis 131
  in tuberculous meningitis 196
Stokes–Adams attack 287
Streptomycin, effect on vestibular nerves 75, 78
  in tuberculous meningitis 196
Strokes, little 152
  treatment 159–162
  see also Transient ischaemic attacks
Stupor, examination during 26, 45–46
Sturge–Weber syndrome 255
Subacute combined degeneration of the spinal cord 236–237
Subclavian steal syndrome 151
Sulthiame, in epilepsy 280
Supranuclear bulbar palsy 157
Sweating, control 28
Syncope 286–287
  cough 287
  micturition 286
Syphilis, meningo-vascular 204, 206
  see also Neurosyphilis
Syringomyelia 251–252
Systemic lupus erythematosus, CNS involvement 167

Tabes dorsalis 205–206
Takayashu's disease 149, 167
Taste, examination 38
  neuro-anatomy 12
Tay–Sachs disease 246
Tegretol, see Carbamazepine
Tendon jerks, functions 20
Tensilon, see Edrophonium chloride
Tetanus 208–209
  treatment 209
Tetany 244
Tetrabenazine in chorea 262
Thalamic syndrome 156
Thermal sensation 42
Thermo-receptors, functions 29
Thiamine, see Vitamin B_1
Thiethylperazine in vertigo 76
Thigh, lateral cutaneous nerve, meralgia paraesthetica 88–89
Thomsen's disease 126–127
Thrombophlebitis, cortical 162
  infective 162
Thrombosis, cavernous sinus 162
  of posterior inferior cerebellar artery 157
  in vascular disease of the spinal cord 168
  venous 162–163
Thyrotoxicosis 133–134
Tic douloureux 70, 71
TOCP, see Triorthocresyl phosphate
Todd's paralysis 273
Tofranil, see Imipramine
Tonic pupil 68
Torecan, see Thiethylperazine
Torticollis, spasmodic 229
Touch, sense 41, 42
Toxic myopathy 135
Tranquillizing drugs in anxiety 299
Transient ischaemic attacks 149–152
Transmission in nervous system 1–3
  role of chemicals 3–6
Traumatic lesions, peripheral nervous system 83–86
  spinal cord 101–103
Tremor, essential 224, 230–231
Treponema pallidum 204
Tricyclic antidepressant drugs in anxiety 299
Trigeminal nerve (Vth cranial), affected by tumour 69
  distribution 9–11
  sensory fibres 9–11
  motor fibres, function 16
  progressive sensory loss 69
  syndromes 69–71

Trigeminal neuralgia, characteristics, and treatment 69–71
  pain 70
Trigeminal neuropathy 69
Triorthocresyl phosphate, causing peripheral neuropathy 113
Trochlear nerve (IVth cranial)
  functions 16
  lesions 68
Tuberose sclerosis 263
Tumour, causing raised intracranial pressure 169–171
  cerebral, see Cerebral tumour
  clinical features 169–178
  of spinal cord 184–185

Ulnar nerve palsy 86–87, 92
  after trauma to elbow 92
  tunnel syndrome, symptoms 91–92
  treatment 92
Ultrasound in tumour diagnosis 180
Unconciousness after head injury 139
  causes 56–57
  and epilepsy 56
Unsteadiness 54–55
Uraemia 243
  and peripheral neuropathy 117–118

Vagus, distribution 16
  paralysis 79
  pseudo-bulbar palsy 80
  syndromes 79–80
Valium, see Diazepam
Vascular disease of the nervous system 147–168
  ischaemic 148–158
    cerebral infarction 152–158
    pathogenesis 149
    pathology 148
    transient cerebral ischaemia 149–152
  of the spinal cord 167–168
Venous thrombosis, cerebral, clinical features 162–163
Ventricular asystole 242
  fibrillation 242
Vertebral artery 29–30

Vertebrobasilar syndromes 156–157
Vertigo, in cerebral ischaemia 150
  clinical features 76–78
  epidemic 77
  labyrinthine 76
  postural 77
  treatment 76
Vestibular division of the VIIIth nerve 13, 14
  destruction 78
  effect of streptomycin 75, 78
  and Ménière's disease 76
  nuclei, diseases 78
  and semicircular canals, investigations 78
  syndromes 76–79
Vibration sense 41
Virus infection 202–204
  see also individual diseases
  slow 203–204
Vision, neuro-anatomy 12–13
Visual acuity, examination 36
  in infants 47
  measurement 61–64
Visual fields, defects, syndromes 61–64
  peripheral, examination 36
  recording 61–62
Vitamin B_1 deficiency 111, 112, 114, 235
  metabolism in nervous system 3
Vitamin B_{12} deficiency 236–237
  and optic atrophy 59
  and peripheral neuropathy 114
  in presenile dementia 268
Voluntary muscle diseases 123, 136
Vomiting, control 29

Walking, examination 35
  unsteadiness 55
Wallerian degeneration 83
Weakness 54
  hysterical 301
Weil's disease 197
Werdnig–Hoffman's disease 266
Wernicke's encephalopathy 111–112
Wilson's disease 238–239
Writers' cramp 231

Zarontin, see Ethosuximide